Moving Beyond Core

Moving
Beyond Core

A Somatic Exploration
Through Whole Body Relationships

Wendy LeBlanc-Arbuckle

Forewords by
Mary Bowen and Carol M. Davis

HANDSPRING
PUBLISHING

First published in Great Britain in 2026 by Handspring
Publishing, an imprint of Jessica Kingsley Publishers
Part of John Murray Press

1

A CIP catalogue record for this title is available from the
British Library and the Library of Congress

ISBN 978 1 91342 647 7
eISBN 978 1 91342 648 4

Printed and bound in Great Britain by Ashford Colour Ltd

Jessica Kingsley Publishers' policy is to use papers that are natural, renewable
and recyclable products and made from wood grown in sustainable
forests. The logging and manufacturing processes are expected to conform
to the environmental regulations of the country of origin.

Handspring Publishing
Carmelite House
50 Victoria Embankment
London EC4Y 0DZ

www.handspringpublishing.com

John Murray Press
Part of Hodder & Stoughton Limited
An Hachette UK Company

The authorised representative in the EEA is Hachette Ireland, 8 Castlecourt
Centre, Dublin 15, D15 XTP3, Ireland (email:info@hbgi.ie)

This book is dedicated to:

Awakening our innate biointelligence

Acknowledgments

The process of writing this book has grown me in so many ways, and has taught me so many things, including meeting my old perceptions and fears and moving through them. It's been deeply inspiring to dive ever more deeply into bodies of work that I have studied over many years. It's also been a labor of love to create, on the written page, a space of awareness and support that inspires readers to discover how amazing they are through exploring their direct experience of their innate biointelligent wisdom.

I am so honored to thank the many mentors and also dear friends, family, and colleagues who have contributed so deeply to my personal growth and embodied approach to movement and bodywork. First and foremost, a deep bow of gratitude to my husband, Michael, my soulmate and the love of my life, brilliant woodworker, toymaker, and artist. Over our 39 years we have been partners in both life and business. Through so many twists and turns and ups and downs, he has selflessly coached and supported me over many decades to find my embodied voice. You, Michael, are the wind beneath my wings!

These next "golden threads of relationship" have touched my life at pivotal times and in many ways, inspiring me, collaborating with me and walking this journey by helping me weave a tapestry of rich life experiences that enabled this book to emerge:

My writing coach, Will Daddario, thank you for your full presence, brilliant guidance and support which empowered me in writing this book: https://invitingabundance.net

Gifted writer and editor, Dr Airdre Grant and inspiring and dedicated project manager, Amanda Greene—thank you both for your masterful skills in helping to edit the word count and hone details of organizing the many components of the manuscript

I'm so grateful to these five Pilates Elders, who I had the privilege of studying with, for their inspired teaching and for carrying the torch that supported keeping Joseph Pilates' vision alive: Romana Kryzanowska, Kathleen Stanford Grant, Ron Fletcher, Lolita San Miguel. With a deeply heartfelt embrace of love and gratitude, thanks to my dear friend, colleague and mentor, Pilates Elder, Mary Bowen, who is an extraordinary expression of living life to the fullest. I thank you for your deep love, guidance, sisterhood, and support of me discovering my true self.

And to Marcos Apodaca, who, after 18 years on staff at Pilates Center of Austin, has now taken the reins. Thank you, Marcos, for your unflagging dedication and passion for continuing the vision at PCA that has inspired this book. We have passed our 30 + year-old visionary studio into trusted hands!

A special thanks to my dear friends and colleagues, Amy Taylor Alpers and Rachel Taylor Segal, and to so many dear Pilates Colleagues, nationally and internationally, who have touched my heart and assisted with my growth in countless ways through support, their own creativity, and our collaborations.

For your commitment to sharing the birthing of my embodied vision as it emerged in its early stages, a deep thanks to Kristi Cooper of Pilates Anytime and thanks to Jennifer and Angelo Gianni at FusionPilatesEdu., for continuing to build on that vision.

A deep bow of Gratitude to all my Passing the Torch Mentoring Program Graduates (2010-2025)—and A Very Special Thanks to these Graduates who volunteered their time and energy to support my process with this book: Dena Tarpley, Kristen Luppenlatz Grech, Marcia Brenner, Elaine Economou, Sybil Shearburn, Jenny Barnack, Iris Cheung, Camila Raeder, Joann Hutcheson, Gary Calderone, Walter Zhang...

and so many others who have been cheerleaders for the vision of this body of work and this book.

To the Pilates practitioners in my CoreConnections® Pilates Teacher Training Program—Graduates (1996-2006)—thank you for being part of the birthing of my embodied approach to Pilates in the early years, and special thanks to dear friends, colleagues and physical therapists, Karen Sanzo and Mark Uridel

A deep bow of gratitude to so many mentors and educators of Somatic Studies, especially Emilie Conrad, Bonnie Bainbridge Cohen and Judith Aston, who opened the world of listening for my fluid body's intelligence and language being evoked within the field of gravity. This book is all the richer for the contribution that your visionary work has made in my life.

I'm deeply thankful to colleagues in the Rolf Structural Integration Community and Embodied Biotensegrity and Fascial Matrix Communities, especially Carol Agneessens, Caryn McHose and Kevin Frank, John Sharkey, Stephen Levin, Joanne Avison, Carol M. Davis, Susan Lowell de Solorzano, Graham Scarr for contributing to my evolving vision in so many ways.

Words cannot express the gratitude I feel for my studies with Jaap van der Wal, Hubert Godard, and Phillip Beach and what awakened in my life and teaching through archetypal and preverbal embryological awareness, gesture, perceptual orientation and so much more.

Thank you to the dedicated Continuum Teachers in our regenerative community. Deep gratitude to Susan Harper, Gael Rosewood, Robert Litman, Bonnie Gintis, Bobbie Ellis, Prue Jeffries (thank you for sharing your gorgeous photographs!), Suzanne Wright Crain, Elaine Colandrea, Mary Abrams, Robin Becker, Beth Riley, Marcella Bottero, Sabine Mead and Sharon Weill—for the space of honoring fluid intelligence that you hold, and for your loving guidance and support.

Thanks to Buteyko Breath Awareness Teachers, especially Patrick McKeown and Robert Litman for a foundational understanding of breath awareness. Your work helped me to deepen mine.

A deep bow of thanks to Raul Garza who supported and inspired me in the early stages of my writing and evolving vision, and to Jan Hutchinson, my generous friend and soul sister who supported the creation of the Glossary and this book in so many ways.

Another deep bow of thanks to dear friends, Scott and Prema Sheerin, whose sacred music and ancestral life coaching has touched my heart and life so deeply and who generously contributed a transformative meditation in Chapter Six, inviting breath awareness and the nature of the elements.

This book could not have been completed without the extraordinary skills with illustrative drawings, photoshop, editing photos, videos and so much more! A deep thanks to Sybil Shearburn, Amanda Greene, Leah Rees, Robert Haden, Diane Strickland and Cecelia Colome.

I'm so grateful to so many yoga mentors and colleagues and macrobiotic, ayurvedic and Traditional Chinese Medicine communities for my healing and energetic journey and a life changing understanding of food as energy. Thank you. Thank you.

Thank you, Richard Miller and IRest yoga nidra teachers for a profound awareness of welcoming the wholeness of who we are as full presence, which so supports my teaching and mentoring approach in this book.

For a deeper awareness of the energy of our bones, the power of a fulcrum and understanding of myofascial release and embodied touch, thanks to Fritz Smith, David Lauterstein, Zero Balancing Health Association and Yamuna Zake

A deep bow of thanks to my late dear friend, Perch Ducote, for supporting my mentoring and book project—and thank you Ted Ducote, Perch's brother, for your loving support

I am deeply grateful to my loving family who have given so much support, especially my extraordinary parents and cheerleaders, Audrey and Milton LeBlanc, and my four fabulous sisters who have always had my back, Peta Anne LeBlanc, Susan LeBlanc Dill, Jan LeBlanc Cranner, Erin LeBlanc and dear friends, family and colleagues in Asheville, Austin, New Orleans, in the U.S., and around the world...you know who you are. Thank you!

And finally to Serena Wolfaard and the team at Handspring Publishing and Sarah Hamlin and the team at Jessica Kingsley Publishers—thank you for your patience, support and perceptive invitation to write this book.

Models for the book: Sybil Shearburn, Jenny Barnack, Amanda Greene, Shela Anmuth, Iris Cheung, Will Daddario, Michael Arbuckle

Contents

Foreword

It is an honor to be asked to write a foreword for Wendy's new book *Moving Beyond Core*...a book to marvel at for sure, but also to live...to learn...and to grow from...much more than just to read.

In this period of time we humans are living in, working with our bodies is a more creative process than ever before. We are learning to recognize and learn that the greatest source and teacher of all is the body itself!

Having known Wendy for over 30 years, I have been a witness to her growth as an individual and especially to her endlessly creative way of living with and teaching the incredibleness of the human body with its wisdom and depth of meaning that will never end or be fully achieved.

Joseph Pilates had a vision of "wholeness." He actually taught that we should use the whole body in every movement. Wendy's book brings us into a deeper awareness of moving and teaching to the whole person, more than just doing exercises. It is a book that will support any movement or bodywork discipline and what our body offers us "beyond what we think we know."

Wendy's description and explanation of this process is many-sided: historical, highly intellectual (don't be scared off), multifaceted with videos, many suggested movement patterns, and especially full of her deep understanding and enthusiasm for what she is sharing with the world via this book.

Moving Beyond Core is a gift of learning to better appreciate that each one of us lives, learns, and heals from...*our body itself*!

I have noticed that the older we get, the more learning is available to us. Aging with awareness makes Pilates or any discipline better since we have a deeper understanding of how to help ourselves. This book speaks of that process.

Are you curious? I hope so. This knowledge of our humanity is here! Let's dare to go deeper. Let's continue to grow. What a gift to give yourself or anyone else. This book is more than wise. It is a treasure that can last!

Mary Bowen
Pilates Plus Psyche, Jungian psychotherapist,
and most Senior Pilates Elder

Foreword

Richard Rohr, in *Just This*, writes:

Every once in a while, we need to switch gears to better be able to perceive what is about to come to us.

When I have sent people into the woods on a retreat, I tell them to draw a symbolic line in the sand somehow and truly expect things on the other side to be special, invitational, or even a kind of manifestation.

It always works.

On the other side of that log, or lawn, or "line in the sand," they start *beholding*.

Someone who is truly beholding is, first of all, silenced with the utter gratuity of a thing, a tree, a bird, even an insect. You find yourself giving it voice, allowing it to have an inherent dignity, and you let it give you a leap of joy in the heart and in the eye.

What has happened is that you have begun to meet reality subject to subject instead of subject object, I and Thou instead of just I and It. Once you can change your actual expectations, the resonance between you as seer and what you can see will also change.

To behold is to allow and to taste the awe and wonder of the world. (Rohr 2017, p.99)

Wendy LeBlanc-Arbuckle has given us, the readers of *Moving Beyond Core*, a deeply meaningful invitation to *behold*, to change our perception, to undergo an entire shift in understanding about how our selves within our biointelligent bodies function, and about how we might move and breathe in concert with nature, with ease and joy.

This book is designed to inspire and instruct movement practitioners from various backgrounds who were taught from an incomplete model of science. As a physical therapist, for example, I was taught from a framework that saw the body with dysfunction as something that needed to be trained and fixed by correctly identifying parts that were not working correctly. "Strengthen the core abdominals to support the lower extremities when climbing the stairs," for example.

Physical therapists often aren't instructed in the verbal and touch cues necessary for patients to enter the "feeling state" of the body. Little focus was given to viewing the moving body as energetically interconnected with an inner self, and with others in our lived environment. The critical importance of fascia as our ubiquitous fluid structure fueled with biotensegral energy was not yet discovered.

Wendy teaches us to tune in to the wisdom of our Inner Guide, to the relationships at the heart of our wellbeing. We can then move forward from what we were taught, to embrace a new awareness, a paradigm shift fueled by the author's precise new language that invites us to a more wholistic, artful way of practicing.

In Wendy's words:

- We begin our journey in our embryonic

beginnings and speak about how we are *held* in the field of gravity, finding our backing, sensing the emergence of our primordial midline that supports us in resonating with the natural living world.

- Then, we behold our whole-body human nature with Core as Relationship—shifting from controlling ourselves and seeing our bodies as machines to be trained and fixed to sensing ourselves as biointelligent beings, in relationship with gravity, ourselves, one another, and our living environment.

- In Breath as a Healing Bridge, we discover that *we are breathed* —wow, once again being held!

- When we approach Movement Beyond Doing, we are exploring the *huge* difference it is to move from a pieces-and-parts, isolated muscular approach to a fluid, fascial approach—which, as we know, changes everything!

Wendy LeBlanc-Arbuckle has given us, the readers of *Moving Beyond Core*, a deeply meaningful invitation to *behold*, to change our perception, to undergo an entire shift in understanding about how our biointelligent, biotensegral bodies function, and about how we might move and breathe in concert with the laws of nature seen and unseen, with ease and joy. We transform "functional exercises" into meaningful inner exploration of what it means to be alive and moving with purpose, engaged in relationship with gravity, with nature, with our loved ones. Little is more important than this gift of self-inquiry that is shared so eloquently in these pages.

And we, and our patients and clients, experience ourselves as deeply changed.

This book is a compelling invitation to each of us to *behold*; not only to learn, step by meaningful step, how to feel ourselves fully alive, present in our wholeness, but then also how to pass on these lessons to our students and to our loved ones.

Carol M. Davis, DPT, EdD, MS, FA
Scarborough, Maine, USA

REFERENCE

Rohr, R. (2017) *Just This: Prompts and Practices for Contemplation.* Albuquerque, NM: CAC Publishing.

Introduction

I was inspired to write this book to shine a light on our innate biointelligence and highlight the work of brilliant somatic pioneers who have contributed profoundly to my transformational growth and body of work. This book tells the story of how when we come from the study of *principles of movement*, rather than exercises, we discover that *Core* is all about relationship. This relationship sits at the heart of our wellbeing: an interconnection with gravity, ourselves, one another, and our living environment.

In the first 25 years of my practice of yoga and Pilates, I was guided by an instructor to follow directions. But I was hungry for more of a first-person, lived experience and sought that out in the somatic field. Here I became aware of the difference between a body-as-machine-to-be-trained-and-fixed approach and a biointelligent, body-as-a-living-process approach to movement and bodywork.

Then I discovered the world of fascial research and reawakened patterns of developmental, psychosocial movement. I discovered that, as babies, we learn to solve physical challenges with gravity, stability and instability, momentum and equilibrium, and more. This knowledge shaped and transformed the way I moved within my own body and the way I mentored students of Pilates, yoga, Gyrotonic, and many other movement and bodywork disciplines.

I am dedicated to fostering awareness in our global movement and bodywork communities, honoring our innate biointelligence and the cross-pollination between disciplines. This approach, which I call *living systems awareness*, enriches daily life practice. It resists rigid adherence to the teachings of a discipline's founder, and instead promotes openness and curiosity among practitioners and students. This dynamic process allows disciplines to evolve, letting innate wisdom emerge, and fosters a collaborative relationship between student/client and teacher/practitioner.

I often ask myself: am I being right or am I being human? Our bodies and the universe are interconnected within a single energy field, as Einstein's assertion that "the field is the only reality" suggests. Engaging consciously with this field enables us to fully participate in reality, navigate the world's complexity, and heal. Einstein also said, "We can't solve problems at the same level of thinking that created them." Inspired by this, I aim to create ripples of curiosity, love, compassion, and collaboration rather than exerting control or claiming expertise on what's "right."

I am inspired by so many colleagues who have studied complementary movement and bodywork disciplines and brought their findings to their Pilates and yoga practice and teaching. This is why I speak, in Chapter 3, of creating a Living Roots Bridge relationship with who we are and how we practice and teach. What I have noticed in my own practice and in mentoring educators over many decades is that teaching from embodied awareness, rather than doing exercises the "right" way, helps us grow as compassionate, porous self-humans in a complex world.

A major takeaway of this approach to life is that, as I age, I am not angry that I can't do what I did ten years ago. Instead, I have compassion for myself and know that I am in my elder years, sharing wisdom gained over decades. That awareness enables me to listen to my body and help myself and, in turn, enable others to help themselves.

Moving Beyond Core aims to help you access the fountainhead of wisdom within, which is innate. Some fundamental principles on which this book and my practice is based are as follows. We are ecological beings in relationship with gravity, ourselves, one another, and our environment. Our body does not perceive separate body systems. While I may mention particular systems or muscular connections throughout this book, I do so only for explanatory purposes aimed at highlighting the philosophy that your body is whole, that it is a continuity with internal organs and external features, and it extends into and entangles with the world. In other words, *we are one muscle*, from foot to head and hand within our fascial matrix body.

My perception of myself and my teaching was transformed when embryologist and MD Jaap van der Wal shared, at his "Embryo in Us" workshop many years ago, that in our embryonic beginnings, *the forces that form us* are the same forces that allow us, as biointelligent beings, to self-heal, self-organize, and adapt till the day we die.

I began to see that my cultural beliefs were based on brain-centered over-thinking. Studying with treasured mentors who awakened my "orientation within the gravitational field" created a seismic shift in awareness. Vestibular internal balance came alive in a way that transformed my relationship with gravity from one of "balance" as an activity or exercise, to an ongoing conversation with my body's relationship between earth and sky. A continually emerging aliveness awakened that was so distinct from doing something perfectly—my relationship with the world shifted. These mentors and many others mentioned in *Moving Beyond Core* all helped me see facts as fluid knowledge and embrace an ever-changing reality in which the body plays a part.

Nature is non-linear and so are we. We are much more than the defined biomechanical directions of flexion/extension/sidebend/rotation. We are multi-dimensional beings who can explore micro dimensions of weight shift within our helical fascial feet and hands in relationship with our spatial orientation. Your spiralic fascial matrix body craves nuance and exploration through connection and relationship.

Gradually, over the course of my life, everything became related—being a teacher and being in the world or with family, friends, and colleagues. As I look back, I see myself as a child playing for hours in our yard noticing how dragonflies landed lightly on my fingers and, with no effort, flew freely into the air, and how hummingbirds hovered magically before a flower, while squirrels seemed glued to a tree before running upside down from canopy to root. I was fascinated with the movement of life. But brushes with death were equally valuable. As I'll explain more in Chapter 3, I was once forced by an automobile accident to lie down and move very slowly for long periods of time in order to heal. In that state, I was surprised by the amount of effort I was using to make the smallest movement. The experience encouraged me to study micromovement from my body's perspective. In asking my body how far and how fast to move, I noticed that I was learning to listen for how gravity was supporting the healing of my tissues. This sensory awareness also influenced my teaching. It invited me to put my hands on people in a way that felt like the act of touch was a presencing event of meeting someone and being met by that person at an interface with curiosity that was collaborative and devoid of any desire to fix. That act of touch would spark questions in me, such as how can we rediscover a sense of grounding, centering, and suspension? My clients told me that my touch was *so gentle yet so powerful*, enlivening their awareness such that the experience of the lesson became integrated into their way of being. My goal with touch became to inspire each person in awakening to their deep biointelligent wisdom—their Inner Guide!

The vision with *Moving Beyond Core* is to explore with readers, both curious students and practitioners alike, how our approach to movement and interaction with gravity and its partner, ground reaction force (spatial orientation), shapes our way of being in the world. When we let go of external validation and discover our innate omnidirectional relationship with our body's fascial matrix, we awaken to a deeper awareness of our body as a living instrument which is tuned by our unique shape-shifting biointelligence. As we explore this way of being with how we are living in our bodies, deeply held tension patterns begin unwinding. They unwind thanks to the embodied approach outlined in this book, one that supports readers in feeling more physically grounded, mentally centered, emotionally calm, and spiritually oriented.

In Chapter 1, I discuss how we embody our embryonic awareness of receiving breath, finding our backing, emergence of our primordial midline and proprioceptive innerness, modes of awareness that support us throughout life within the gravitational field.

In Chapter 2, we compare and contrast a (core control) biomechanical, body-as-machine-to-be-trained-and-fixed approach to movement and bodywork with a (Core as Relationship) biointelligent, body as a living process, one that teaches individuals how to be aware of their self-healing, self-organizing, and adaptive nature.

In Chapter 3, we explore the nature of Breath as a Healing Bridge, which grounds us in the here and now and, through nervous system co-regulation, connects us more deeply to one another and the world in which we are interwoven. We explore various methods of breath awareness, beyond the instructional "how-to" language we most often encounter and toward an embodied experience that requires enabling the power of breath to meet our metabolic need and shift acute and chronic conditions.

Chapter 4 goes into Movement Beyond Doing, which is a deep listening to our biointelligent wisdom, our Inner Guide, as a guide for embodied awareness in movement, where movement becomes a "nutrient" like food. In Chapter 5, we explore Communicating from Our Way of Being that occurs in concert with Movement Beyond Doing. In Chapter 6, we see how the perceptual shifts we have cultivated over the course of the previous chapters lead to Self-Care as Context for Community Service and Resilience. In Chapter 7, we see that It's All About Relationship. When we cultivate a biointelligent approach to movement and life, we ground ourselves in the magnificence of who we are within the gravitational field. We become more porous, able to sense our physical, mental, emotional, and spiritual selves and merge with collective consciousness by partnering with the innate resilience of the natural living world.

A large part of this book is made up of principles of practice through movement explorations. I invite you to explore each of these movement sequences, consider the embodied ideas supporting the movements that I articulate in this book's pages, and then be back in touch about your experience. I wish for this book to be a living document that sparks new ideas and changes, and grows each time readers use it to further engage the wisdom of their Inner Guide.

CHAPTER 1

Cultivating Your Inner Guide

ENVIRONMENT AS SHAPING OURSELVES

Our Inner Guide is critical to who we are as it operates in direct response to our environment and influences the way we think, feel, and move in the world. We understand that the places we live in influence our lives, yet have you deeply considered that every environment you've been in has played a part in shaping who you are and how you move and think? Think about the first time you visited a large body of water, like an ocean, and the way the ebb and flow of the slow tidal shift pulled at your feet. The smell of the salt water permeated your bones. A sense of the landscape stays with you, transforms you, and the experience forever shifts the way you perceive the world. When I hike in five-finger shoes, my feet sense every rock, each nodule of every root. I merge with the trail, sense the forest bathing me. Which environments have been most crucial in shaping you?

Physical space is always entwined with emotion. Remember the emotional tenor of your childhood. Perhaps you sought out certain people, ones who gave you safety, nourishment, and support. It's possible that your first memory takes you to your earliest experiences, being in the womb and the rhythm of your mother's heartbeat. The work of phenomenological scholars like Jaap van der Wal (www.embryo.nl/en) helps us to understand what happened in this womb space. For example, there was a time when you were equally shaping yourself and being shaped by the life-support system surrounding you. At a certain point, about a month into your becoming, your fingers and toes began to *emerge*, thereby introducing extension into your physical world. Whatever memory your body has of that first experience of extension and emergence, that same memory is completely integrated with knowledge of the womb space that enabled the movement in the first place. That environment is where you were introduced to gravity, to the sensation of backing (into the womb), and the coordinated movement, spiralic, mobius-like, between your legs, arms, head, and spine. What action is being called forth in the present to recall and utilize the knowledge we embodied of ourselves and our surroundings in that space?

The focus of this chapter is threefold. First, to draw attention to this Inner Guide. Second, to illustrate how the type of knowledge presented by this practitioner is viewed by inquiring scholars. Third, to transpose this renewed awareness and scholarly information into a map that invites curiosity and awareness which can chart our course through this book.

We come into the world as fluid beings. The midline forms fluidly, where oral and anal portals emerge in concert with our other fluid systems. These fluid resonances continue to communicate throughout our life. The Inner Guide, our body's innate ability to know what to do in order to survive and thrive, is emergent within this fluid environment. Once we tune in to our Inner Guide, a world of possibility unfurls.

My studies of the embryonic journey led to an understanding of the earliest forms of knowledge in general and of Inner Guide. As an embryo, I understand that I was self-organizing within a fluid environment, coupled with the bodily knowledge produced through the act of expanding into the womb space, which carries with it an ability to heal and find equilibrium. Living and health are synonymous in these early days. In the present, when we either fully acknowledge these earliest experiences and/or return to them through fluid movement explorations, we reconnect both with the knowledge of that space and with who we were in that space. We revitalize our wholeness, and the extent to which our selves are fully supported by, healed by, and integrated with our environments.

Bonnie Gintis, osteopath and Continuum teacher, explores this knowledge. She writes:

A miracle began at the moment that the sperm met the egg, and that miracle became you. That miracle hasn't ended yet. The mystery that propelled the growth and development of an embryo continues after birth and throughout life as the forces of adaptation and healing. The movement of embodiment is the vehicle for the expression of this life force. There is no spiritual path without a physical body in which to have it; and there is no physical existence without the presence of the mysterious nonmaterial life force, often referred to as "spirit." (Gintis 2007, p.4)

I propose that we understand Gintis's word "nonmaterial" to mean something too great to be explained in words. Read this way, "spirit" is surely present in the womb space as a kind of traveling partner that is deeply entwined in our physical becoming. If we can at least momentarily understand "nonmaterial" and "spirit" in this way, then we can get at an important insight there, which is that our ability to adapt and heal in the present begins in this embryonic stage. As such, to revisit that stage is to reconnect with our innate healing and adaptive powers. Such powers include breath, touch, movement, sound, and intuition.

My fascination with embryology helps me go deeper in re-knowing myself and re-imagining the ways in which my body/mind/emotion/spirit collaborates with other beings and forces of the natural world.

Embodiment requires accessing and listening to our Inner Guide, understood as an initial reservoir of knowledge that implants the wisdom of the womb environment in our being. This helps guide all our extensions into and through space as an embodied way of being in life. This is bio-intelligence, the innate, fluid knowledge of your somatic architecture and its relationship within the field of gravity, which includes other beings and your environment.

WHY SENSING OUR EMBRYONIC BEGINNINGS IS IMPORTANT

When teachers of body and movement education think of the body as a bunch of static bones or as a machine to be trained and fixed, it ignores the wisdom of the Inner Guide. In contrast, when we understand bodies to be fluid fields of bio-intelligence in relation with the field of gravity and endowed with an innate wisdom gained through our earliest experiences, the difference is palpable. We perceive ourselves as a living process, always healing, always adapting, and, most importantly, as a deeply intelligent organism that is innately regenerative. The challenge becomes learning to listen to our inner wisdom as we encounter various philosophies of movement and look at supporting the unique nature of each human being, by coming from a fluid-dynamic understanding of body awareness.

There are times when anatomical photographs, diagrams, or cadaver-based studies can be useful to study the body's internal mapping. I recommend the whole-body fascial awareness taught through Thiel soft embalming dissections with pioneers like John Sharkey, Gil Hedley, and Tom Myers. At the First International Fascia Research Congress in 2007, my whole world changed. That conference marked the first gathering of fascial researchers dedicated to the study of the continuity of *living* fascia in all its forms and functions. This congress made real the relationship between the cadaver-based anatomical parts and their embedded relationship within the fascial matrix. We were awed when French hand surgeon Jean-Claude Guimberteau showed images of living fascia in his film *Strolling Under the Skin*. He had used a special endoscopic camera during hand surgery to study our *living* architectural tissues and discovered that the fascial continuity is global, fascial matrix.

The fascial matrix, especially the living fascia, had been largely unacknowledged in conversations about the "whole body." I have come to realize that a biomechanical, "pieces-and-parts" approach to movement and bodywork gives a limited perceptual awareness of our whole living body. The images and diagrams I relied upon became important as jumping-off points into the body's dynamism and concert of relations. Cell biologist James Oschman, author of *Energy Medicine in Therapeutics and Human Performance* (2003), inspired deeper studies into the structural and energetic, vibratory continuum of our living fascial matrix and how this body-wide communication system supports and influences every other system.

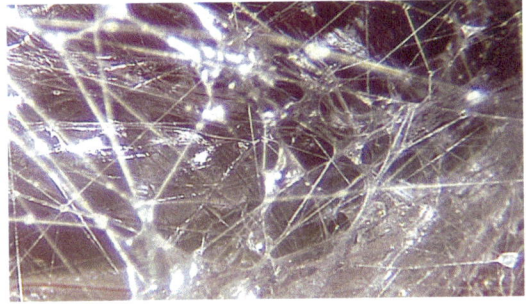

Figure 1.1 Fascial matrix
REPRODUCED FROM *ARCHITECTURE OF HUMAN LIVING FASCIA* (HANDSPRING PUBLISHING 2015, P.18, FIGURE 1.8). GRATITUDE TO JEAN-CLAUDE GUIMBERTEAU

Where do I see this knowledge that we are born into our embryonic beginnings *in action*, and how does it age with us over time? Through many sources, including the work of Dr. Rollin Becker, I have understood our Inner Guide as an innate and resilient health-seeking force:

> The seeking of health from within is a continuous time, tissue, and tidal effort from conception to the final moments of physiological life. Within every trauma and/or disease entity, there is an effort on the part of the body physiology to deliver health mechanisms through the local area of stress to full functioning health capacities. (Becker, cited in Kern 2005, p.101)

The body asks for support through the conscious incorporation of grounding, centering, and uplift in each movement. When I listen to my body, I begin to utilize my body's intelligence to experience each movement in the way that is most suited to my whole-body health. From observing nature, I know that life springs up at every opportunity: after a forest is ravaged by a fire, between the cracks in cement, in injured bodies and minds. Life finds a way. The same must be true in my body. Nature's health-giving forces are always present as an intrinsic part of our lives, and those forces constitute an ongoing dialogue you can utilize when you establish communication with your Inner Guide.

Think about which aspects of nature are the best guides for instructing me in how to connect and communicate with my Inner Guide. I see that fluidity is key. Rachel Carson, marine biologist and author of the pioneering book *The Sea Around Us*, prompted me to think about the similarities between my physiology and the intelligence of the oceanic environment. She wrote, "There is no drop of water in the ocean, not even in the deepest parts of the abyss, that does not know and respond to the mysterious forces that create the tide" (Carson 1961, p.142).

Through studies, I learned that the cerebrospinal fluid is like the ocean in that its motion and subtle pulse are supported and stirred by its interconnection with the body's other fluid systems. Also the movement of the cerebrospinal fluid protects the central nervous system and stimulates our body's healing abilities. Gintis wrote in *Engaging the Movement of Life* (2007) about the fluid nature of our earliest self. She cites an experiment by anthroposophist and engineer Theodor Schwenk that reveals how water of one temperature moves when poured into a container filled with water of a different temperature. Schwenk's images of the experiment show that the poured water charts a specific course through the other liquid. The stream divides into two nearly symmetrical halves as it reaches the bottom of the container. Each half spirals upward toward the right and left sides of the container before turning back toward the center point. The resulting movement closely resembles the emergence of the human midline, with a brain at one end and a canal running through the center within our early embryonic development.

Gintis's inclusion of Schwenk's experiment affirmed my deeper knowing to honor the fluidity of the midline and its spiralic nature. This required thinking beyond a notion of the spine as a rigid column. By understanding the meeting of the fluidity of the spine with the fluidity of my breath, I can engender spinal movements that support my nervous system's co-regulation.

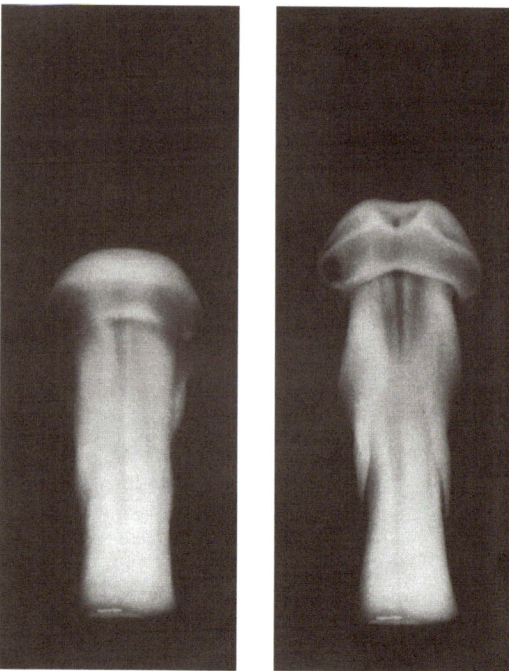

Figure 1.2A Experiment using water poured into a container to simulate movement, causing a mushroom effect

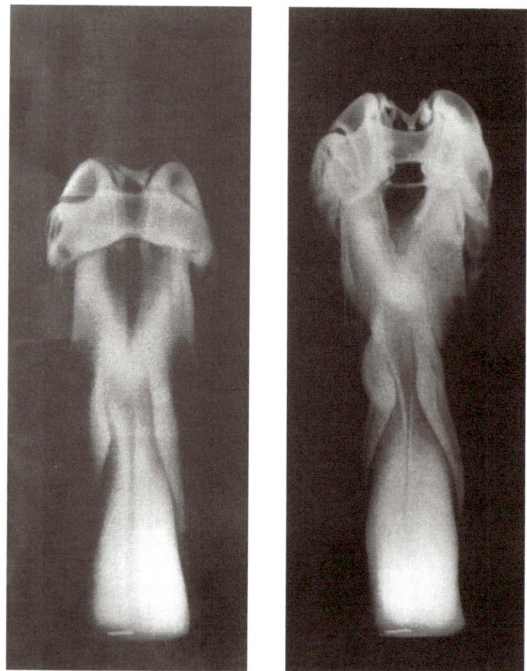

Figure 1.2B The mushroom effect turns into two spiral columns of water within the container

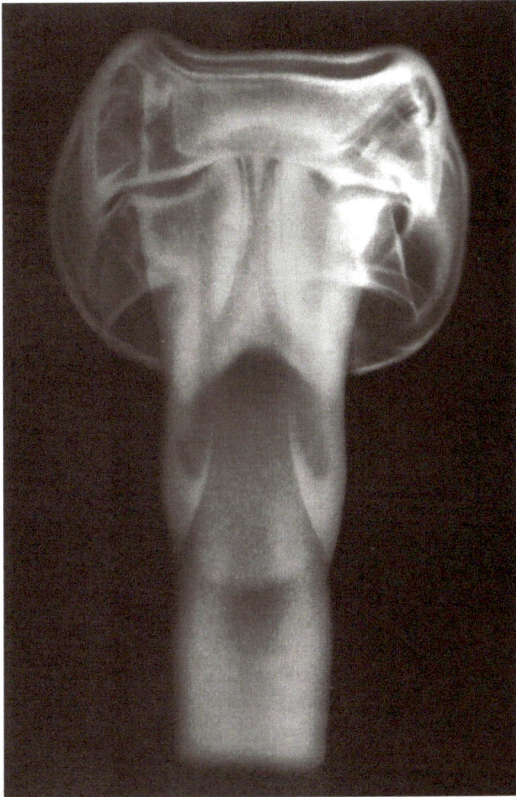

Figure 1.2C The two columns of water turn back toward the center looking like a jellyfish

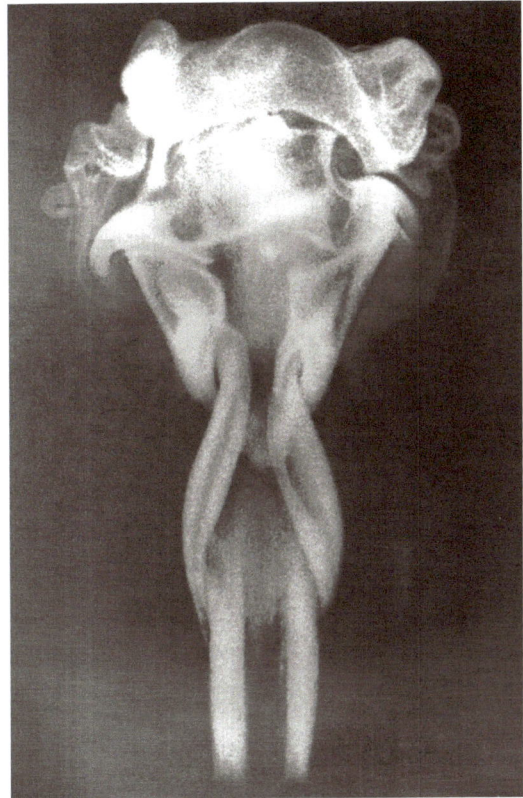

Figure 1.2D The final fluid nature of the water experiment resembles the emergence of the human spine

IMAGES IN THEODOR SCHWENK, *SENSITIVE CHAOS (1996),* PLATES 49–54

Somatic approaches, such as Continuum, Body-Mind Centering, Alexander, and Feldenkrais, informed me how to bridge models of spinal movement based on biomechanical approaches and shift to a biointelligent approach.

I learned that biointelligence and inner wisdom, those of the body's fluidity, are central to my practice changing. The earth's surface and our human body are both approximately 70 percent water, with 97.5 percent salt water (blood and body fluids) and 2.5 percent relatively fresh water (cerebrospinal fluid) (Gintis 2007, p.78). This *should* also be enough to drive home the microcosm/macrocosm symbiosis of self and planet. But, again, demands of lived reality get in the way of this insight. Patterns of stress and trauma are usually approached through the nervous system. It can also be helpful to think about underneath the nervous system to the circulation of our blood. Embryologically, blood develops before the nervous system is formed. *Nerves follow the pathways laid down by the blood* (Bainbridge Cohen 2023).

As I write about the potency of the Inner Guide, I do not *fully* know it, because complete knowledge of it is impossible. We *are* this Inner Guide. Knowledge of the Inner Guide really starts to become audible or sensible through engagement with *a way of being with ourselves.* This means a process of being through which we discover our innate connection with the natural and social world.

ENGAGING WITH EMBRYOLOGY

According to embryologist Jaap van der Wal:

> The forces that formed the body are continuously at work throughout life, carrying the blueprint of health into manifestation at every moment. (van der Wal 2018)

These forces, the embryonic field of pure potential, are like a primordial soup. The complex being we call our Self begins here.

Within you is a wellspring of knowledge about how you relate to gravity, and how you feel in social and natural environments. Often, our movement practice is dissociated from this knowledge, so we turn to movement or bodywork "experts" to fix something. Our natural instinct to move our bodies can be separated from our everyday lives. When most people think of movement, they think of "exercising," and even where exercise has become a form of therapy, prescribed like a drug.

DISCOVERING CELLULAR AWARENESS

In January of 1996, I attended a weeklong immersion with Bonnie Bainbridge Cohen at Mont Marie Center in Holyoke, Massachusetts, called "Embodying Cellular Consciousness." What we weren't expecting to happen was the "blizzard of 1996" that paralyzed the Eastern Coast with up to four feet of wind-driven snow the entire week! What an awesome experience. We explored our inner landscape, as snow blanketed the world.

I was familiar with the image of a cell and its contents, a more brain-centered knowing. What emerged from this immersion of embodied explorations was a deeper knowing of cellular awareness. One particular moment of the workshop, as we were being guided into yielding to the support of the earth while exploring breath, was when I became aware of my breathing wholeness, of breathing beyond doing. My body fluids felt porous, making contact with the air, and as I gently sensed my inner and outer environment, my state of consciousness shifted. I became hyper-aware of my embryo body, breathing in the potency of amniotic fluid, sensing the constantly flowing dialogue between conscious and unconscious awareness. This stunning moment of awakening my Inner Guide was a conversation *with* my body that has continued to emerge and unfold over these years. It supports what my mentor, Emilie Conrad, founder of Continuum, has observed that movement is who we *are*, not something we *do*.

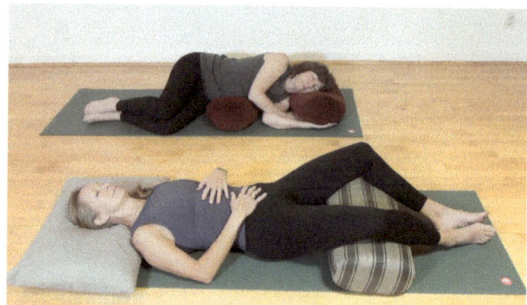

Figure 1.3 Sensing breathwave

My purpose in sharing it here is to invite you to draw on your Inner Guide and begin an exploration of your body's biointelligence. **See Video 1.3 for full exploration.**

Using the floor and pillows as support, see which set-up feels best to you:

▸ Lie on your back with a small pillow under your head, your knees resting over one or two pillows so your back and hips feel relaxed. Place one hand on your low belly, below your navel center, and the other hand on your mid-chest to support your deeper sense of whole-body breathing.

▸ Lie on your side with a small pillow under your head and another pillow under your ribs for gentle support. You may also want a pillow between your knees. Relax your shoulders and arms so that they are resting comfortably.

Close your eyes and notice if you can sense the weight of your body as it meets the floor and the pillow. You might also sense the floor and pillow meeting you. This sensing allows your body to feel more grounded and supported. Grounding and support here are related, as each of them invites a "letting go" that is not about collapse. Rather, it is like actively inhabiting a "restful resilience."

Without attempting to "do" something, begin noticing the movement of your breath as it flows gently in and out through your nose.

If you can allow your belly to soften—neither pushing your breath in and out nor tensing your abdominal muscles—you may notice the movement of your belly expanding slightly on your natural inhale and gently melting back down as you exhale.

There is no need to control the belly movement. You are allowing your body to move freely with your breath. By releasing more of your body weight into the floor and pillow, you may notice that your body responds to your soft breathing as your sense of grounding and support increases. This support may allow you to sense your spaciousness—your connection with the space around you.

It is possible to let go of excess tension by allowing your eyes to rest in the sockets and your tongue and jaw to soften.

You can continue to sense this letting go, and when you are ready, notice if you can begin to sense your *breathwave* through the exploration of the fluid movement of your inhale and exhale, supported by your cerebrospinal fluid. The grounding and support you feel is in coherence with the architecture of your whole body and creates a pathway for the wave of this fluid resonance. Although I speak of it as a wave, the movement may register in the moment as extremely subtle. Consider, however, the same movement taking place as a baby. There, the wave is profound as you are growing your body. Give yourself time to play with the fluid motion. You may notice that your waist floats away from the floor in a tiny wave-like movement that is beyond gentle as you sense your body inhaling. Also, you may notice that your waist floats toward the floor as you sense the movement of your body exhaling. This very gentle rocking motion between your sphenoid (yellow), occiput (green), and sacrum (blue) (see Figure 1.4) is a fluid spinal motion and the birthright of your omnidirectional breathing spine—a way of being that your body knows from the very beginning.

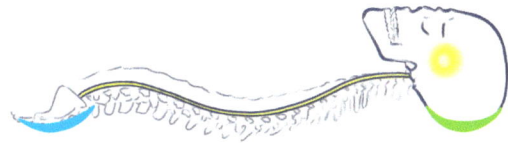

Figure 1.4 Cranial spine—sphenoid and sacrum/coccyx relationship
GRATITUDE TO LEAH REES, ARTIST

Fluid awareness changes everything. As we explore the balancing act of sensing our autonomy and our relationship with the world, we sense our fluidity, the creative intelligence at the heart of existence. It reminds us of our primal connection with the natural living world and the relational "breath" we share. This is in stark contrast to sensing ourselves as a biomechanical machine where the mind controls the body.

Experiential workshops and personal explorations of movement have been crucial in my ongoing exploration and embodiment of my Inner Guide. I have found it important to engage with scholars of embryology who understand the science behind our embryonic beginnings.

STILL, SUTHERLAND, AND BLECHSCHMIDT

In 1899, a student at the American School of Osteopathy in Kirksville, Missouri, William Garner Sutherland, observed a model of a skull mounted and floating in a position where the bones were separated. He wondered why these bones would be so intricately shaped unless their shape reflected a function. The rest of his life was dedicated to exploring and understanding that question. During his explorations in the cranial field, he had an insight and was the first to claim to *feel* a rhythmic shape change in the bones of the cranium. He could "sense" a subtle movement. (He claimed that this biodynamic potency is resonant within all body tissues. He also proposed that the cerebrospinal fluid, potentized and transmuted by an invisible bioelectromagnetic field, originating of its own kind in the early stages of embryonic self-organization, is the chief ordering principle of the embryo.) He later named this felt sense motion the body's "primary respiration" (Sutherland 1990).

Sutherland was deeply influenced by Andrew Taylor Still, the founder of osteopathy, who stated that life is matter in motion. He advised his students to look beyond the study of the structure of bones, and their adjustment, to enhancing the "freedom of the movement of fluids and open the space for the body to function better and heal itself, which he called 'connected oneness'" (Gintis 2007, p.178; Still 1902). When there is a spatial freedom of the movement of fluids, what becomes available is increased vitality, health, and a sense of wellbeing, in addition to a deeper connection with the fluid resonance of the natural world. Creativity, greater body awareness, and trust in one's body wisdom becomes available.

Erich Blechschmidt, an anatomist and embryologist, pioneered 40 years of research into our embryonic beginnings. This resulted in more than 120 scientific papers, numerous books, and a Carnegie collection of human embryo development, focused on evidence presented from the embryo's perspective, rather than the previous findings from the field of zoology used to describe human development. Blechschmidt speaks eloquently about how human nature is still a puzzle, in that it concerns not only the metaphysical aspects of an individual, but also the somatic—the study of the form and the forming of the body. He was concerned about the growing tendency to "molecularize" the human being and to study human function in increasingly isolated "specializations," so the whole gets lost in parts, especially with the aid of the electron microscope, where more than 200,000-fold magnifications are possible. His vision was to obtain a coherent, holistic understanding of the body, "creating a clearer understanding of how the body's form and structure are developed and maintained by the metabolism of living cells" (Blechschmidt 2004, p.1).

Anatomist and embryologist Brian Freeman, a student of Blechschmidt's, shares:

> The sustained investigation of this wealth of material led to a totally new way of looking at early human development, which compels us to re-think older interpretations based mainly on molecular biological studies. It is possible to see how adult functions arise naturally and consistently from the embryo's earlier growth functions. (Blechschmidt 2004, p.1)

Studying Blechschmidt's original ideas and embodied approach to embryonic growth movements, growth forces, and metabolic fields helped me to embody a deeper appreciation of the biodynamics of our emerging form.

ROHEN AND VAN DER WAL

Dr. Johannes W. Rohen's remarkable book *Functional Morphology* (2007) further inspired my deeper appreciation of our human organism as a self-organizing dynamic whole. Rohen's *Color Atlas of Anatomy* (2007) is just one of his series of cadaveric anatomy books used in European medical schools. In his final book, *Functional Morphology*, he speaks of how deeply satisfying it is to shift from the accepted biomechanical anatomical approach and shares his lifelong passion for understanding a "living way of thinking" around the science of the human being with phenomenological studies on human morphology and functional anatomy. This inspired my vision in *Moving Beyond Core*.

Another inspiring scientist whose teachings evoke interoceptive participation is Jaap van der Wal, a phenomenologist and embryologist, who brings the voice of the embryo to life. In his workshops, he expresses this inspiring insight as where biology meets biography. This perception of self as embryo, whole and complete from the very beginning, and self-organizing, self-healing, and adaptive throughout life can be life-changing.

According to van der Wal, our embryonic existence is not merely a passing phase of human life. The embryo still exists in us, throughout life, carrying the blueprint of health into manifestation at every moment.

In his workshops, van der Wal creates a potent space of exploration and curiosity, where accepted theory can be questioned. For instance, there is a theory in embryology that an individual adult human arises from a single fertilized egg, which creates a belief that the dominating sperm fertilizes the passive egg. What van der Wal proposes from a phenomenological perspective is a very different story. Emily Martin, PhD, in the Department of Anthropology at Johns Hopkins University, highlighted this concept in her article "The egg and the sperm: How science has constructed a romance based on stereotypical male-female roles" (1991).

Van der Wal's research on embryology completely rewires the language we use to talk about human conception and the sperm dominating the egg. There is no talk of the sperm "penetrating" the egg, and therefore no privilege given to the male sex in the procreative process. Rather, he highlights a moment of receptivity and a dialogue between sperm and egg in creating a union. This is a paradigm shift. Rather than the sperm dominating the egg, it is more like pollinating a flower. The dialogue shifts away from one of domination. This creates a ripple effect, of what could be possible if we understood life as a respectful, collaborative, reverent approach.

BEING BREATHED VS. "TAKING" A BREATH

I started wondering whether babies actually "breathe" in the womb. The answer is a mixed one. Babies do not breathe in the womb, at least not by inhaling and exhaling air through the lungs, but oxygen travels through the mother's lungs, heart, uterus, and placenta, making its way through the umbilical cord and into the fetus.

As adults, or even as children, we rely on the language of taking a breath to cultivate an active breathing practice. But this word "taking" creates an impulse of thinking we have to do something in order to breathe correctly. The body *receives* breath. We are, in a sense, *breathed*. Think how your body exhales, pauses, and allows your inhale to happen, quite naturally. The ethereal quality of air is swapped out for a more viscous and river-like understanding of the blood/oxygen relationship. Breath supports all of our explorations. This innate wisdom is biointelligence and a movement practice which completely reorients the ways we understand "body," "breath," "uprightness," "health," "wellness," and "relationship."

BACKING INTO THE WOMB

Jaap van der Wal introduced the concept that supports the embryo's "backing into the womb" as the first yielding to gravity (LeBlanc-Arbuckle 2014).

Ignoring the yield to gravity in the present moment allows us to silence the fluid bodily knowledge and relationship that began during that action of backing into the womb. Silencing that relational knowledge has the negative effect of also silencing gravity's role in our movements. Ignoring gravity's role in movement can trick us into thinking that we are doing something ourselves, that movement is something we make happen without any assistance from our environment. But movement with ease begins with a yield to gravity, earth's support, and the embodied action of yielding is a foundational power of support that we already accessed in the womb.

I was introduced to this sense of "bonding" in the womb while studying developmental movement with Bonnie Bainbridge Cohen. Constructive rest, a somatic exploration that involves lying on your back with knees bent and feet on the floor, enabled me to sense a potent experience of what Bonnie referred to as the *yield* to gravity. Yielding is not collapse. Rather, it is a resting aliveness, allowing ourselves to sense our primordial relationship between earth and sky, the foundation of embodied movement. When I yield to gravity's support, I cease fighting against gravity. With this resonant support, I can then move with more ease, even in the most difficult movements. The yield always comes first because with yielding to gravity, our innate reach, uplift, and spatial orientation, ground reaction force, gravity's partner, is evoked. Often we can tune out the process of yielding in order to "do" the movement.

EMERGENCE OF THE MIDLINE

You may remember the experiment conducted by Schwenk earlier in this chapter that revealed the dynamic path of liquids in a container, simulating our midline emergence. Bonnie Gintis uses images to show the intelligence of fluid and the intelligence of our fluid midline. To benefit from these insights, we must understand that the midline moves through breath, sound, and fluid movement.

Around day 15, a mysterious quivering pulsation marks the emergence of the midline.

Throughout this chapter, we avoid referring to the spinal "column" to honor the fluid dynamism of this pulsation. In these early stages, the midline is a fluid function rather than a structure, around which the developing embryo organizes itself. Therefore, what we label as the midline can also be thought of as our "field of influence." In Gintis's words, this field of influence supports

the creation of an orientation, not just for development, but also for the rest of life through adulthood. From this point on, the top, bottom, right and left sides of the body are established. The reference point for the development of the brain, spinal cord, the rest of the nervous system, vertebral column, arms, legs and all the systems of the body is in place and is establishing functional relationships throughout the whole body. (Gintis 2007, p.123)

The two ends of the embryonic midline represented in bone are the tip of the coccyx and the center of the body of the sphenoid bone (Gintis 2007, p.178). These two directions will eventually come to orient themselves as grounding and uprightness (refer back to Figure 1.4), our relationship between earth and sky which I call our "breathing spine."

These orientations, however, are never statically holding a grounded or upright posture. The fluid spine is always moving from these two directions. The resulting bidirectional movement creates a fluid pathway in the shape of a *torus* (a donut shape that folds into itself), which is omnidirectional. This insight allows for us to sense our bodies as spiralic instead of linear, as more closely related to the movement of an octopus than to that of a biomechanical robot. To move in such a way as to support the torus shape of our omnidirectional midline requires rethinking what models we use to assist our movement practices.

In the world of embryology, we become aware that our fluid, dynamic midline is less a column or thing, and more of an *event*, one that takes place within the matrix of the womb. These insights help us recognize not only the spiralic/mobius/torus movement of our midlines but also the relational dimension of these movements. The intelligence of our midline emerges within the environment of the womb and is supported by the fluid architecture there.

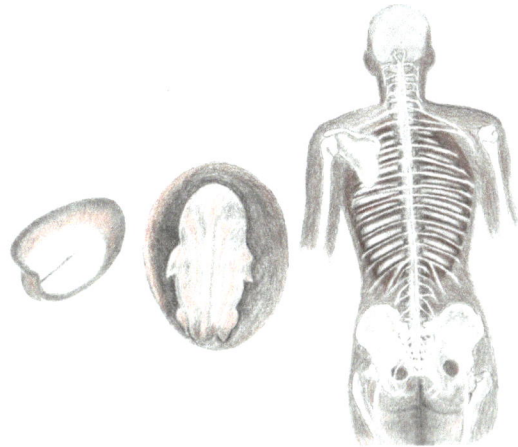

Figure 1.5 Primitive streak, emerging embryo, adult spine
GRATITUDE TO CECILIA COLOME, ARTIST

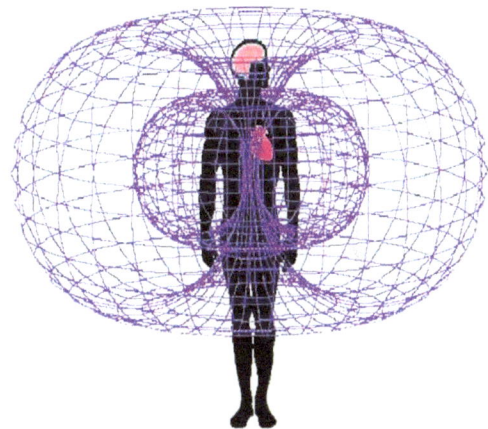

Figure 1.6 Heart field—torus of spine
This image depicts the omnidirectional biomagnetic field projected by the human heart. Notice that our spine functions as the bridge between earth and sky.
WIKICOMMONS IMAGE. https://commons.wikimedia.org/wiki/File:Heart-field.jpg

MOVING FROM MESO

Prior to the emergence of our midline, as we are self-organizing in the womb, two "outside" body walls and an "in-between" emerge. The two outside body walls are our Ectoderm, which forms our back body and gives rise to our nervous system and outer layer of skin and the amniotic cavity, and our Endoderm, which forms our front body and gives rise to the yolk sac, and forms our digestive and respiratory organs. The third "in-between" is our mutable Meso.

> The tissues that develop from embryonic mesoderm make up a very large proportion of the body and compose the capsules or containers of everything else that is not made of it. Tissues in this family can be viewed as "structural" or "non-structural." The tissues with an obvious structural role include: muscle, fascia, bone, cartilage, tendon, ligament, joint capsule, scar tissue, intervertebral discs, subcutaneous tissue and fat. Another category of structural tissue support is provided by the walls of blood and lymph vessels, the capsules surrounding organs such as the liver, kidneys, heart, and gonads, the fibrous dividing sheaths inside organs, the mesenteries that support the abdominal organs, the muscle of the heart, the smooth muscle of the respiratory tract, the sheath around nerves, the microglial cells of the brain and the spinal cord. The non-structural mesodermal elements encompass the blood and lymphatic components: red and white blood cells, bone marrow, lymph nodes, the thymus, and the spleen. (Gintis 2007, p.157)

Jaap van der Wal distinguishes what he calls the *Meso* as manifesting itself as connective tissue *mesenchyme*, the intermediate layer and tissue of innerness, which creates our three-dimensionality, and the *matrix fabric* of our body organization, which he calls "our proprioceptive innerness."

Van der Wal reminds us of our embryonic beginnings when he speaks of *blood as primitive connective mesenchyme tissue*, through which the motion of the levity of capillaries and blood pressure returns blood to the heart. This updated research allows us to sense that "the heart is not a mechanical pump but actually a sensitive integrator of all our experiences" (Chitty 2013, p.404). Understanding the blood as specialized connective tissue and that its fluid resonance with our spiralic heart develops *before* the nervous system forms is a deep shift in thinking.

Van der Wal's research offers a dialogue between the "in-between" emerging Meso and its interrelationship with the boundary-like epithelial tissues of the Ectoderm and Endoderm as what births the *quivering pulsation* of the midline primitive streak, the origin of our future perineal body. He uses the term "Meso" to emphasize that it is not a matter of three layers, but a "'triune' body with an inner dimension" (van der Wal 2018).

The whole notion of proprioception is also revolutionary. It refers to the body's ability to sense movement, action, and location. Typically, people talk about the external dimension of proprioception. The skin, for example, senses approaching bodies and reacts in specific ways to familiar surroundings. In each case, proprioception defines a kind of bodily seeing and sensing. As van der Wal shares, *proprioceptive innerness* is a kind of bodily seeing and sensing from the inside. Here our fascial architecture supports spatially, connects globally, and informs kinesthetically through postural orienting, balance, and locomotion. We shift our attention from external motion (e.g., walking, dancing, jumping) to an internal concert of motion. This is what is referred to as *interoception*. Interoception is our ability to sense our internal workings. Proprioceptive innerness is the inside's ability to sense where "I" am in space and the impact on my internal systems.

The practice of rekindling our *listening* relationship through interoceptive awareness of proprioceptive innerness heightens our attention to our Inner Guide. This, in turn, becomes a wake-up call and conversation with our body and sends messages such as you are thirsty, tired, and so on. Your Inner Guide begins speaking with you on a regular basis and even questions habitual actions as if to ask, "Are you going to ignore me or nurture me?"

In Blechschmidt's view, all cells are always kinetically or metabolically linked to each other through the transport of substances. This activity is biotensegrity, or living tensegrity, a tensional balance between cells and the fascial matrix, the continuity of our living architecture from nucleus to skin. When we integrate the sensation of this tensional balance into our external movements, we no longer over-stretch, we minimize our tendency to lose relationship between earth and sky, collapsing our posture, and we activate our body's fluid dynamism which honors our bio-intelligence. Through attuning to our proprioceptive innerness, we enhance our knowledge of our body in space, illuminating the awareness that we are influenced by many unseen forces, such as gravity.

Biotensegrity is a self-organizing, tension-compression, fluid process. It is our living architecture, but unlike rigid steel construction in a skyscraper, it is an ongoing conversation within the fascial matrix that results in a regenerative organism. The components of our inner landscape are always regenerating and reshaping their place within the concert of internal activity. There is no fixed thing called fascia or Meso. There is our living fascial matrix movement in communication with all aspects of body function. Muscles. When we engage the embryonic field of Meso through fluid movements, such as relaxed, rhythmical, and spontaneous

walking, we are no longer in the orbit of biomechanical models. Instead, we access the body in relationship with the environment. The connective tissue fascial matrix links cells to each other and to other tissues and structures in a complex communication system. Spiralic, figure-eight patterns are inherent in our embryological becoming. There is something vital to bodily development bound up in figure-eight lemniscate patterns. The most rhythmical of all geometric forms, lemniscate patterning is expressed in the swirling vortexes of a running stream, the spiralic growth of plants. Legendary mystic and educator Rudolf Steiner observed in a lecture to his students:

> Yesterday I showed that wheresoever we may look in the human body, we shall find the formative principle of the looped curve or lemniscate...so, for example, when you are tracing the bony system or the nervous system in man, even the blood circulation can be traced in this way. You must imagine it all not in a plane but in space. The figure eight—you are dealing with geometrical figures of rotation. The forms of our inner organization, in the nerves and senses system and in the metabolic and limb system respectively, are mutually related upon the principle of a lemniscate of rotation. (Steiner 1921)

Jaap van der Wal spoke of the helical, migratory dance of the emerging arms and legs through growth gestures. Our hands and arms reach forward and around in a grasping, giving/receiving gesture, like an embrace, and then come to rest in external rotation. Our feet and legs grow out in a more extended gesture, pre-exercising to standing and kicking in the womb, where the hamstrings and calves spiral internally to the posterior thigh, which in our Meso movement patterning "allows our leg musculature to act like a pogo stick, coiling and uncoiling in our later gait pattern" (Beach 2010, p.46).

OUR LEMNISCATE BODY

Phillip Beach spoke about the *Wolffian ridge*, a remarkable intermediate structure in our embryological morphology that appears around day 28 in the womb space, which "links the precursor tissues of the nose, eyes, and ears with the vagus nerve, the upper limbs, the nipples, the lower limbs and genital tip into one cohesive interconnectedness" (Beach 2010, p.17).

Just as the fins on fish develop in response to the evolutionary demands of fluid dynamics, which allows fish to move through the water in many directions, our upper and lower limbs are positioned on our bodies to optimally amplify and inhibit whole-organism movement. Reaching, pulling, pushing, and walking are all enabled by the lemniscate patterning of the body. We rely on this deeply ingrained pattern each day.

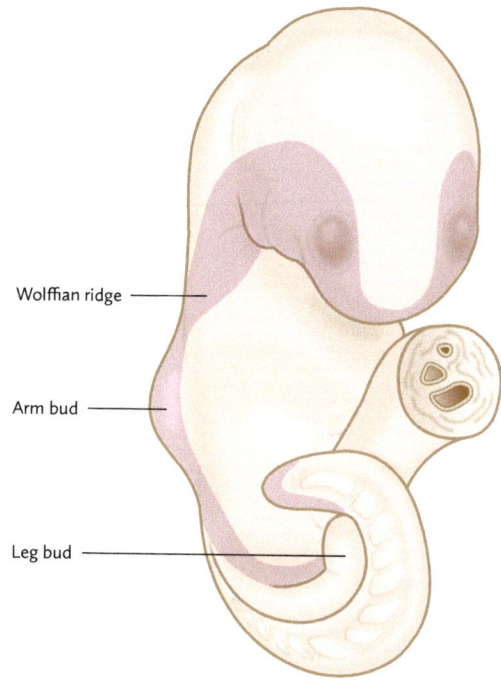

Figure 1.7 Wolffian ridge

AND THE JOURNEY CONTINUES

All of these insights from the work of pioneering embryologists provide a deep dive into the generative and emergent fluid processes within our embryonic beginnings. This informs how we continue to self-assemble the manifesting blueprint of our adult lives. This is cultivating our Inner Guide.

As students of movement education and/or structural or energetic bodywork, we can renew and regenerate ourselves, and thereby support our clients and ourselves in both unraveling patterns of dysfunction and enhancing our health and vitality. Learning to listen to our Inner Guide leads to important changes in the most fundamental principles of movement and bodywork. When I speak of listening to the Inner Guide, I am talking about reconnecting to a kind of

listening that was present in our earliest beginnings. The Inner Guide alerts us to new kinds of embodied sensations. It does so by drawing on sensory experiences that our bodies have been processing since we were embryos.

There are signs that you are connecting with your Inner Guide. You may find yourself more and more willing to slow down. You may choose to listen to yourself from a place of curiosity instead of judgment. You may have an entirely new relationship with the notion of difficulty. Rather than a hurdle or obstacle, movements or events now show up as opportunities for growth. The notion of finishing a task can be replaced by a love of process.

You begin to suspect that "whole-body awareness" is even more amazing and dynamic than you knew... Each "part" of you feels like the "whole" of you because even "small" movements have a tremendous ripple effect and feel supported by your entire fascial matrix body.

Here we begin, with a tingling of curiosity and excitement which is linked to the conscious acknowledgment of the mystery that is *your* Inner Guide.

In the next chapter, we explore how the concept of Core ceases to be defined by abdominal strength and the control of the body, and becomes, instead, Core as Relationship, a relational way of being that evokes a fluid dynamism functioning within an equally dynamic natural and social environment.

Use the following QR code for the video in this chapter:

REFERENCES

Bainbridge Cohen, B. (2023) "Supporting the nervous system through exploring the weight and flow of blood." Body-Mind Centering®. www.bodymindcentering.com/supporting-the-nervous-system-through-exploring-the-weight-and-flow-of-blood

Beach, P. (2010) *Muscles and Meridians: The Manipulation of Shape*. Edinburgh: Churchill Livingstone.

Blechschmidt, E. (2004) *The Ontogenetic Basis of Human Anatomy*. Berkeley, CA: North Atlantic Books.

Carson, R. (1961) *The Sea Around Us*. New York, NY: The New American Library of World Literature.

Chitty, J. (2013) *Dancing with Yin and Yang*. Boulder, CO: Polarity Press.

Gintis, B. (2007) *Engaging the Movement of Life*. Berkeley, CA: North Atlantic Books.

Guimberteau, J.-C. (2015) *Architecture of Human Living Fascia*. London: Handspring Publishing.

Kern, M. (2005) *Wisdom in the Body*. Berkeley, CA: North Atlantic Books.

LeBlanc-Arbuckle, W. (2014) "Wendy Interviews M.D., Embryologist, Jaap van der Wal." YouTube. www.youtube.com/watch?v=2KsO-U66sVs

Martin, E. (1991) "The egg and the sperm: How science has constructed a romance based on stereotypical male-female roles." *Signs 16*, 3 (Spring), 485–501.

Oschman, J. (2003) *Energy Medicine in Therapeutics and Human Performance*. Oxford: Butterworth-Heinemann.

Rohen, J. (2007) *Color Atlas of Anatomy*. Hillsdale, NY: Adonis Press.

Rohen, J. (2007) *Functional Morphology*. Hillsdale, NY: Adonis Press.

Schwenk, T. (1996) *Sensitive Chaos: Creation of Flowing Forms in Water and Air*. Forest Row, East Sussex: Rudolf Steiner Press.

Steiner, R. (1921) "Lecture XII—GA 323. Third Scientific Lecture-Course: Astronomy." Rudolf Steiner Archive. https://rsarchive.org/Lectures/GA323/English/LR81/19210112p01.html

Still, A. (1902 [1892]) *Philosophy and Mechanical Principles of Osteopathy*. Kansas City, MO: Hudson-Kimberly Publishing Company.

Sutherland, W. (1990) *Teachings in the Science of Osteopathy*. Portland, OR: Rudra Press.

van der Wal, J. (2018) "Embryo in US" [workshop]. Boulder, CO: Colorado School of Energy Studies.

CHAPTER 2

Core as Relationship

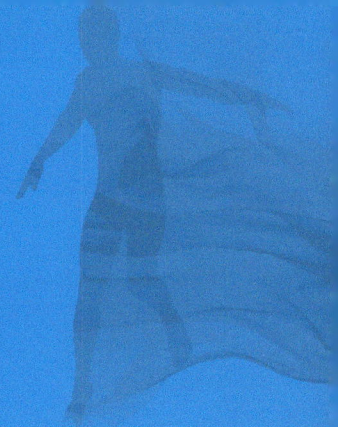

This chapter looks at the essential difference between a biointelligent and a biomechanical approach to movement and bodywork. There is a subtle and vital difference in the way a practitioner or student approaches the body and works with what is referred to as the Core.

There is a tendency in some circles to speak of biointelligent approaches, but then focus on biomechanical exercises. Some writers and practitioners, such as Bonnie Gintis (*Engaging the Movement of Life*, 2007) and Joanne Sarah Avison (*Yoga, Fascia, Anatomy and Movement*, 2015), have discussed this distinction. It means we look at how the physical body is innately supported by regenerative forces that are relational within our environment.

Chart 2.1 compares biomechanical and biointelligent approaches (the left column describes a biomechanical approach to the body; the right column reveals a biointelligent perspective).

Chart 2.1 Comparing and contrasting "biomechanical" and "biointelligent" approaches to movement

Biomechanical	Biointelligent
	Nuclear Envelope, Nucleus, Cytoskeleton, Extracellular Matrix
Closed cell theory...cell as a bag...membrane as a barrier	Open cell theory...cytoskeleton/living matrix...emerging embryo to adult to cosmos as tension-compression biotensegrity
Body as object	Body as living process of biodynamic fields
Dissective view...mind controls body... Isolating: muscles, bones, fascia, psoas... Brain as computer...heart as pump	Whole Ooganism Interrelationship view... Mind in every cell of body... Biotensegrity...no part more important than another
Core control...abdominals as area of concentration	Core coordination...abdominals in spatial relationship with whole body
What's right/wrong...coming from judgment, convincing, competition	What's working/missing...coming from inquiry, listening, cooperation
Problem local	Problem global

Biomechanical	Biointelligent
Alignment	Orientation
Old view of autonomic nervous system *Sympathetic* "mobilization...flight/fight" *Parasympathetic* (dorsal vagal complex primarily system for "calming")	*New view* of autonomic nervous system... *Polyvagal theory* (ventral vagal complex serves "empathy, mobilization and calming")
How "should" I breathe?	Being "breathed"
Doing	Non-doing...being present
"Tell me what to do" approach...downloading information	Evoking inner teacher...direct experience/primary perception
Fighting gravity...effortful	Partnering with gravity...effort with ease
Doing something *to* the body	Conversation *with* the body
Being broken...need to be fixed	Deeply intelligent organism that knows how to heal itself
Teacher as expert	*Client as expert* in their own body

3CoreConnections® Embodied Perspective of Living Architecture with Wendy LeBlanc-Arbuckle

A biomechanical concept speaks about "doing something *to* the body." In terms of core in the Pilates or fitness world, we notice what a workout routine is doing *to* your core, your abdominal area.

The cue of drawing the navel to the spine is to "recruit" the proper abdominal muscles and achieve the aesthetic goal of a flatter abdomen. This form of core stabilization has infiltrated the belief systems of so many fitness disciplines, including yoga, which comes originally from a tradition based in "wholeness" rather than the current over-stabilizing "fitness" trend. For example, the abdominal core might indicate that it has a strong connection to another part of the body, one that might not be addressed through typical exercise.

A biointelligent approach invites a "conversation *with* the body." This phrase is holistic and looks at the inherently complex qualities of our "self."

The biointelligent approach respects that the body's innate intelligence has something to say before the brain instructs it to action.

The image on the left in Chart 2.1 presents the cell-as-bag, a concept that was arrived at from studies with the light microscope, which at the time—the early 19th century—seemed to show a barrier at the cell surface (Pollack 2001, p.5). The image on the right presents the cytoskeleton's relationship with the whole body's extracellular living matrix as a continuum (Oschman 2003, p.65).

The image on the left emerges from the reductionist thought process of myself as a separate entity from the expression I perform as movement—I move my legs, I twist my spine, and so on. In contrast, the image on the right embodies a sense of self that emerges *as* movement; there is no outside agent doing the movement.

These images present two different philosophies of how we exist on a cellular level. Here, it is important to notice that the image of the cell bag on the left is missing the cellular communication that exists in our living architecture, where all of the systems of the body are co-mingling, embedded in and partitioned by connective tissue.

Cell biologist Bruce Lipton noted:

the cell membrane, which is the brain of the cell, through its receptors picks up signals and translates them into biology which then sends signals into the nucleus which controls the genes. Therefore, a change in perception of an individual can change their biology, virtually immediately. (Gustafson 2017, p.16)

The image of the cell, with a membrane as a barrier, allows no room to visualize cellular communication, the conductivity of electrical pulses, or the body's fluid intelligence.

Another cell biologist, James Oschman, transformed my contextual understanding of our living architecture through sensing the connective tissue as a liquid crystalline matrix. According to Oschman, our *living matrix* has semiconductor properties, one of which is piezoelectricity—from the Greek, meaning "pressure electricity"—where every movement of the body, every pressure, and every tension anywhere generates a variety of oscillating bioelectric signals or microcurrents through the whole body:

> These signals are precisely characteristic of those tensions, compressions and movement and because of their continuity and connectivity, the signals spread throughout the tissues, into the cell's interiors. If the parts of the organism are cooperative and coordinated in their functioning and every cell knows what every other cell is doing, there is coherence, which is vital to injury repair and defense against disease. (Oschman 2003, p.61)

In Figure 2.2, Amanda is sitting with hips above knees, in order to access her body's natural uplift from foot to head.

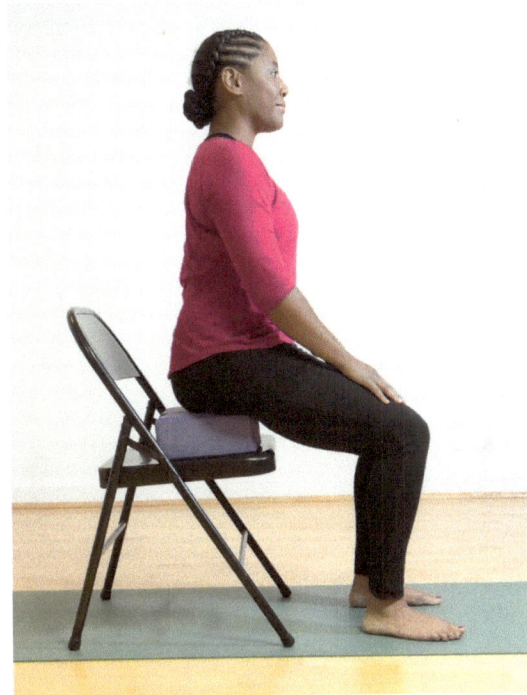

Figure 2.2 Perching on a chair to access ground reaction force (GRF)

Sitting on a chair, with hips higher than knees, the conversation between feet, abdominal area, and spine deepens. See Video 2.2 for full exploration.

WHY IS THE CONVERSATION BETWEEN THE BODY AND INNATE INTELLIGENCE IMPORTANT?

This matters because it shifts the way I think about the shape and tone of my abdominal area, the exact parameters of which begin to expand, as influenced by how I ground with earth's energy through my feet and sitting bones.

Another answer has to do with gravity and its "partner" ground reaction forces (GRF). In the biomechanical approach, my abdominals are isolated through muscular compression—like driving your car with the parking brake on. In the biointelligent approach, my abdominals are in relationship with the fascial continuity of my whole body from foot to head and hand, so pressing into my feet wakes up whole-body core coordination.

Having access to that feeling of uplift is both

noticeable and important when one sits with hips and knees level in a chair or hips below the knees on a low stool or in a squat. The idea of "lumbar support" exists to solve the problem created by right-angled seating. Move toward a perch position and the lumbar curve comes back on its own and the spine finds its natural extension. The right angle between legs and spine is hard on the lumbar spine (rolling it backwards), so for most people, sitting with the knees lower than the hips in a perch position, with feet flat on the floor, will take strain off the lumbar curve.

BUILDING THE RELATIONSHIP BETWEEN CORE COORDINATION AND THE BIOINTELLIGENT SELF

Sitting with the feet as support is not focused on stabilizing and controlling, but on becoming more aware of the role of gravity. Core is now in a relational context that includes your abdominal area, feet (the receptors of your feet that meet the ground and the minute activities of bone, tendon, muscle, fascial matrix), and gravity.

Let's explore two other distinctions as we look more deeply into the world that our feet awaken. In Chart 2.1, we find the terms "alignment" and "orientation." In exploring "alignment," it is common for the client to stand up and be appraised by the instructor, an expert in the discipline, whose trained eye will be able to tell whether or not the person is properly aligned. In this assessment, the instructor is looking for an aligned head, chest, pelvis, knees, and feet, consistent with one's relationship to an *external*, static plumb line. In that configuration, the role of core is the dominating abdominal center from which the upward and downward extensions unfold.

The biointelligent perspective has a more interoceptive approach, one that embarks from the relationship with the field of gravity. The word "orientation" actually refers to multiple things at once. This includes discovering the relationship between ankles, feet, and ground, and to begin to sense what range of motion their stance supports and encourages.

Consider: I am standing up, barefoot, asking myself the question "What is the connection between the floor and my feet and ankles?" My ankles become a facilitator of a certain range of motion that I sense first on the surface of my feet as I rock back and forth, side to side, and around the circumference of my feet. I begin to notice how much surface there is on the bottom of my feet, and how much movement is possible simply by playing around with this orientation. The multilayered bones of my feet and toes begin to receive impulses from the floor as I explore. From here, the orientation of my feet and ankles continues up my legs into my knees and hips, pelvis, spine, and head as I explore all these connections. As my range of movement becomes a bit more expansive, I can begin to sense an invitation to walk or move off this center stance.

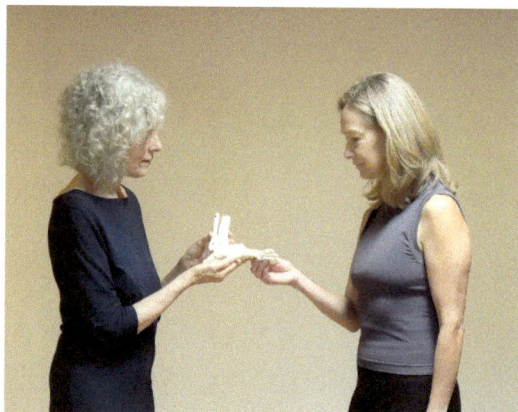

Figure 2.3 Bones of the feet

In contrast, a biomechanical approach to alignment comes from a static place and needs to control the organization of every body part in order to move. The orientation in the biointelligent approach builds a proprioceptive and/or interoceptive map of your body's natural movement. By building a map, it brings your attention to your body in a new way and reveals that the whole body is always involved in movement. That interconnectedness between parts of the body is much more dynamic because everything is always interrelated and in motion.

In this orienting movement, I could sense a core within each of these zones that I just explored. These core zones are like dynamic centers of gravity that help me create a deeper awareness of my body and its surroundings. As I explore these relationships, awareness expands throughout my whole body through biointelligent curiosity. **See Video 2.3 for full exploration**.

Pioneering somatic educator Emilie Conrad (2007) says, "We don't do movement, we are movement."

When we open to an internal dialogue that grows from cellular dynamics, breath, and sonic vibrations, we can evoke a deep wisdom that expresses itself as an embodied experience of our exhale. In this experience, grounding through your feet (standing) or sitting bones (sitting) supports your low belly and pelvic diaphragm following the upward lift of the respiratory diaphragm, naturally drawing the abdominals inward and upward, as the lower ribs melt down toward your navel center.

As we put all these comments and explorations about Chart 2.1 into action, we are able to notice ways of being with ourselves that emerge as either objectifying or embodying.

Think of two ways of moving through a Bridge Pose. The first demonstrates how biomechanical approaches to movement understand the body as an anatomical structure formed by isolated muscle groups that perform certain actions. The second exploration demonstrates how biointelligent approaches to movement broaden the scope of the body beyond anatomical terms, acknowledging other relationships in even the most minute of movements. Some of these relationships include, but certainly are not limited to, gravity, ground reaction force, fascial connections through your whole body from foot to head and hand, and the ongoing influence of our habitual movements. Many biomechanical exercises, even if they don't state this explicitly, presume that the body's core is a corset of muscles around your mid-spine and that this core is fundamental to the success of the exercise. By distinction, the biointelligent approach invites a consideration of fluid and dynamic core *relationships* that exceed the perceived boundaries or limits of the physical body.

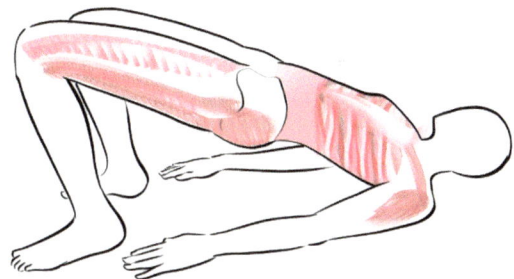

Figure 2.4 Biomechanical bridge
GRATITUDE TO LEAH REES, ARTIST

BRIDGING (BIOMECHANICAL APPROACH)— DOING SOMETHING *TO* THE BODY

When performing Pelvic Curl and Bridge Pose with the muscular focus from the beginning, a reader's focus may zoom too easily in on the isolated muscle groups targeted by the exercise.

There is often a listing of muscle groups followed by a brief step-by-step "execution" of the exercise. It's possible that confusion may arise here, though, because readers are sometimes being asked to keep track of a list of targeted muscles, lists of accompanying muscles, and possibly even notes that supplement the description of the exercise, all this while trying to do the exercise. See Video 2.4 for full exploration.

If I use my thinking mind to execute the exercise by fitting my body into the idealized picture, I will often exert extra effort to figure out how to do the exercise "properly," which is different from exploring the sensations that arise. I am likely to believe that the key to the movement is my body's isolated muscle groups.

What does a typical biomechanical instruction leave out? What is often omitted is the support of gravity as the tail curls as a response to, and in relationship with, the action of pressing gently down through the feet. If this cue is only mentioned later in accompanying notes, a reader attempting to perform this exercise would tend to overthink in order to progress. In turn, this isolated muscular approach often separates the mind from the body and can lead to more difficulty with exercise progression from fundamentals to flow. The disconnect between mind and body visible in the description of exercises like the "Pelvic Curl" is from the tendency to target specific muscles to move distinct parts of the body. This distinction stems from an approach to the body that has as its goal the desire to *idealize*, *train*, or *fix* the body. The presentation of the exercise assumes that a teacher-expert, someone with enough experience to understand how to interpret the instructions, will help a client to do the exercise properly.

To bridge several problems that can arise from this biomechanical approach—from its quiet idealization of the perfect pose to the notion that certain muscles do certain tasks in isolation of one another—I would like to explore the "Bridge Pose" from a biointelligent perspective.

BRIDGING (BIOINTELLIGENT APPROACH)—A CONVERSATION *WITH* THE BODY

This movement exploration utilizes a conceptual framework called "Waterfall Down the Back," or relationship with gravity. I was guided to develop this distinction in order to allow a deeper sense of grounding to encourage a conscious awareness of how earth's energy supports us. The "waterfall" is the fluid, widening movement of your clavicles (collarbones), the softening of your front lower ribs, and the gliding sensation of your shoulder blades Down the Back, responding to your exhale. The feelings of widening and gliding continues to flow down your spine to your sitting bones/tailbone to the tripod of your feet, all the while supported by gravity and your relationship with earth's energy.

Allow yourself to explore and experiment this felt sense of your shoulder blades gliding Down the Back and your low belly suspenders responding to your exhale Up the Front.

Placing one hand on your low belly, below your navel, and the other hand behind the base of your skull, you may notice that, as you soften your knees, allowing your *inhale*, your feet take your weight. Then, as you press into your feet and *exhale* as you straighten your legs (without hyperextending your knees), your head floats up as your shoulder blades glide down your back on your exhale and your low belly "suspenders" move in and up your front. We call this distinction "shoulder blades to internal belly suspenders" which is listening to the language of your body's internal connection—what Pilates teachers would call a natural powerhouse. See Video 2.5 for deeper exploration.

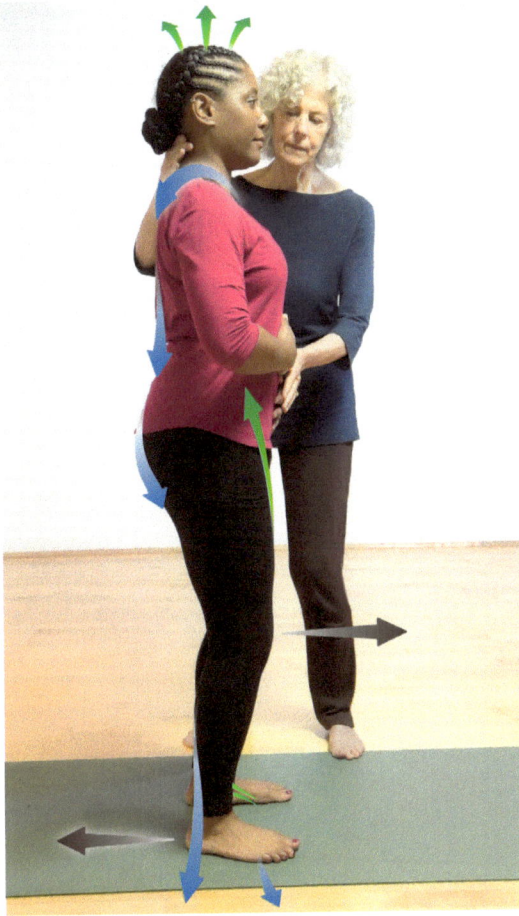

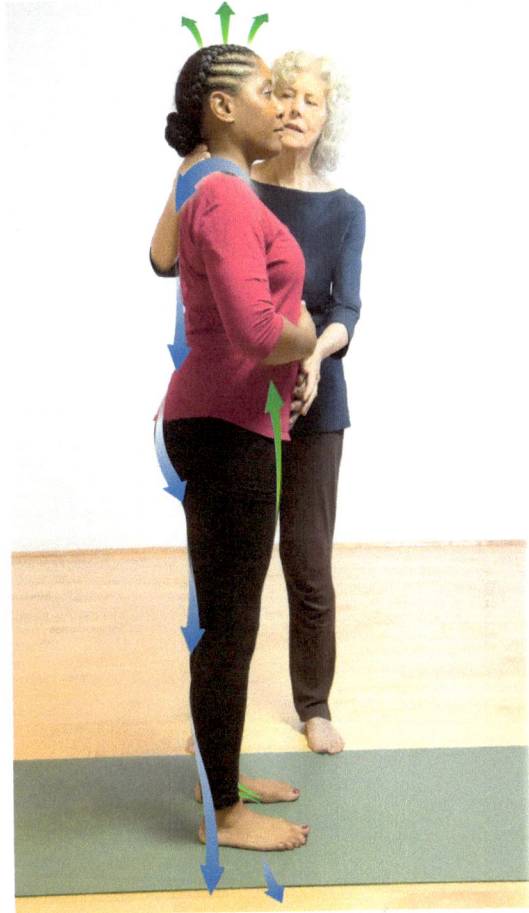

Figures 2.5A and 2.5B Waterfall Down the Back and internal lift Up the
Front as "shoulder blades to internal belly suspenders"

The emphasis here is on *your experience* of bridging, which is an embodied, relational approach, and will change each time you explore, becoming more integrated with your natural movement.

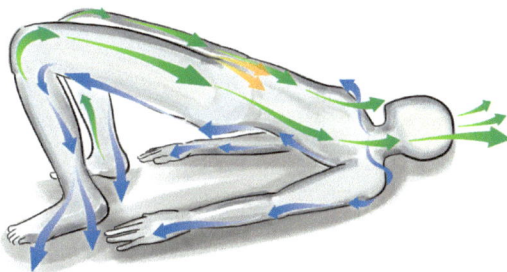

Figure 2.6 Biointelligent approach to bridging—evoking Core as Relationship

As you begin your practice, you are creating a baseline awareness of how your body is meeting the floor and how the floor is meeting you. You may notice the ways in which gravity is always participating in your movement by sharing how your weight shifts through your body, allowing a sense of grounding and uplift, as you press gently into your feet, before sensing the curl of your tail and the lift of your hips. What is important is the shift from a mentality that says there is a right and a wrong way to do the movement, toward an inquisitive awareness that wonders what's working and what you can become aware of that might be missing and that you can provide in the way of support (foot position, strap, pillow, etc.). **See Video 2.6 for deeper exploration**.

- As you are lying down, allowing your breath to move you, can you sense your feet grounding, which allows your tail to curl, supported by your knees reaching toward your feet, which gives space for your belly wall to fall back toward your midline? These actions evoke gravity's partner, the uplift of ground reaction force (GRF), your low belly suspenders, "Up the Front."

- This awareness accompanies the sense of grounding achieved through "Waterfall Down the Back." Together, these two felt sensations constitute a dialogue your body has with gravity and GRF that speaks of the ways in which grounding evokes uplift.

- What may surprise you, as you sense what we will come to call your *breathing spine*, is that your feet, legs, hands, arms, and head are invited to move with your spine, if you allow them to communicate. As you practice, you will notice that your body knows these relationships and will flow through the movement more easily each time. This bodily knowledge is guided by your Inner Guide, and your body's innate "knowing" of its living architecture through the interrelationship of Lower Core (grounding), Central Core (centering breath connection of lower and upper body), and Upper Core (suspension and uplift), and your breath's relationship with your body's metabolic need.

In the biointelligent bridge, the cueing is an invitation to be aware through the movement of what is needed in order to sense a whole-body approach that creates *effort with ease*.

As you explore a movement often cued as the "Pelvic Curl" leading into the "Bridge," the biointelligent approach encourages individuals to embark on a personal journey. This journey symbolizes our role as a "bridge" between the grounding force of the earth and the spatial orientation of the sky. It invites people to explore and become aware of their movement in a non-judgmental manner, meeting them where they are. From this place of acceptance, the focus shifts to identifying what's needed, rather than labeling something as "wrong," and learning how to discover what is missing to find support.

This fluid approach brings about a transformative connection within the Upper Core, particularly with the arms, as they rediscover their embryonic relationship with the doming nature of the feet. This embodied, biointelligent approach engages not only the physical body but also the mind, emotions, and spirit of the whole person.

We are a biointelligent organism, a living process, who knows how to self-heal, self-regulate, and adapt. This biointelligence is a resonance in coherence with other beings and the living world, flowing all the time. We discover how to meet ourselves, like a best friend, and be curious about how we can ask for support with an injury, illness, or emotional difficulty. Studying an embodied approach teaches us to explore movement as a lived experience of our relationship with gravity, spatial orientation, one another, and our living world. This lived experience, in turn, increases presence, vitality, empathy, joy, and wellbeing.

From this approach, we begin to sense our body as a relationship of tension-compression spatial forces and movements. When we become acquainted with our body's innate biointelligence, we "remember" the elastic integrity that we had as children—we were fluid beings, rolling, jumping, running, throwing. As we age, we tend to stiffen and collapse by sitting too much or holding on to emotional stress. When we rediscover moving from our biointelligent wisdom, we turn on the lights of our innate connection with the river of all life as flowing, coherent motion. We move away from an isolated muscular approach to movement and begin sensing our whole body's extracellular fascial matrix, which supports and communicates with every system in our body. We engage our body's tensional integrity which includes a resting tensional tone, rather than collapse. With this seismic shift, our body remembers its fractal nature, where grounding, centering, and uplift supports *effort with ease*.

Ultimately, "Core" shows itself in both exercises. But, the "core" of the biomechanical approach is an isolated set of muscles that is used to fit the body into completed postures. The biointelligent approach is always about evoking a coherent relationship:

- between gravity and ground reaction force (spatial orientation)
- between my fascial elastic recoil breath and my whole elastic body
- between self and other beings, including our living environment
- between trauma and perception
- between body, mind, emotion, and spirit.

ARRIVING AT 3CORES

My vision of the 3CoreConnections® embodied awareness emerged as an evolving, biointelligent process that raises awareness of the complex ways our bodies function and shape themselves internally, and how we are shaped by our environments. What has emerged, over these decades, is an embodied approach to teaching/mentoring that enables students and practitioners of any discipline to discover their wholeness by cultivating their own voice through the portal and brilliant guidance of their innate biointelligent wisdom—their Inner Guide.

This body of work came alive for me as I studied with treasured mentors, along with Core as Relationship. This perspective developed organically out of the process of my explorations with gravity, movement, sound, and sensory and structural awareness as relational forces. Their interactive relationships support our postural orientation and ways of being in life. What emerged is an embodied, perceptual approach that can be applied to any discipline; meeting ourselves or clients where we are, developing awareness of our innate intelligence and ability to help ourselves at any age.

Whereas many movement arts and bodywork disciplines highlight *the* body, as if the body is an isolated entity, we explore how bodies form and shape themselves through relational networks that are formed in equal part by unseen external forces and our bodies' many internal activities. When we learn to *yield* into the support of gravity, we cultivate a relationship with gravity's partner, ground reaction force, the *uplift and reach* of spatial orientation. This relational way of being releases and frees the back of the body from gripping and cultivates a deeper relationship with the front of the body from inner ankle to inner ear and hand. When we allow ourselves to be supported by gravity, by "yielding" our weight into the earth through our feet in standing, or our back/front or side body in lying down, we access "embodied awareness" and Core becomes a relational context.

Letting go is an important principle that affects our perceptions, emotions, and behavior. When we let go of judgment and right/wrong thinking, we enhance our presence with ourselves in the moment. We shift from the binary "what's right" and "what's wrong" to a resourceful perspective of "what's working" and "what's missing." Letting go becomes a non-judgmental way of being that opens us, through deeper listening skills, to provide what is needed, and allows discovery, curiosity, and adaptation.

Finally, the name 3CoreConnections is a contextual way of sensing your body within the gravitational field so the learning is innately yours. This concept shows that through grounding, centering, and uplift, it is possible to explore the complex network of forces that exist, so that movement becomes fascial unwinding—*movement as bodywork.*

THE JOURNEY TO CORE AS RELATIONSHIP BEGINS

At the beginning of my journey, the relational way of being with myself that dynamizes the heart of this biointelligent perspective was a sporadic experience, at best. As many people do, I relied on the insights of biomechanical—isolated *muscular*—approaches to movement and bodywork. Now I invite colleagues to explore their own biointelligent nature, and think about how we relate to gravity, ourselves, one another, and our environment. Underlining some of the main realizations I made between biomechanical approaches and the biointelligent way of being that would become the heart of my explorations, I would like to share a brief story of the path that brought me here.

To begin, let's zoom into a scene where I was studying yoga at the Himalayan Institute, in my mid-20s. I'm in one of my favorite poses, Wide-Angled Seated Forward Bend. As I extend my torso and the rest of my upper body forward between my legs, feeling a deep release in my hips and groin, my arms reach forward, to help me draw closer and closer to the floor. I continue to breathe deeply into the pose, allowing my spine to soften and lengthen, and finally reach a fully prone position with arms widening toward my feet and head turned to the side on the wooden floor. It wouldn't, at the time, have occurred to me that I was over-stretching my hypermobile body, or that there was anything problematic about my "go as far as you can" approach to movement.

DISCOVERING PILATES

Fast forward to the mid-1980s when I met some dancers in New Orleans who had studied Pilates. They were telling me how profoundly this method contributed to their body awareness and technique, but it wasn't until the early 1990s, when Michael, my husband, and I moved to Estes Park, Colorado, that I had the opportunity to experience the method myself. The Pilates Center (TPC) had just opened in a small studio on Pearl Street in Boulder, and as it was close, I booked a class to learn about the Pilates Matwork. Straight away, I loved learning the flowing movements of the method, where the rhythmic inhales and exhales led my body to discover deeper connections.

Coming from a longtime yoga practice, I looked at the Pilates spring-based apparatus and thought, "Why would I want to be on a machine? I know how to be in my body." For six months, I rejoiced in practicing and understanding the brilliant levels of the Pilates Matwork. Eventually, I accepted a friend's invitation to join her in a session learning the Pilates Reformer.

That experience opened a whole new world. Lying on the sliding carriage of the Reformer, I felt an "internal conversation with my body" from the power of the springs, through the simple action of bending and straightening my legs. There was a moment where I knew something was different, but I couldn't quite put words to it at the time. As I look back through the 3CoreConnections lens, I understand that experience as the communication between my foot-to-head, connective tissue fascial matrix and the springs' tensional resistance. It seemed as though the springs connected with my fascial body's interoceptive awareness. The external assistance of the apparatus provided such a sharp contrast to the internal awareness of my yoga practice.

I was so excited about all of this that I participated in the first certification program at TPC with Romana Kryzanowska, who had studied directly with Joseph Pilates. The training was powerful, because Romana was amazing, and TPC's excellent approach to teaching helped me grow my understanding of the Pilates method and its many strengthening and stretching benefits. And yet, at the time, the teacher-as-expert approach often prohibited an adventurous exploration of movement based on what my body was curious to learn. That curious voice got turned off because the teacher-as-expert voice was so dominant.

A TRANSFORMATIVE DISCOVERY

The next phase of my life took me to Austin, Texas, where Michael and I opened the Pilates Center of Austin in 1993. I had made a decision when I started studying Pilates to pause my yoga practice so that I could fully understand the mental and physical conditioning of Pilates. Here I was, three years later, noticing that something felt very different within my body than I had felt in 20 years of practicing yoga. I didn't have words for the feeling at the time, only that I felt very "held" throughout my entire torso. What I finally discovered was that I was "over-stabilizing" in my Pilates practice. I had see-sawed from over-stretching in yoga to over-stabilizing in Pilates by over-recruiting my abdominals.

PARTNERING WITH GRAVITY

Part of me was longing for a deeper awareness as I had experienced in yoga. As luck would have it, Judith Aston, somatic pioneer and creator of Aston Patterning bodywork, offered a workshop on deepening our relationship with gravity and ground reaction force. During a private session I had with Judith, all of those ideas about gravity and ground reaction force landed. I was lying prone on the massage table, and Judith's hand was gently probing the deep tissue of my calf muscle, which was very tight. I said to her, "Judith, you can go deeper, if you choose." She paused and said, "I'm actually right on your bone. Now, I'll come out and re-enter the tissue without honoring the direction of the tissue, so you can feel the difference." I nearly came off the table in pain and could not believe the huge difference. The major embodied realization I gained here had to do with the nature of support and deep listening.

As I returned to my studio, I knew I had experienced something profound with this potent relationship with gravity as a relational force field. I started experimenting with approaching gravity as a teacher—inspired by Ida Rolf's visionary statement "Gravity is the therapist."

As I studied more about my relationship with gravity, I began to sense that *core from my body's perspective* begins with vestibular awareness. I was inspired to learn that the inner ear is our first sense to awaken in the womb, and discovered it is through that awareness that we embody our relationship with gravity and our sense of balance. I also discovered that when we have a befriending relationship with gravity, we awaken a deeper perceptual and receptive way of being in the world.

After years of searching for ways to articulate these distinctions so they come alive for clients and mentoring teachers, I began creating images with lines of energy "Down the Back" (blue arrows) and "Up the Front" (green arrows),

that evoke ways of moving that are engaged, gesturing, and connected with spatial orientation (see Figures 2.7A, B, C). In the side walking position, I show the powerful spiralic relationship of the hamstrings innervating with the adductors and the front of the pelvic diaphragm and spine (orange arrows), as the hamstrings move from the front of the thigh to the back of the leg in our embryonic beginnings. This gives us a deeper understanding of why sensing your feet with soft ankles and coming off the back foot to step into the front foot as we walk is so powerful in our whole-body movement awareness.

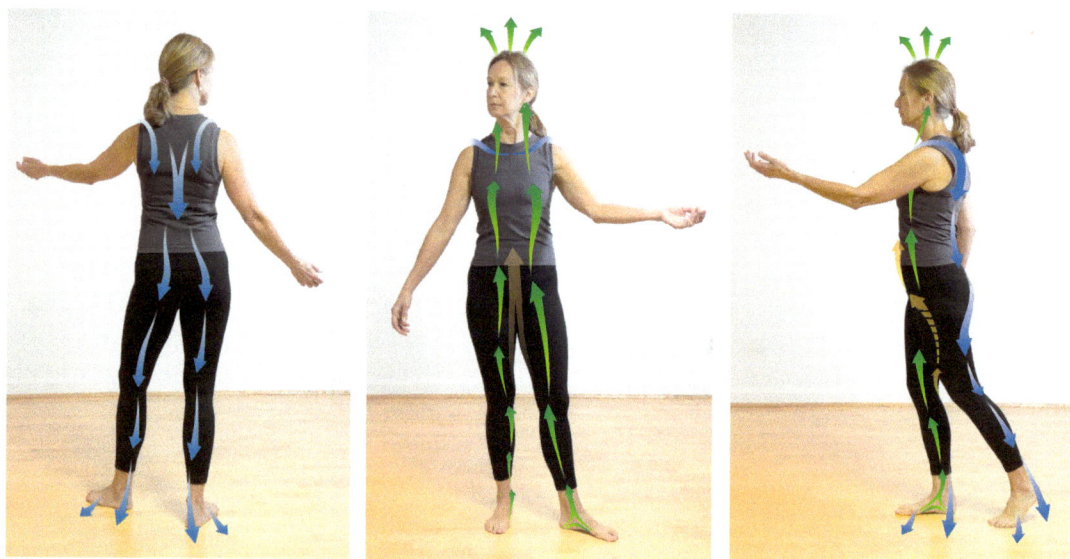

Figures 2.7A, 2.7B, and 2.7C 3CoreConnections exploration of grounding, centering, and uplift

My vision, through this embodied approach, has been to evoke our living architecture's relationship with gravity and spatial orientation within any movement or bodywork discipline. This allows each person to discover and embody their own voice and vision.

The following story relates to how an embodied awareness can be accessed by a small child and help him find his Inner Guide. It is from Alena Goodman, the mother of a young boy who was referred to me by another Rolf Structural Integration practitioner, about 15 years ago:

I was referred to Wendy LeBlanc-Arbuckle in 2008, when my son Aleksey was about 20 months old. Previously, he had been diagnosed with cerebral palsy and was not able to sit, crawl with his lower body helping, or walk on his own. His lower body was very low toned. When we met Wendy, Aleksey was crawling by pulling his lower body around with his upper body. During our sessions, Wendy showed me how we can stimulate Aleksey's lower body and his development by placing my hands on the bottom of his feet and pushing from the bottom of his feet through his spine to the crown of his head in a supine position, and also play with him with balls to support his rolling. I would do this regularly at home during the day. It was a breakthrough moment when Aleksey was able to sit up! Wendy advised me to let his body use his inner intelligence and let him kick with his heels on the hard surface or a ball which would help legs' strengthening. One day, Wendy tickled him while he was lying on his back and he rolled toward one side and pulled his knees in, laughing—and more began changing. We were excited when Aleksey was able to begin crawling on hands and knees, alternating right and left sides. Through playing with balls and sound, Wendy encouraged his natural curiosity to crawl up to a door and push up into standing to open it and see what was behind it. Finally, Aleksey was able to walk in a walker independently!

Aleksey's discovery of his Inner Guide helping him to yield, reach, fold, and unfold is an example of how deep our relationship with yielding to gravity is, in order to discover our ability to sit, stand, and walk. These big realizations with gravity and ground reaction force have sparked my practice and teaching on so many levels. I have also been influenced through my studies with so many brilliant somatic movement and bodywork educators, and five of the Pilates Elders who studied directly with Joseph Pilates: Romana Kryzanowska, with whom I studied originally, and Ron Fletcher, Kathy Grant, Mary Bowen, and Lolita San Miguel.

Each of these teachers shared a unique perspective on their relationship with the method known as Pilates; each of those perspectives influenced me immensely, through their dance and teaching careers and Mary Bowen's Jungian analysis.

In the very early years of my study, learning the classical Pilates method, I was taught that props were *not Pilates*. However, being informed by yoga studies, Alexander technique, and Feldenkrais,

along with Pilates Elders Mary Bowen and Kathy Grant, who both used props in such nuanced ways, and becoming a Rolf Structural Integration practitioner, I felt a freedom to explore with each client according to what their body needed. I discovered that a seemingly inflexible shoulder can release when a pillow or a soft ball is placed under a client's armpit in side-lying (bringing support of gravity *up* to the tense area). When a client is lying on their back with knees bent, I noticed how I can support with my hands in Core-to-Core whole-body cueing. This meant my hands might choose to be closer to the upper or lower thighs, to allow their legs to relax and their feet to make deeper contact with gravity. This would allow the entire head, spine, and pelvis to release into support, often leading to softening, widening, and awakening the relationship between their *breathing spine* and *pelvic diaphragm*, creating a ripple whole-body effect, like dominoes falling.

Over 15 years, I re-imagined the concept of core from one of control to Core as Relationship. The breakthrough was a gradual sequence of revelations, and my somatic studies along with studies with bodywork and breathwork pioneers were essential in the process.

I began to question the principle of Contrology, *uniform development*. This term can create a critical external assessment of the body and its alignment with perfect symmetry, a concept that doesn't exist, and can keep teachers locked in a judgmental paradigm. To step outside of an unreal march toward uniformity allows practitioners to develop a movement plan that meets the uniqueness of each individual. I sensed a deeper understanding of my abdominals as being in relationship, not only with my entire body, but also with the field of gravity. It felt limiting to control my center, to sense core as predominantly tense and localized. I understood that there is no *whole-body health* unless we are considering our fascial matrix continuity (our connective tissue *fascial matrix*, from foot to head and hand). This is primordial. This awareness is what I call "Core as Relationship."

CORE COORDINATION AND BIOTENSEGRITY

Core is a dynamic, biointelligent expression, an effect of sensing earth's energy through the gravitational field, and a spatial, enlivening, social, and physical relationship with ourselves, others, and our living environment. To sense this, explore a basic movement of bending your knees slightly, while you are standing up.

At first, this seems like such a simple movement, because we are so accustomed to seeing and approaching the body in parts. When we look beyond the body as a collection of parts, sensing our body's wholeness, we move away from isolated core control.

When I soften my knees in a gentle bending motion, I am aware of connection with the ground through the vital receptors of my feet, and sense that internal lift is evoked through the domes of the body (more about this in Chapter 4) to prevent me from falling. My feet, ankles, hips, pelvic diaphragm, and primordial midline are relational with my knees, so they also soften in response to the softening knees, in order to give my knees more tensional spring-like support, so my knees do not take the entire load of my body as they soften. The *sitting bones to heels connection* comes alive to support buoyancy and uplift through the softening ankles, knees, and hips. This tensional spring-like integrity is related to a concept called *biotensegrity*, which supports my body responding as a whole elastic organism. "When one thing moves, everything moves" (Tai Chi classics as cited in Lowell de Solorzano 2021, p.1).

When I sense the ground beneath my feet as my knees soften, along with that awareness, my breath deepens, my nervous system relaxes, I experience a connection with the space around my body. This connection opens me to a concert of deeper relationships. The "simple movement" of softening/bending and then straightening the knees without hyperextending is an activation of an entire network of relationships: knees moving in response to ground, evoking support through feet, ankles, hips, and spine, motivated by breath and the body's fluid resonance from feet to head and hands. The core of knee bending evokes these interconnected relationships between grounding, centering, and uplift—a relational way of being with ourselves and our environment. **See Video 2.8 for deeper exploration**.

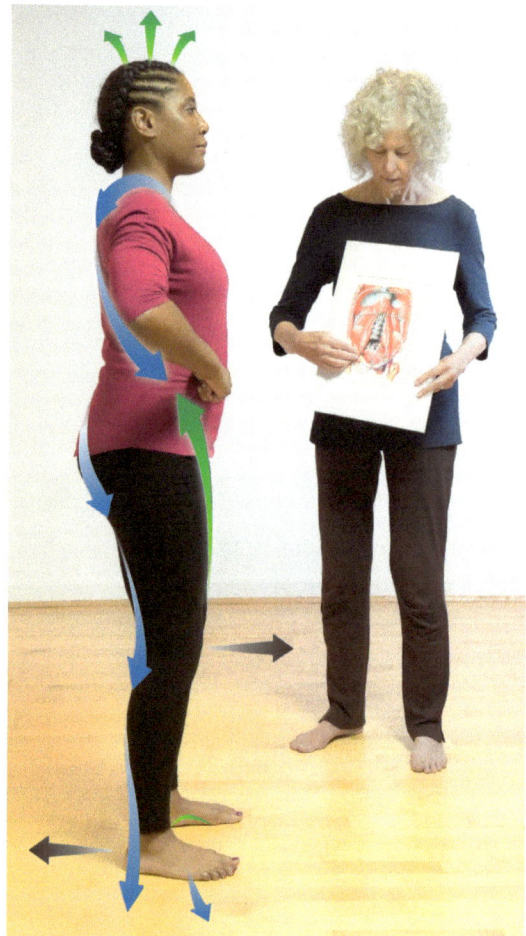

Figure 2.8 Softening the knees-to-spine relationship—soft ankles with heels releasing back as knees move forward

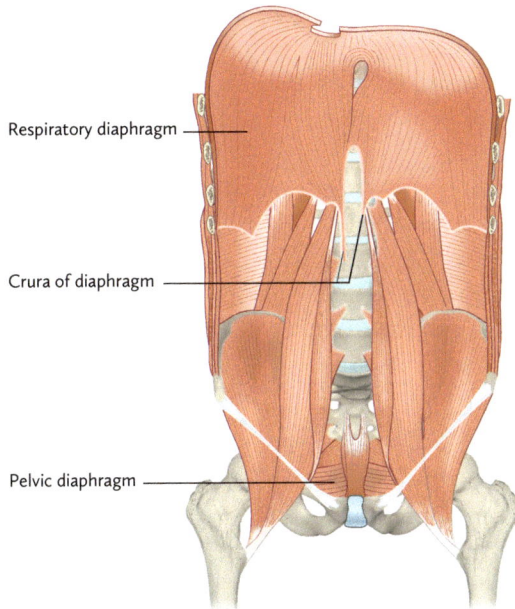

Respiratory diaphragm

Crura of diaphragm

Pelvic diaphragm

Figure 2.9 Front of the back—how legs root to front of spine

Building on this fluid resonance, notice in Figure 2.9 the relationship between the pelvic diaphragm, primordial midline, respiratory diaphragm, and front of the spine, which I refer to as "the front of the back." When we allow our back to widen and lengthen with breath as we soften/bend our knees in standing, we allow the psoas and belly wall to release toward the front of the back. Our embryonic connection between the back of the leg and the front of the pelvic diaphragm and spine is also awakened—the rooting of the legs to the front of the spine. Remember that the hamstrings internally spiral to the back of the leg as we are self-organizing in the womb. **See Video 2.10 for full exploration**.

AWARENESS OF EMBODIED SELF

This revelation of Core as Relationship is about our cellular awareness and embodied self. This embodied self sees the body as an organ of perception, where the whole body, the extracellular fascial matrix, skin, muscles, bones, nerves, and the internal organs are sensitive to changes, to *messages*, from the environment.

> We inhabit an ecological body, a feeling body, which extends beyond the skin and is constantly exchanging information and meaning with its surroundings. (de Quincey 2005, p.159)

The process of broader knowing of self emerges from the communicating relationship of each cell to another and to the extracellular living matrix in which the cells are embedded.

That is why I feel it is important to be aware that, as bodywork and movement therapists, we can help individuals connect to their interoceptive awareness; this helps them feel the way the body knows its internal landscape. Proprioception tells us where we are spatially and helps us strengthen and coordinate our body as we grow and develop by telling us how much force to use when we are holding, pulling, pushing, or lifting something.

> According to a recent article by Schleip et al. our myofascial web actually has a much higher concentration of interoceptors vs. proprioceptors. 80% of the peripheral nerves found in fascia are actually free nerve endings—with 90% of those being interoceptive! This puts the fascial innervation at 1:7 ratio [of] proprioceptors to interoceptors. (Splichal 2017)

This interoceptive network is often referred to as our *primitive skin* as it is what drives our need for social touch and also promotes the release of oxytocin. Slowing down and developing a foundational, somatic approach to movement calls forth our interoceptive awareness, and that builds a proprioceptive and kinesthetic foundation for everything.

This relationship between our cells and our connective tissue living matrix generates a resonance that originates in the womb, but tends to get tuned out as our rational minds come to dominate our daily life and we look to external cultural guidance in how to live. The notion of Core as Relationship builds directly on the notion of embodiment as a living process we are emerging within, rather than a seemingly finite and static state that we occupy while alive.

Body-Mind Centering creator Bonnie Bainbridge Cohen says the following:

> Cells resonate in relationship to each other. As more cells within us become aware of themselves and are responsive, there is a fuller resonance between them, and we experience inner balance and self-knowing. (Bainbridge Cohen 2023)

What we experience as self-knowing is not a rational process that begins with the ability to conceptualize a self and a world through language, but is the outgrowth of our fluid nature which mediates our cellular activities. Cells know their functions and are aware of their relationships with other cells. There is a *fluid intelligence* that seeds the microscopic cellular process that is self-knowing. Self-knowing is a resonance, a vibration. We will never actually experience the processes of balancing or self-knowing if we think of ourselves as a biomechanical mass with a separate soul or mind. To sense resonance and embrace the body's biointelligence, it serves our deeper awareness to let go of mechanistic images of the body and turn instead to images of our fluid, fascial nature.

Emilie Conrad, the creator of Continuum, sums it up:

> In resonance all fluid systems are united... [N]o matter where in the galaxy they may be, all fluid systems function as basically one body or organ of intelligence. (Conrad 2007, p.262)

We often think of fluidity as an adjective or adverb, such as in the desire to dance more fluidly. Fluidity is much more like a medium in which we grow, shape-shift, and change. We begin our embryonic phase, as fluid beings, as we self-organize and grow ourselves in the womb. We don't *have* a body, we *are* a body. When we reconnect with our primal, fluid nature, we access a deeper relationship with ourselves, one another, and our living universe. We connect with the *pulse of life*. Emilie suggests that though we may not be fully aware of it, cellular resonance vibrates along with the larger resonance, the galactic matrix, meaning that our selves resonate with the stars. To begin sensing this connection with the galaxy, we start with something much closer to home—the notion of core.

BIOTENSEGRITY—"LIVING TENSEGRITY"

I would like to share with you about biotensegrity, our "living tensegrity," and how it relates to this notion of Core as Relationship.

In 1948, Kenneth Snelson, a young art student at Black Mountain College, North Carolina, met R. Buckminster Fuller, inventor, designer, philosopher, poet, and visionary, who was exploring geometric architectural construction based on his understanding of "energetic geometry" (Martin 2016, p.3). The result of their collaborative venture was a new construction which Snelson spoke of as *floating compression* and from which Fuller later coined the word "tensegrity," meaning tensional integrity, or the dynamic interplay of tension and compression (Snelson 1999).

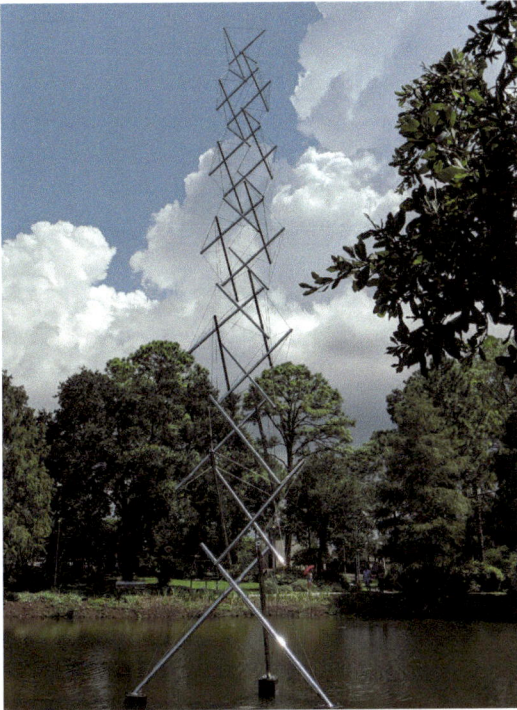

Figure 2.11 Kenneth Snelson's Tensegrity Virlane Tower in New Orleans Museum of Art City Park Sculpture Garden
PHOTO BY WENDY LEBLANC-ARBUCKLE

In her book *Living Biotensegrity*, Daniele-Claude Martin discusses how orthopedic surgeon Stephen Levin adapted Snelson and Fuller's work to the realm of medicine in orthopedics. She tells the story of Dr. Levin visiting the National Mall in Washington, D.C., where the Needle Tower was on display in proximity to the Obelisk of the Washington Monument. It occurred to Levin that the Needle Tower might provide answers to questions he had been struggling with that remained unresolved through a biomechanical perspective. He studied the floating tension-compression of the Needle Tower, and later, at the National Museum of Natural History, he saw how dinosaur tails never dragged along the ground and are described as being able to be used like a whip.

Through these observations, he was inspired to re-envision biologic structures through the tensegrity model. Eventually, Levin introduced the term "biotensegrity," which he used to describe "biological structures from viruses to vertebrates at every level of their hierarchical systems" (Martin 2016, p.4). For Levin, the tensegrity of the Snelson and Fuller architecture was more able to account for the intra-articular space between the articular spaces in joints. Dr. Levin was clear that he did not have all the answers, yet the more he learned, the more he was perplexed by how living organisms function with the distribution of forces through the whole system.

By applying Levin's biotensegrity into the world of movement and bodywork, we start to learn how movement is always a concert of tension-compression, a "living tensegrity," an ensemble of interrelationships produced by your body's innate intelligence.

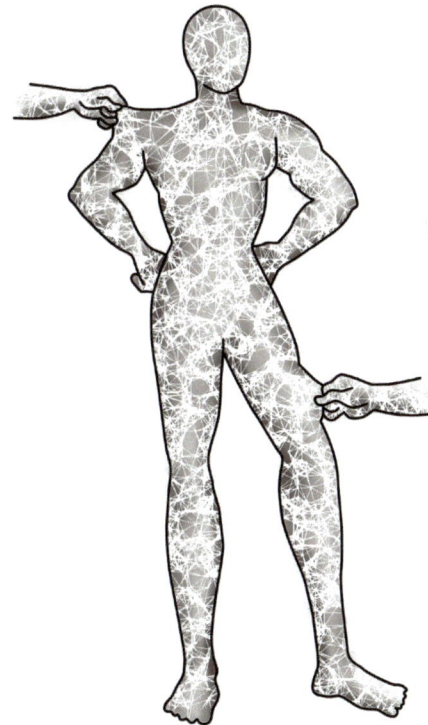

Figure 2.12 Fascial matrix person showing elasticity of whole body and Domes of Uplift

Another way of thinking about biotensegrity is as the living architecture of your body, which is shaped in part by your internal and external environment and is always responding to multiple stimuli. *Biotensegrity* validates the existence of multiple core zones within your body—we call them *Domes of Uplift*. These are cores within your primordial midline, from the inner ankles of your feet to the pelvic diaphragm through the respiratory diaphragm, the thoracic inlet, the palate, the cranium, and the hands, which are resonant with the relationship between your body's tensional-compression forces and the forces around you. *Biointelligence* is a term that speaks to the fact that your body knows this living architecture as its reality. *Inner Guide* is our biointelligent self that learns through movement and communicates its needs, likes, and dislikes to our body/mind/emotion/spirit. Core as Relationship is a portal that gives us access to these other terms and helps us to constantly reframe our thinking to a whole-body fluid, dynamic organism, thereby developing a resilient dialogue with gravity, ourselves, one another, and our environment.

COMING FROM WHOLENESS

This next section further develops the notion of Core as Relationship in more detail by exploring wholeness. The whole body is present in the softening of the knees as this gives access to our primordial midline, which puts us into connection with the fluid and electrical forces that shape us, including gravity. The wholeness of the person is also enlivened through the action of bridging if we approach bridging from a biointelligent perspective.

Many established disciplines offer language to help us tune in to the whole body, but do they encourage approaching the discipline as a living system? This approach fosters a felt sense awareness of the present moment, addressing the wholeness of the person rather than just the body in front of us. As a practitioner of several somatic disciplines, I believe we need to be well grounded in the principles that underlie each discipline. This grounding allows us to play lightly with the sheet music of movement, sound, and breath, sensing our bodies like musical instruments in relation to the gravitational field. This holistic perspective enables us to dialogue with out-of-tune areas.

The gravitational field acts as a therapist, and our role is to prepare the body to receive its support, enhancing overall wellbeing. However, there's often a tendency to mold individuals into the fixed framework of a discipline, which can overshadow the biointelligence that originally inspired it.

By attuning to our Inner Guide in relation to the dynamics unfolding in front of us, we can perpetually deepen our listening practice and maintain the vitality and relevance of the discipline.

> The gravitational field is the therapist. What we do is prepare the body to receive the support from the gravitational field which gives a greater sense of wellbeing.[1]

How do we honor the vision of a discipline so that it is a "living system," one that is always growing, one that is always guided by our own biointelligence and, if we are teachers, that of the whole person in front of us? One way is to approach technique as a form of deep listening, and attune to our Inner Guide in relationship to whatever

---

1   Widely attributed to Ida Rolf.

dynamic is unfolding in front of us. Here are some examples of how we can either miss or *listen for* that moment of deep attunement:

- Not Being Present with what is needed:
  - Teaching a client without having the client develop awareness of how their movement patterns can help them correct old habits—just doing exercises and not becoming aware of how they are moving.

- Being Present with what is needed:
  - By sensing yourself as a vital part of your client's environment as they move, so they become aware of how to set themselves up in their environment to move with more ease and apply what is happening in the session to their activities of daily living. This is a felt sense, awareness-building approach that the client can use as a healing reservoir in their life. In this approach, the client leaves the session with a new way of being with themselves.

In uncovering the contextual notion of Core as Relationship within my own body, I have found the ancient traditions of meridians and chakras incredibly helpful. These traditions inform so many movement systems and invite us to embody the whole body relationally.

I find it helpful to consider that the insight of the chakras, glands, and meridians is always at play. They are important because they help us be aware of our energy body, which can have blockages that manifest later as physical problems.

CHAKRAS, MERIDIANS, AND MORE

Within the biomechanical notion of core, there is little discussion of energy or emotions in consideration of the whole body. From the biointelligent perspective, my body records a huge variety of life experiences, which are imprinted and help me to shape and form my body. This physical, mental, and emotional record of life history accumulates from the deepest structures to the surface, creating our personality, behavior, and persona, which operate as a way of being in the world.

Core as Relationship can be further explored by the examination of two ancient Eastern descriptions of the human organism, which offer maps for understanding energy and emotions holistically. They are the Chinese medical model of the acupuncture meridians, and the Indian yogic map of the chakras, which relates to our endocrine glands.

By offering glimpses of the insights gained through working with the meridians and the chakras, I hope to open a door to a wider field of study. I invite you to engage your "beginner's mind" and consider what happens to your awareness and your knowledge of movement and bodywork once you overlay the language of the meridians, the chakras, and the glands atop the images we've produced up to this point.

The chakras are located along your primordial midline, from your tail to head, at root, sacral, navel, heart, throat, brow, and crown centers, and can be envisioned as spinning vortices of energy that support our physical, emotional, and mental experience.

In her book *Yoga, Body, Mind, Spirit* (2000), Donna Farhi reminds us that aligned with the chakras are a series of endocrine glands which secrete hormones into the bloodstream. The glands work in relation with the nervous system to help create balance in the body. The interplay between the chakras and these glands is interesting, as is the fact that the emotional resonance of the chakras is harmonized with physiological bodily processes. For example, the root chakra at the base of the spine relates to our primal needs, food, sleep, sex, and self-preservation, where we cultivate our sense of security, stability, and safety. This chakra is often related to our adrenal glands and our kidney health, which work together in determining how we respond to stress, are able to regulate blood pressure, and generally feel at home in our body.

We might think of the chakras as a new way for understanding the complexity around what Western medicine calls the endocrine system. Remember that physical problems first show themselves through our energy body, so a study of our fluid pelvic diaphragm and its relationship to our neuroendocrine glands becomes an embodied activity. Let's revisit and explore the grounding and internal lift of Bridge again to see the natural, fluid massage which can occur along our fascially nested midline to tone, balance, and co-regulate the endocrine glands, chakras, and our emotional selves as we move.

Before, you explored the Bridge by sensing the movement of your tail as you pressed gently into your feet, moving through the Lower Core to the Central and Upper Cores. You explored the language of "Down the Back/Up the Front" to sense the facial flossing of your spine's relationship with your feet and head, and how that may have created a more open sensation in your hips and chest.

Let's overlay the chakras. The energy of the root chakra helps to soften and widen the tail bone, your relationship with earth and a sense of grounding. Likewise, the sacral chakra can energize and relax the hips and is related with our sexual and creative energy. Together, root, sacral, and solar plexus chakra energy supports the lift of the Bridge along the front of your breathing spine, while also providing a sense of grounding linked to the flow of respiration. This awareness provides support for the upper, more spiritual chakras, so you still feel a sense of groundedness. By grounding the Lower Core (the epicenters of

which, here, are the solar plexus/diaphragm, pelvic diaphragm/tail, and inner ankle/feet), the body's other cores awaken and resonate with each other. The activated root, sacral, and solar plexus chakras create grounding, nourishing, supportive energy for the upper body and for our emotional expression in life. Here is some feedback following a session, that speaks to this awareness, shared by Patricia, a Certified Rolfer:

> I have a sense of feeling my back as I am standing and walking, feeling not only my back but my spine in relation to the space behind me (a very tactile sensation too!), and the backs of my upper arms are heavy and feel "weighted," as if being pulled slightly posterior and down. I am aware of being more connected to ground, yet with a sense of uprightness and ease. I am realizing what it feels like to *not* pull, squeeze, throw back, or otherwise arrange myself in my body—I just am.
>
> I feel whole—as if everything is where it should be in gravity and deeply relaxed. I feel a flow of energy in all my chakra channels as a stream of moving light. I feel a deep sense of "this is my body" and how easy it is to be in it.
>
> One of my new realizations is how grounding an embodied approach to a Pilates Bridge can be. With my feet on the wall and curling gently along my midline, I could feel energy come into my pelvis, and into my first, second, and third chakras. I was not standing up connecting to the earth—I was on my back with my feet on the wall! It is easy for me to stay in the fourth chakra and above in my body and not reside or connect with my first three chakras.
>
> I am a bit chagrined to say I have been leaving the first three chakras out of my life and body for years. Now I am learning the importance of being in my body while staying connected to my spiritual body. This is what "wholeness" is to me. Prior to this, I tried to "mentalize" being in my first three chakras,

but in our session, I did not get into my body through my brain. I got there by feeling and sensing my connection to ground, and four days later this "being in me" is continuing to unfold between my body, mind, and spirit.

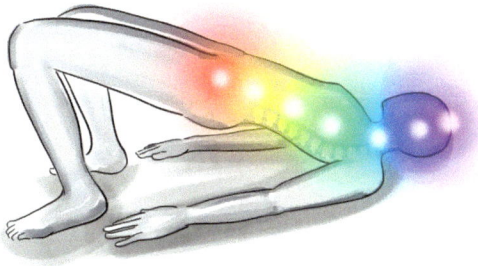

Figure 2.13 Bridge with chakras from root to crown of head
GRATITUDE TO LEAH REES, ARTIST

Meanwhile, your endocrine system is buzzing with dynamic activity. When your Lower Core glands—the coccygeal body, sex glands, adrenal glands, and pancreas—soften and widen in response to embodied awareness, a new type of toning occurs. This is more than muscular toning; it's a synchronization of the continuity between endocrine glands, chakras, and meridian channels, grounded through the bones from foot to head and hand. Consider the meridian point Kidney 1, located in the hollow below the ball of your midfoot, which activates the Kidney meridian. This point acts like your body's battery, managing stress response and energy levels daily.

In the bridge position, there is a concert of chakra, glandular, and meridian activity. As you ease into a fuller bridge, you may notice a smoother transition into inversions like a Pilates Rollover or yoga shoulder stand. Your thyroid gland at the base of your throat becomes more energized, empowering your entire endocrine system.

This biointelligent Bridge exercise, infused with the language of the meridians, endocrine system, and chakras, emphasizes the full-body communication happening constantly. The core is no longer something to tense and control but a relational embodiment maintained through active releasing and supported by the communication from foot to inner ear and hand.

The logic in the biointelligent Bridge Pose includes the 12 meridians governing the energetic expression of each internal organ which begin or end at most fingers and toes. As explored in Chapter 1, during fetal development, our fingers and toes initiate our body's evolution. By softening and widening your feet and hands, and yielding your body's weight into gravity, these meridians receive attention.

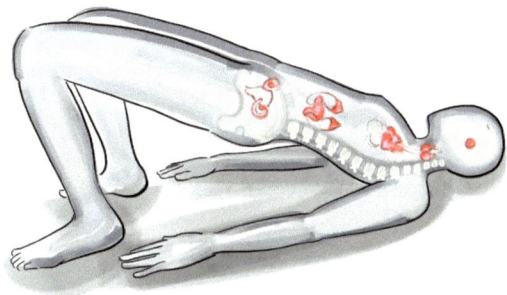

Figure 2.14 Bridge with glands, from perineal body along the front of the spine to the pituitary and pineal within the center of the skull
GRATITUDE TO LEAH REES, ARTIST

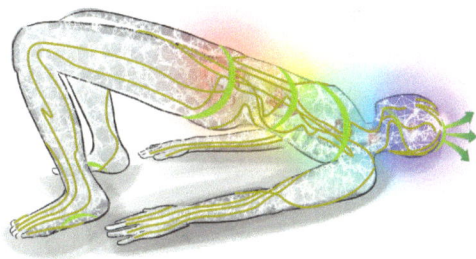

Figure 2.15 Embodying fascial matrix—embedding meridians, chakras, glands, and so much more

Here, it becomes possible to see how discovering the coherent relationship between the extracellular fascial matrix that embeds the meridians, the glands, and the chakras creates a seismic shift from core control to Core as Relationship. Our energy flow through this global fascial matrix affects how we feel, how we think, and the over-all condition of our internal organs and health, allowing us to move fluidly, breathe deeply, and digest and eliminate food. The meridians, glands, and chakras embedded in the fascial network and grounded through the bones are critical pathways that support Core as Relationship through the body's interrelated systems.

THE FASCIAL DOG FLOW SERIES

Let's explore together a variation on the Sun Salutation Series that Dr. Martha Eddy and Shakti Andrea Smith share about in their book *Dynamic Embodiment of the Sun Salutation* (2021). Here, they looked at the dynamic relationship between the meridians, chakras, glands, and whole-body fascial matrix awareness. I learned the bones of this practice from my mentor, Hubert Godard, which he called "Flight of the Eagle." I came to call it the "Fascial Dog Flow Series," with Phase One, Two, and Three, which I developed further over time to meet the needs of clients. Many years ago, a client renamed the series, as she was having difficulty weight bearing on her hands in her yoga practice with Downward Dog. I took time to guide her in sensing how she could begin to have a felt sense of her fascial flossing spine supporting foot to head and hand. She exclaimed "This is like a Fascial Dog!" as she felt more grounded and fascially supported through her hands and feet to her breathing spine. This valuable Phase One, Two, Three approach, especially with a wall for foot to head and hand support, is an embodied, transformative, biotensegrity-inspired practice that surprises clients with its regenerative results. See Video 2.16 for full exploration.

- **Phase One:** Finding your *hover* as you straighten your legs, sensing your rounded, spring-like spine.
  - Becoming aware of your perineural nervous system (your connective tissue nervous system), the pre-tensed biotensegrity that embeds muscles, bones, internal organs, glands, chakras, and meridians in a living fascial matrix.
  - Softening your solar plexus/crura, allowing soft eyes (peripheral vision) and inner ear support to float and "hover" your spine.
  - Awakening core coordination where sensory receptors in your hands and feet ignite whole-body perceptual awareness, a sense of grounding, and your Domes of Uplift.

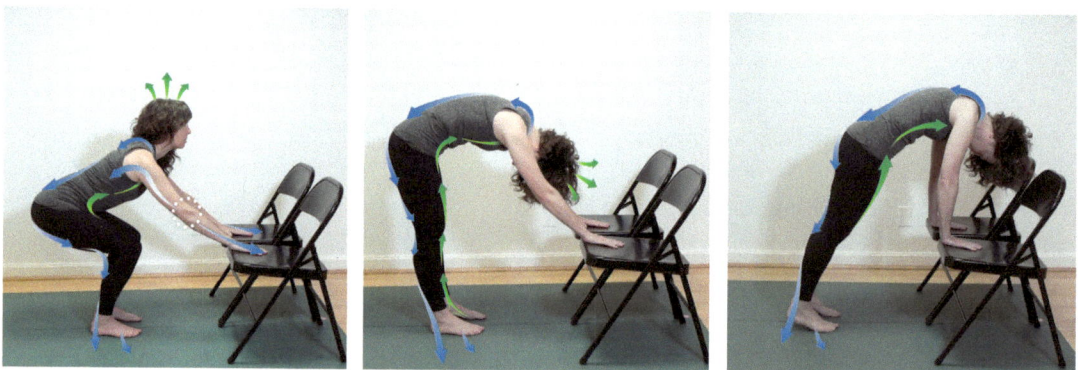

Figures 2.16A–C Phase One

- **Phase Two:** Evokes Core as Relationship through grounding, centering, and uplift with inner ear and eyes leading breathing spine rather than abdominal gripping.
  - Strengthens and releases tension patterns in the hands, wrists, neck, and shoulders of the Upper Core, from the shoulder blades to internal belly suspenders relationship (Down the Back and Up the Front).
  - Supports the embryonic relationship of the front body (yolk sac nourishment), supporting the back body, sensing what is just enough support.

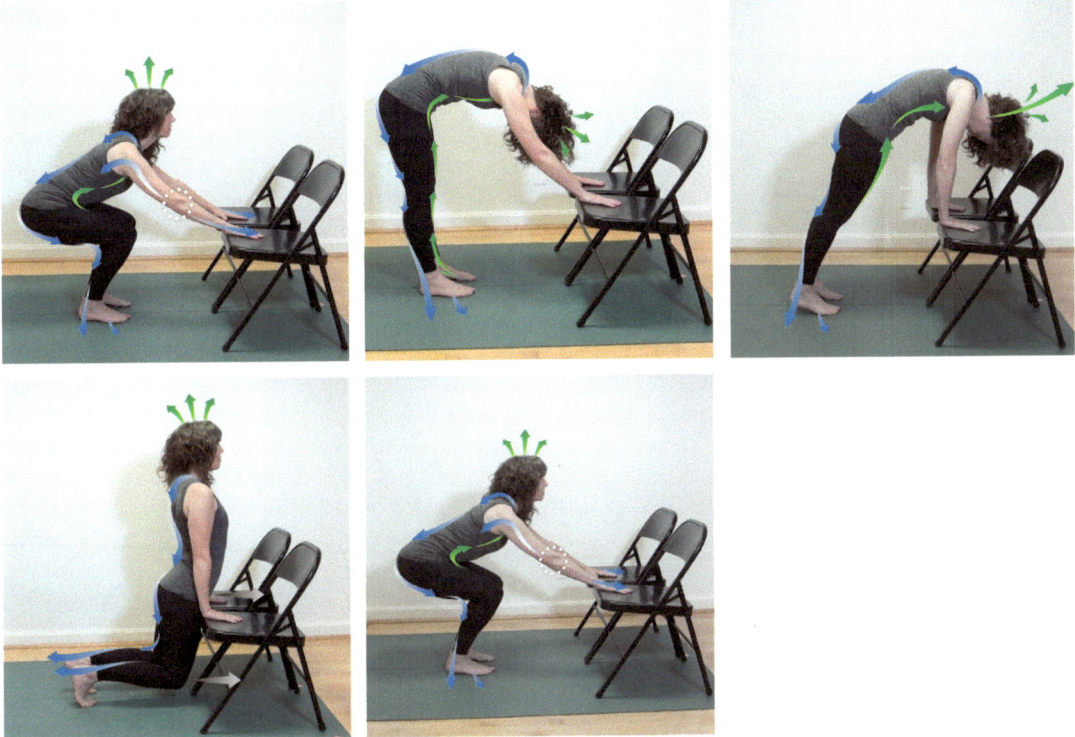

Figures 2.16D–H Phase Two

Important awareness: Be sure to look up *before* bending your knees, so you are moving from your internal lift at your inner ears and eyes, allowing your waterfall Down the Back and "shoulder blades to low belly suspenders" to support your Upper Core in extension.

- **Phase Three:** Evokes a deeper relationship with the vectors of the two directions of the spine through the portals of the hands and feet, within the field of gravity.
  - Cultivates the body's innate, contralateral coordination for natural walking.
  - Utilizes the wall to strengthen and balance the body's natural stability—gravity-based tonic function through foot to head and hand relationship.
  - Deepens interoceptive, proprioceptive, adaptive, and perceptual awareness.

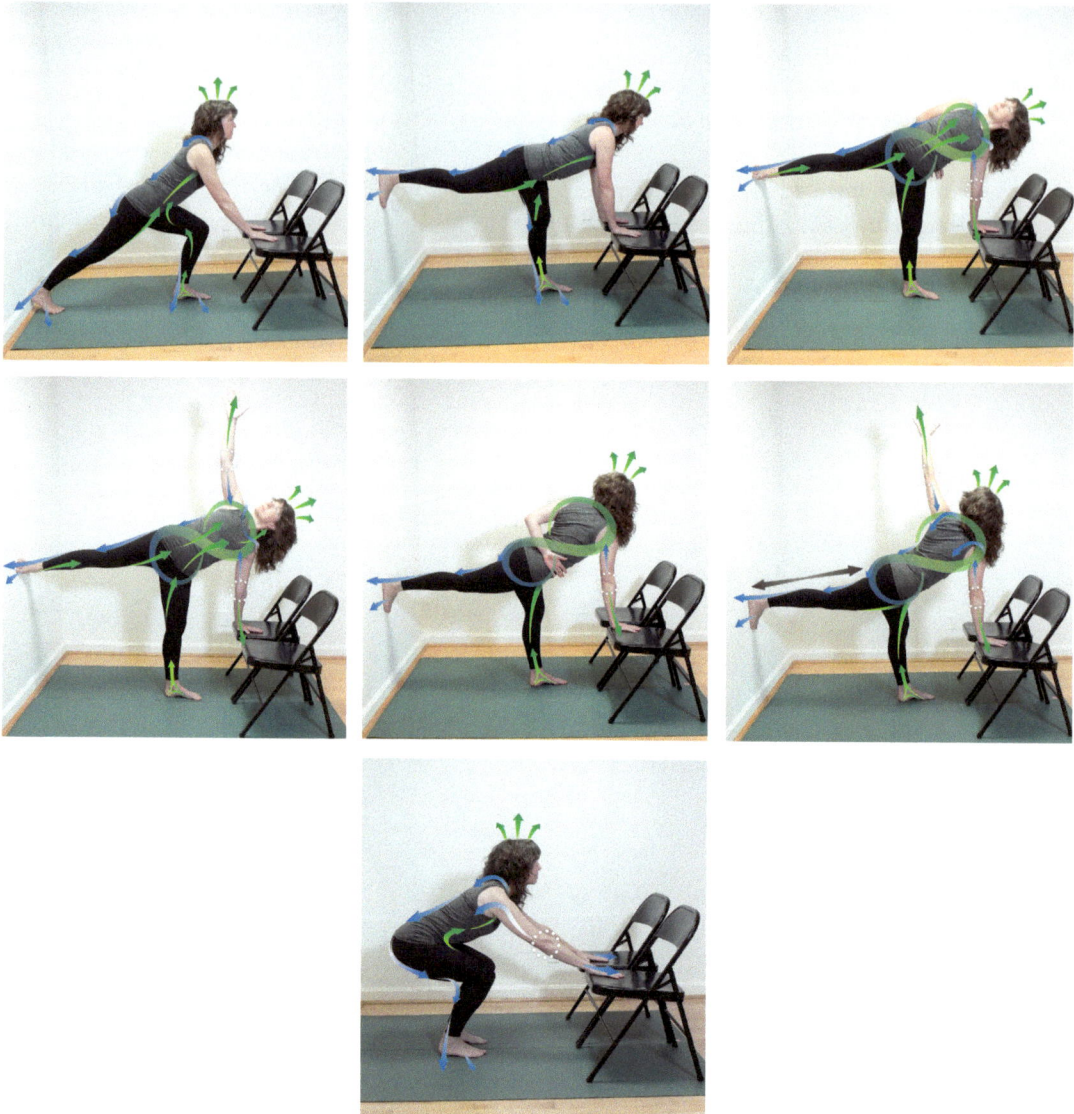

Figures 2.16I–O Phase Three

Your body is supported by the many vectors of limbs reaching and your head and tail reaching in many directions into the ground and space. This Core as Relationship support awakens us to our body's natural coordination as *effort with ease*.

As you move forward with this biointelligent approach, I invite you to consider that there may be a big shift in your understanding of "grounding." As with this new relational understanding of core, grounding also becomes a relational act. Your fingers and toes collaborate with the earth, and this collaboration is coherent with your sense of locating yourself in time and space. Consider the thought that *we can't know who we are till we know where we are located*. So, sensing where we are becomes a vital portal to a practice that continues to grow our perceptual awareness as we age. Grounding/ yielding is a perceptual action which leads to a clearer sense of presence with ourselves and one another.

Additionally, you may investigate your understanding of practice generally. For example, do you automatically equate your movement practice with *doing*? Core as Relationship invites us to consider how, prior to any action, all individuals are acted upon. We are a mixture of action and being acted upon, of meeting and being met. If we give attention to the ways that the natural and social environments shape our movements, our thoughts about movements, our sense of safety, then we learn how our movement practice is always taking place. This chapter helps to draw awareness to the potency of meeting and being met that is taking place at all times. Down the Back informs and evokes Up the Front, and this support is happening all the time, even as you move in the simplest task. Your body doesn't care what you call what you are doing—yoga, Pilates, Alexander, Feldenkrais, sitting, walking, or washing the dishes. What it cares about is *movement with awareness*. In general, you may discover how practice always entails more than doing. Practice becomes equally about sensing and listening to how our body/mind/emotion/spirit is shaped by the forces within and around us.

As we continue to explore the contrast between biomechanical and biointelligent approaches to movement, I hope it's clear that I'm not saying biomechanics is wrong. All of my experience has taught me that practitioners from both fields of study benefit from collaborating with one another and engaging in dialogue about the specific way that ideas from various artistic and scientific disciplines inform our collective understanding of what we mean by "bodywork" or "movement arts." While biomechanics is not wrong, I do think it tends, in practice, to be incomplete and encourages a right/wrong approach. As I mentioned in this chapter, biomechanical narratives and exercises tend to objectify the body, defer to an "expert" outside of oneself, and almost always exclude discussion of our felt sense emotional intelligence. So, how do we understand the role of the breath in all of this work? Clearly, our breath is linked to our emotional states.

Historically, breath has been considered equal to and even synonymous with spirit. But we cannot exclude the emotional and spiritual dimensions from the breathwork and the way it underpins movement. The next chapter—Breath as a Healing Bridge Between Matter and Spirit— explores these questions directly.

Use the following QR code for all videos in this chapter:

REFERENCES

Avison, J. (2015) *Yoga, Fascia, Anatomy and Movement*. Pencaitland: Handspring Publishing.

Bainbridge Cohen, B. (2023) "About Bonnie Bainbridge Cohen." https://bonniebainbridgecohen.com/pages/about

Conrad, E. (2007) *Life on Land: The Story of Continuum, the World-Renowned Self-Discovery and Movement Method*. Berkeley, CA: North Atlantic Books.

Eddy, M. and Andrea Smith, S. (2021) *Dynamic Embodiment of the Sun Salutation: Pathways to Balancing the Chakras and the Neuroendocrine System*. Pencaitland: Handspring Publishing.

Farhi, D. (2000) *Yoga, Body, Mind, Spirit: A Return to Wholeness*. New York, NY: Henry Holt and Company.

Gintis, B. (2007) *Engaging the Movement of Life*. Berkeley, CA: North Atlantic Books.

Gustafson, C. (2017) "Bruce Lipton, PhD: The Jump From Cell Culture to Consciousness." *Integrative Medicine 16*, 6, 44–50.

Lowell de Solorzano, S. (2021) *Everything Moves: How Biotensegrity Informs Human Movement*. Pencaitland: Handspring Publishing.

Martin, D.-C. (2016) *Living Biotensegrity: Interplay of Tension and Compression in the Body*. München, Germany: Christl Kiener.

Oschman, J. (2003) *Energy Medicine in Therapeutics and Human Performance*. Oxford: Butterworth-Heinemann.

Pollack, G. (2001) *Cells, Gels and the Engines of Life: A New Unifying Approach to Cell Function*. Seattle, WA: Ebner & Sons.

de Quincey, C. (2005) *Radical Knowing: Understanding Consciousness through Relationship*. Rochester, VT: Park Street Press.

Snelson, K. (1999) "Kenneth Snelson: Art and Ideas." http://kennethSnelson.net

Splichal, E. (2017) "Interoception: The Emotional Side of the Human Myofascial System." Barefoot Strong Blog. https://barefootstrongblog.com/2017/06/20/interoception-the-emotional-side-of-the-human-myofascial-system

CHAPTER 3

Breath as a Healing Bridge Between Matter and Spirit

The previous chapter discussed a new way of understanding the foundational concept of core in movement and bodywork, one grounded in the perspective of our Inner Guide and innate biointelligence. Now we look into something even more essential: the fluid nourishment that is breath.

Although breathing is an autonomic activity that happens without our control, relaxed diaphragmatic breathing is a skill. Various life tensions, however, especially trauma, create myofascial holding patterns that impede relaxed diaphragmatic breathing. Over time, stress makes the breath shallower, and we may not even recognize this until we encounter yogic breathing techniques or nasal breathing methods. In my early 20s, studying yoga and pranayama was a lifeline to self-healing a chronically hypervigilant nervous system. Since then, conscious awareness of breath-based self-regulation continues to underpin my understanding of how breath patterns sustain whole-body healing.

The skill of natural breathing awareness has direct consequences on whole-body health, as each physiological, psychological, and emotional state has a corresponding breathing pattern. Conscious awareness of how you are breathing is transformative.

At least 17,000 times each day, each time we breathe, we are at a threshold of transformation.

During inhalation, we expand. The taking in of air creates a literal and metaphorical spaciousness. In this capaciousness lies an opportunity to disengage from dysfunction, reorganize, and take on new form. The actual movements of inhalation parallel the movements of growth of a developing fetus. During each cycle of the in-breath we experience a microcosm of growth and development, and in the exhalation phase we dissolve, let go, and reenact our ultimate "expiration." The mutability of our form and function is our true identity as homeodynamic living, embodied beings, and this changeability is recapitulated in each cycle of inhalation and exhalation. (Gintis 2007, p.23)

Dr. Andrew Weil noted that his medical training did not include breathing and its relationship between the conscious and unconscious mind as a doorway to help regulate the autonomic nervous system. Or the possibility that breath could be representative of the movement of spirit in the body and that the study of breathwork could be a primary means of raising spiritual awareness (Weil 2006).

Dr. Konstantin Buteyko devoted his life to studying the human organism. When he monitored the breathing of terminally ill patients, and spent hundreds of hours observing and recording breathing patterns, he was able to predict, often to the minute, the time of death of each patient.

There was an increase in each patient's breathing as they approached death and as their condition deteriorated. Over time, he noticed that mouth breathing bypassed the body's natural breathing wisdom, whereas nasal breathing cleanses and warms the air before it reaches the lungs, while also coordinating the proper balance of oxygen and carbon dioxide.

Dr. John Douillard wrote the pioneering book *Body, Mind, and Sport* (2018). I hosted Douillard for a workshop on the power of nasal breathing at my studio in 2001, and the teaching he gave was a revelation to the many yoga and Pilates teachers in attendance. His paradigm-shifting research revealed that sustained nasal breathing during physical exercise causes the body to make adaptations that are conducive to improving physical performance and recovery.

I was honored to be on the team of track and field Olympic athlete Sanya Richards-Ross for seven years, and accompanied her to the 2008 Beijing Olympics. The Russian team was leading the field when Sanya received the baton as the final runner in the 4 x 400-meter relay. Sanya's focus, nasal breathing, and relaxation from our pre-race regenerative workout helped her to edge out the Russian team to win the gold medal for the U.S. Sanya then went on to the 2012 London Olympics with this mind-body awareness and won her first individual gold medal in the 400-meter race.

Another pioneering breath awareness technique that has transformed my practice and teaching for over 20 years is Carl Stough's Breathing Coordination, which I refer to as the Counting Breath. This is because of how Carl described the way the movement of the tongue influences the diaphragm. He wrote about the importance of exhalation. Stough was able to reverse the effects of emphysema. This was a revolutionary approach when he began working with emphysema patients as a breathing specialist in several hospitals between 1958 and

1962. He had discovered that, by counting on the exhale from 1 to 10 repeatedly to the end of the exhale, and then allowing the inhale as a reflex through the nasal passages, the technique stimulated the phrenic nerve that regenerates the movement of the diaphragm and its innate elasticity. In turn, this relaxing focus on the exhale also supports vagus nerve tone and the elasticity synchronizes with the body's metabolic needs. The result is a felt sense of the interplay between tension and compression that coordinates the many diaphragms of the body, from inner ankles, pelvic diaphragm, respiratory diaphragm, thoracic outlet, palate—which I refer to as our Domes of Uplift. In studying this breathing awareness, I discovered a deeper dysfunctional pattern in my own body of unconsciously holding my breath when stressed. I now experience this tension-compression elasticity as a central component of innate biointelligence/biotensegrity, which can be consciously accessed to create self-regulating healthy habits.

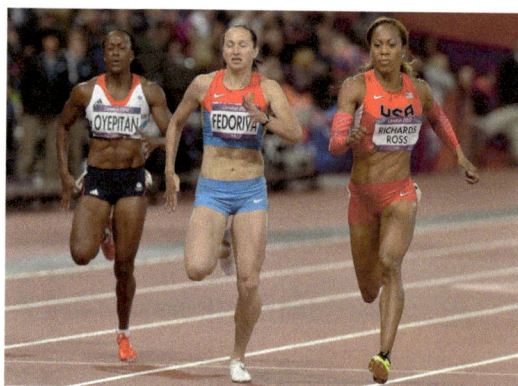

Figure 3.1 Sanya Richards-Ross, nasal breathing in the 400-meter race, 2012 London Olympics

Insightful work on breathing has gained recognition with many writers looking at trauma, breathwork, awareness, and healing: Patrick McKeown's *The Oxygen Advantage* (2015) and *The Breathing Cure* (2021); Bessel van der Kolk's *The Body Keeps the Score* (2015); Donna Farhi's

The Breathing Book (1996); Robert Litman's *The Breathable Body* (2023); Robin L. Rothenberg's *Restoring Prana* (2020); James Nestor's *Breath: The New Science of a Lost Art* (2020); and Swami Rama, Rudolph Ballentine, and Alan Hymes's *The Science of Breath* (2007).

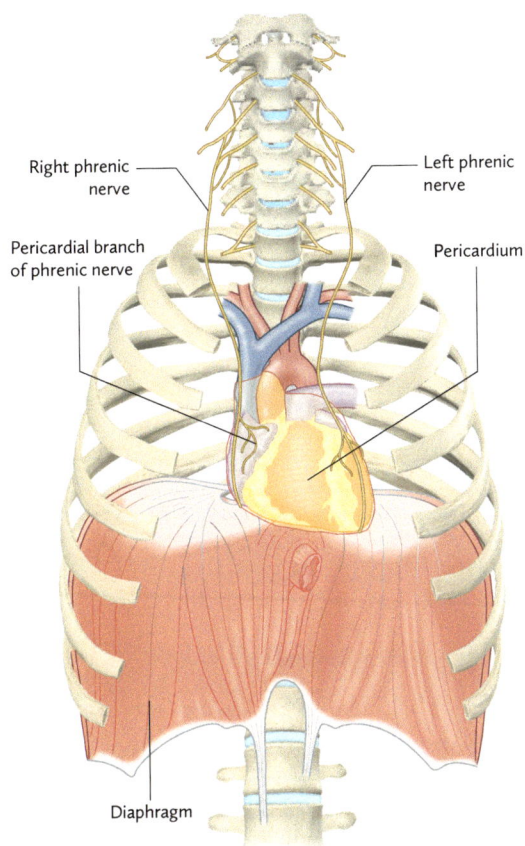

Figure 3.2 Phrenic nerve and diaphragm relationship

My interest here is twofold: first, the reappraisal of what we think we know about breath through vivid imagery and attention to the felt sense of breathing; second, related to that felt sense of breathing, checking in when we are feeling out of sorts to gain access to ways we can alter our body's breathing patterns. Knowledge of this can help lower blood pressure, balance oxygen/ carbon dioxide levels, and stimulate vagal tone which affects the co-regulation of our autonomic nervous system.

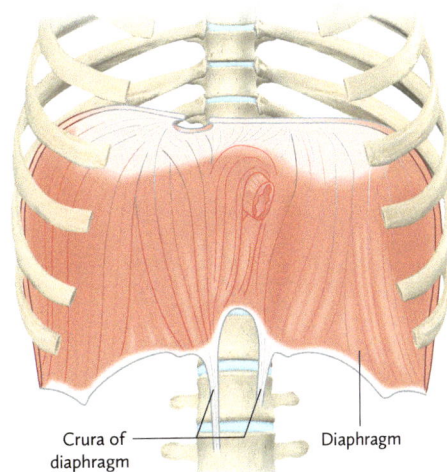

Figure 3.3 Diaphragm's crura/roots

Bonnie Bainbridge Cohen shared her embodied discovery of the crura's link to the entirety of the spine. Bonnie showed that in the literature of classical anatomy, the right and left crura are shown to attach to the upper two or three lumbar vertebrae; however, in her *embodied* explorations, she discovered that this fascial continuity continues along the entirety of the spine. We now know that our fascial matrix is a continuous, crystalline, oscillating communication system, traveling from the dural covering of the brain and spinal cord, through the periosteum of living bone, to the connective tissue wrapping every visceral, internal organ, in support of the glide and function of heart and lungs as well as our superficial fascia as skin.

Your vagus nerve is a living root. It's the longest cranial nerve in your body. It runs down from your brainstem through your neck and chest to your abdomen, co-mingling with other nerves and your major organs along the way.

Living root imagery leads us to a deeper awareness of the expression "a felt sense of breathing," which is different from breathing the right way. A felt sense of breathing is more like a phenomenological perception originating inside breath itself. Through interoceptive awareness, I have been guided to replace the phrase "breath work" with the embodied practice of "*my* breathing body." Living root imagery can support the awareness that the ego has little part to play in breathing well, but, rather, that each cell of our body is breathing, becoming more dynamic and spacious than my psychological sense of self. Root imagery can help us become present to this broader, ecological self. These roots establish a regenerative, lifelong blueprint of health within our embryonic self-healing, self-organizing, self-adaptive nature as we grow and shape ourselves throughout the journey of life.

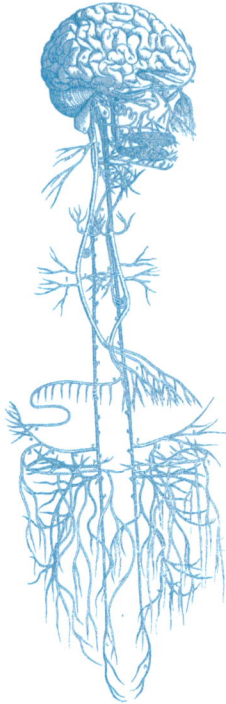

Figure 3.4 Meandering vagus nerve
SOURCE: Wellcome Collection

AN UNEXPECTED INVITATION

Almost 20 years ago, I was involved in a head-on automotive collision. My friend and I were driving along a dark highway between Boulder and Longmont late one evening when we struck a 75,000-pound piece of road-building equipment. We hit it head on, with no airbags. My friend's car, an old Lincoln, absorbed most of the shock. Yet, on impact, I remember feeling like every bone in my body was broken. My friend, who had been driving, somehow lifted me out of the car and laid me on the ground. I could feel my body going into shock. Upon sensing the ground beneath me, however, something deep inside awoke and reoriented my relationship to what was happening. A deep breath of calm comforted me. Something greater was supporting me. A sense of being held, coupled with awe and wonder. I went on

a journey as the stars glimmered overhead, one that sent me back to my embryonic beginnings, an embrace surrounded by amniotic fluid within the womb, where I sensed the entirety of the cosmos. I describe that moment now as "being breathed." Gradually, my awareness returned to the present moment and helped me sense my surroundings. I felt gratitude wash through me. Although my sternum had broken and I had sustained massive whiplash, my embodied insight about breath and being breathed was by far the most significant and enduring part of the entire experience. The journey was a movement both inward toward the world of the past and outward to the present. Breath and a felt sense of being breathed was the map that guided the journey.

BREATH AS A LIVING BRIDGE

I suggest we think and feel the body *as* breath. When we sense this image, breath begins to look like a *living* bridge, a tangible structure that connects and sustains our connection to two primary parts of ourselves—matter and spirit, bridging earth and sky. The felt sense of breathing that I experienced after the accident offered an image of bridging both worlds. I've been inspired by that image throughout my teaching life.

I return again and again to the image of breath as a healing bridge between matter and spirit. It spans and unites seemingly distanced territories through a complex partnership with gravity and various materials. The bridge that is breath *heals*. Health is not attached to illness here. It is, rather, our embryonic baseline, the state from which we are constantly in our living process.

When we think of a bridge, most people likely think of its span. We use bridges to move from one side to another. But that span is only possible because of a downward force (gravity) and its partner (uplift). The interplay of downward and upward forces enable the spanning tension of the bridge. The bridge's resilience allows it to absorb and transform the vibrations, the wind, earthquake tremors, and other forces. Prior to the realization of the necessity of this "resilience," bridges often lacked the structural dynamism to absorb extreme wind force, as in the case of the Tacoma Narrows Bridge. Watching videos of that bridge bend and fold, we could think, wow, that looks flexible for such a massive object. We can understand breath through a similar type of imagery.

Breath travels spiralically down, up, outward, and all around. Like a suspension bridge, the movement of breath enables a span, one which goes beyond the boundary of the physical body. At the level of your body, your inter- and extra-cellular expansions are fueled through breath.

We commune more fully with our porous selves by opening more fully to our living environment. Advanced Rolfer and researcher Hubert Godard described being present as a way to access a deeper relationship between earth's grounding and sky's spatial orientation.

Think of the breath as a *healing* bridge that spans matter and spirit, earth and sky.

LIVING BRIDGES

Since that pivotal experience with being breathed after the accident, my understanding is that breath has more in common with *living bridges*.

Around the world, there are functional bridges that are made entirely from *living* trees. In the mountainous regions inhabited by the Khasi and Jaintia tribes of Meghalaya, India, bridges are woven from living *Ficus elastica* trees, which can stretch across rivers and ravines for up to 50 meters, connecting villages and allowing farmers to access their land. The bridges last for hundreds of years. According to Professor Ferdinand Ludvig:

This type of bridge building could change green urban architecture, where the mainstream way of greening buildings is adding plants on top of the built structure. But this would use the tree as an internal part of the structure. In architecture, we are placing an object somewhere and then it's finished. Maybe it lasts 40, 50 years. This is a completely different understanding. There's no finished objects—it's an ongoing process and way of thinking. (Hunt 2019)

This ongoing process spans generations, allowing descendants to use the knowledge of their ancestors to maintain and utilize a bridge that was traversed by those same ancestors, thus curating a living connection across history.

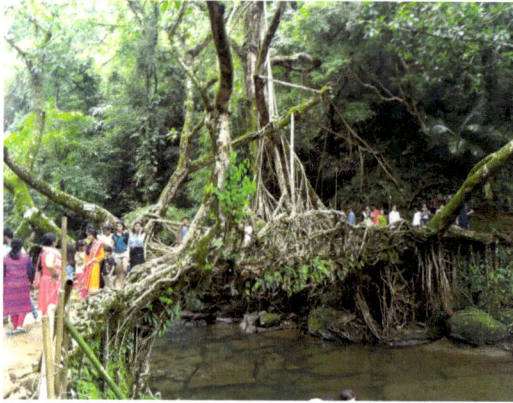

Figure 3.5 Living Roots Bridge, Shillong
PHOTO BY SAHEEN SHEHNAZ BEGUM. REPRODUCED UNDER CREATIVE COMMONS LICENSE. https://commons.wikimedia.org/wiki/File:Living_Root_Bridge,_Shillong.jpg

The *Ficus elastica* grows as fast as it grows tall. This means the strength and durability of the Living Roots Bridge fashioned from this tree are linked to the vitality of the tree itself. Keeping the tree in good health means keeping the bridge functional. Over decades, local engineers intertwine the roots of a single tree on opposite banks and weave tight knots to cultivate each bridge, which gets stronger as the roots grow and eventually has the capacity to span wide chasms.

When I learned about these bridges, I thought this is a perfect example of our regenerative living architecture. The bridge's roots maintain a balance of pre-tensed tension-compression forces, something that activates and energizes the bridge's living nature. Historically, India's monsoon season brings heavy storms and floods, leading man-made bridges (of cut timber, for example) to rot and decay. With the living bridge, however, the bridge rejoices in the waters of the monsoon and uses the precipitation and weather all year round to build itself. Our bodies are similarly self-generative. Our balance of pre-tensed tension-compression forces can be maintained

by hydration within the microfibrils of our living matrix and, of course, through our breath. We tend this breath over the course of a lifetime, and it is one of the forces that helps us maintain our health, to stop rot and decay.

To cultivate these living root bridges, seedlings are planted on each bank of the river or edge of a ravine. Once aerial roots sprout and grow above ground, people weave the roots around frames made from bamboo or palm stems and then direct the roots toward the opposite bank. Once each individual group of roots from one tree reaches the other side of the ravine or chasm that people wish to cross, they are implanted in the soil. The crisscrossing roots of both trees not only tangle with each other but also physically grow into each other, a process called inosculation, thereby creating the strength and elasticity required to carry mechanical loads and the weight of people crossing. Our body's many *nested* systems are similarly inosculated. For instance, our nervous, musculoskeletal, respiratory, lymphatic, and circulatory systems, all typically separated for analysis in biomechanical approaches, entwine with and interweave with each other to create the whole.

There is really so much to say about the teachings available to us through these living root bridges. We could focus on how sustainable farming practices and environmental sensibilities that tend the health of the *Ficus elastica* trees so clearly fold back and sustain the health of the larger society by providing these bridges necessary for transport and communication. We could investigate the similarities between the soil in which the trees grow and our body's fascial matrix.

The main point here is that the notion of breath and bridge between matter and spirit is reflected in the root bridges. The living bridge spans generations. It is a material artifact infused with the spirit of ancestors, spirit that lives on in the knowledge and building practices of contemporary society. Our breath is similar. It doesn't belong to us. Breath—oxygen, nitrogen, carbon dioxide—comes from outside. We breathe in the world every time we inhale. When we exhale, we give a part of ourselves back. Maintaining awareness of this dimension of breath in our movement and bodywork helps us consider the ways we can nurture our bodies and our social landscapes across spans of time.

The bridge also reminds us that spirit can be a word for the internal energy of an organism that has physical properties but also an extra, indescribable quality that provides dynamism. The water coursing through the roots, the nutrients from the soil carried by that water—these elements spawn elasticity in the roots and enable its dual role as a bridge. The life of the bridge is its spirit. The flow of blood creates our spiralic heart in our embryonic beginnings, infusing our connective tissue body with energy that allows us to thrive. Blood is, in this way, like spirit. And of course, the breath in our bodies, partly made up of the oxygen carried by our blood, is similar. Breath is not a mechanical process. The act of breathing is fully entwined with unseen forces that nurture us and give us life. Breath spans matter and spirit.

COMMON MYTHS

Thinking about the importance of breath varies. Some feel that breath is an activity that can be done either properly or improperly. Breath here is seen as a mechanical function.

There are a lot of cultural and perceptual myths about breath. For example, we learn that the *more* we breathe, the healthier we are. "Take a big breath" is a common instruction. Yet, physiologically speaking, big breaths take in an amount of oxygen that is disproportionate with the amount of carbon dioxide in our bodies. Exhaling after a big breath causes a similar problem. We exhale more carbon dioxide (CO_2) than our bodies need to. Instead of seeking out big breaths, our bodies look for a balance of oxygen (O_2) and CO_2.

To demonstrate, I use a "breathing ball." The ball expands omnidirectionally, which parallels the ideal movement of the body when breathing. If I pull the ball open without any relationship to metabolic need, it will expand, but at a cost. That over-exertion of energy equates to overbreathing that feeds hypervigilance. By contrast, we want to imagine that the breathing ball expands from grounding, centering, and uplift, slowly, evenly, outward in all directions. The parallel breathing experience is a gravity-supported slow breath from the diaphragm outward. **See Video 3.6 for deeper exploration**.

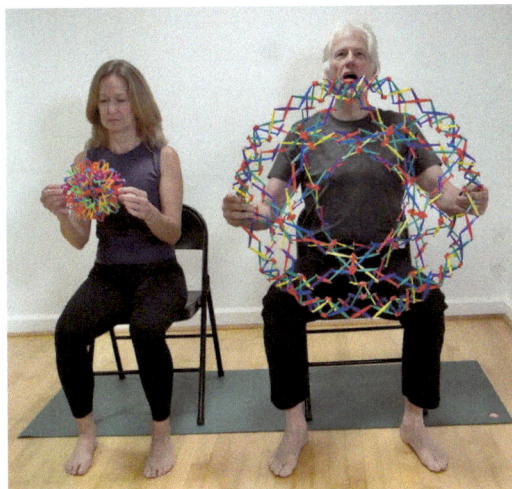

Figure 3.6 Small and large breathing ball expanding on inhale and contracting on exhale

Some consider CO_2 as toxic, a waste gas. This perception is partly true, insofar as CO_2 emitted from cars pollutes the earth's atmosphere. But CO_2 in the body plays a different role. Without sufficient CO_2, we can't actually use the O_2 that we inhale. "CO_2 acts like a hormone, enabling the release of oxygen in the same way that insulin prompts the release of blood glucose" (Patrick McKeown cited in Tracey 2022).

Nasal breathing matters. It is the body's preferential mode of breathing. To self-regulate and self-heal, the body prefers a regular nasal breathing practice over mouth breathing. Also, the awareness-building practices in this chapter help us to develop methods for healthy breathing capacity and learn how conscious breath holding creates a more adaptive, resilient organism.

PHYSIOLOGY OF BREATH AS A LIVING BRIDGE

The entrance to your respiratory passages lies above your mouth (oral cavity) in your nose (nasal cavity). Your respiratory and digestive tracts cross in your throat, at a ring-like muscular tube that acts as the passageway for air, food, and liquid. When air enters your nose, a tiny leaf-shaped flap, called the epiglottis, opens and allows air into your larynx. When you consume food and liquid, the epiglottis closes to allow those substances to enter your esophagus. This configuration makes talking and breathing harmonious activities, but talking and eating are incompatible due to the risk of choking and aspiration.

The dexterity of your epiglottis is quite magical, and it happens without conscious thought. By first becoming aware, cognitively, of the way your epiglottis participates in the respiratory cycle and then, second, by sensing the epiglottal motion, you activate your interoceptive capacities and drop into the world of embodied breathing. "Effort with ease" is the name I give to magical activities like this, which take place without me doing anything. I benefit from my awareness that they are happening, and how I am positioning my body to support or inhibit natural breathing. Sitting in a collapsed posture and eating can be a set-up for choking or poor digestion. The benefit of this awareness is a type of resting into a natural breathing rhythm that adapts to your metabolic needs. Awareness, in this case, can reduce tension in your epiglottis, tongue, throat, jaw, neck, and shoulders.

I'm grateful to my colleague, yoga breath master Leslie Kaminoff, who introduced me to the following awareness in my body many years ago. To turn the awareness on, simply begin by exhaling. Exhale completely without over-exerting—remember, effort with ease—then wait till your body wants to inhale through your nose. You may notice that the inhale just happens by itself, without you having to do anything. When your body functions on its own time, responding to its own needs, your epiglottis opens effortlessly and facilitates the suctioning of air into your lungs. We don't need to take a big breath in order to breathe well.

EXPLORING EFFORT WITH EASE

Our natural breathing is very efficient. Nerve impulses fire from the brain down the phrenic nerve into the diaphragm, which causes it to contract, allowing air to flow into your lungs. The diaphragm stops contracting, and when the diaphragm relaxes, there is an elastic recoil. When we allow an inhale, we are expanding our lung tissue, which is elastic, and expanding the spiralic ribs attached to the sternum. Your flexible ribs, moving elastically, condensing and expanding in concert with your pelvic and respiratory diaphragms and abdominals, massage your upper and lower internal organs and breathing spine.

Here is an exploration of sensing effort with ease in your body. It involves the movement of your ribs. First, picture the spiralic nature of your intercostal muscles supported by your fascial matrix. Your fascia matrix spans each rib to create an elastic recoil when you exhale and inhale. The unique shaping of your intercostal muscles and your fascial matrix is an effect of the relationship between breath and the tension-compression biotensegrity of the bones and soft tissue that orchestrate this spring-like motion. In mentoring and in workshops, I like to use a chiralic tube inside a tube to illustrate this (thank you for the inspiration, Joanne Avison). The tube is a cross patterning and, when spiraled in relationship with one another, closely resembles the interplay between the 3Cores from foot to head and hand. The tension-compression of this chiralic fabric mirrors the bones–muscle–fascia helical connection in the body.

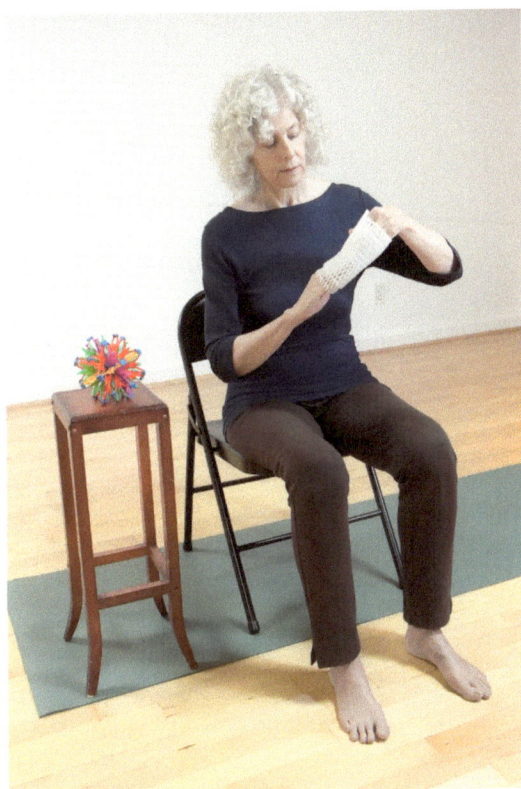

Figure 3.8 Spiralic intercostals and fascia paired with Counting Breath and chiral tubes counter-spiraling to the one inside it—which is how trees grow—with left to right growth rings

See Video 3.8 which shows me engaging my Counting Breath to feel a deeper exhale from pelvic diaphragm to palate, without over-efforting. This distinction of a powerful elastic recoil breath practice that creates effort with ease is what Dr. Andrew Weil is referring to when he illuminates a deeper awareness with this statement:

Breathing is the only function that we do completely consciously and unconsciously. No other function in the body has that aspect to it. You can breathe as a voluntary act or involuntary act, so breath is controlled by two different sets of nerves and muscles: there are voluntary nerves and muscles that can activate the system fully, or involuntary nerves and muscles that activate (operate) the system fully. As a result, *breath is the only function you do that can influence the involuntary nervous system*—that is, you can establish rhythms of breathing with your voluntary nerves and muscles that will affect the involuntary nervous system. Imbalances of involuntary nervous system function underlie many common problems. (Weil 2006)

This is a distinction that is often missing, especially with elite athletes. In relaxed breathing, the exhale happens from the passive recoil of the lungs and the relaxation of the diaphragm—effort with ease. When one learns to come from a state of relaxation to recruit more muscular effort with nasal breathing and whole-body fascial matrix support, the established rhythms of breathing will enable higher performance within the zone.

An image that captures that tension-compression, elastic recoil fascial patterning which affects both the voluntary and involuntary nerves and muscles through the fascial matrix is the lemniscate or figure-eight infinity pattern, which is the energetic blueprint of your body's structure prior to integrating into its actual form. It is the vibratory essence underlying form which embryologist Johannes Rohen writes of as the most rhythmical of all geometric forms, which "can be maintained only through the alternation of sleeping and waking, catabolism and anabolism, inhalation and exhalation, systole and diastole—the rhythmically structured oscillation of form-providing (informational) and materially determined (metabolic) processes" (Weil 2006).

Building on this rich awareness, Biodynamic Craniosacral therapist Charles Ridley writes in *Stillness: Biodynamic Cranial Practice and the Evolution of Consciousness*:

> In its most simple two-dimensional form, a lemniscate is a figure-8, but as a fundamental motion pattern of life, it defies description. As a fundamental fractal pattern of life, the lemniscate is a figure-8 that is non-linear, multi-dimensional, multi-directional and ever-changing. Like a mobius strip, this baffling figure-8 motion expresses a pattern by which formative forces create living organisms. In the center of this complex array of figure-8 patterns is a fulcrum, or point of stillness, that is in a constant flow, always altering its position to accommodate all outside and inside influences that impact its function. The outside forces enter this flowing fulcrum through an unlimited fractal array of lemniscate loops that return from the periphery and touch the center to provide the organism with new information that changes it. The lemniscate, in turn, emanates from the center to the periphery with new information that reflects a changed body, and so this process repeats ad infinitum. This creates an ever-changing fractal matrix that exchanges information between organism (center) and the Breath of Life (periphery). (Ridley 2006, p.199)

When you sense the lemniscate patterning within your body, some of which are the toroidal field of your heart, your elastic recoil breath through cellular respiration, the helical, mobius internal and external movements of your limbs, pelvis, ribs, and spine, you have the capacity to understand the anatomy of your living architecture as a process with regenerative vitality and life. As we move through rhythmic weight shift and force transfer from foot to head and hand, we are returned to our shape-shifting archetypal origins.

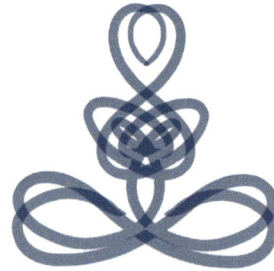

Figure 3.9A Lemniscate breathing body
GRATITUDE TO LEAH REES, ARTIST

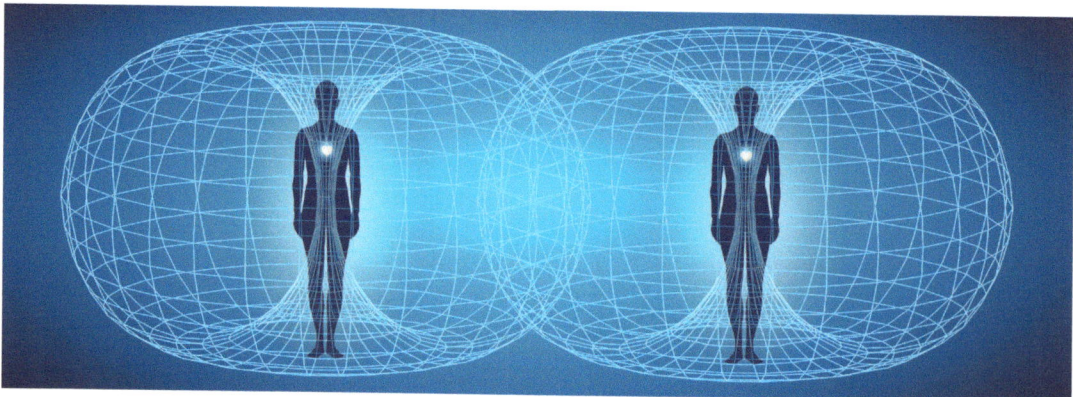

Figure 3.9B Toroidal field of heart
IMAGE COURTESY OF THE HEARTMATH® INSTITUTE—WWW.HEARTMATH.ORG

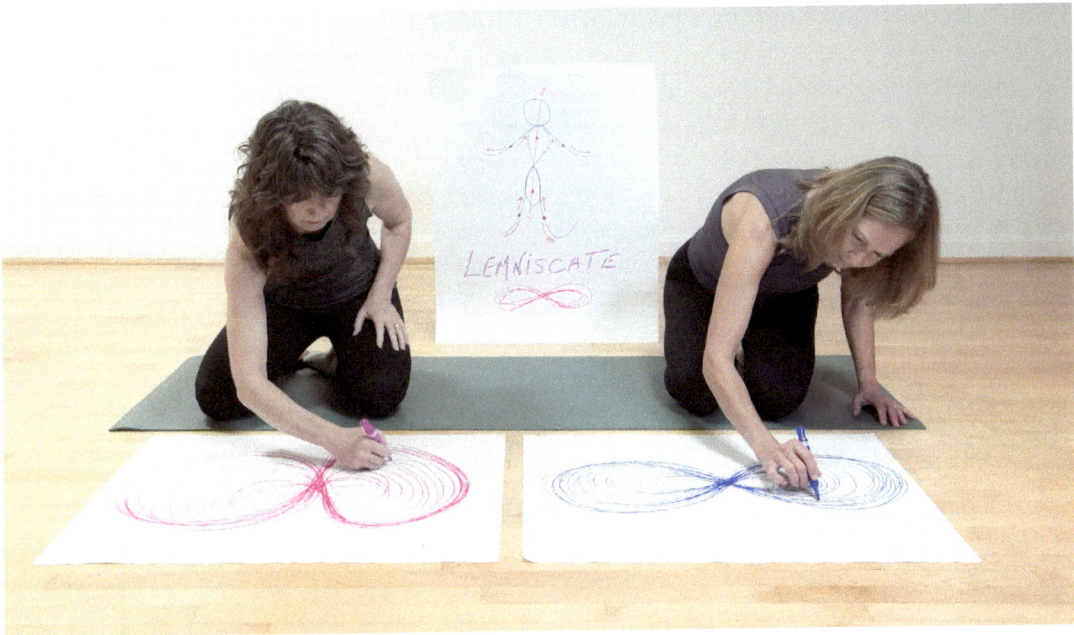

Figure 3.10 Playful drawing with the idea of lemniscate

A powerful exercise that I experienced with embryologist Jaap van der Wal was drawing the lemniscate pattern as a way to sense our fluid continuity and our polarity between earth and sky.

Embody the Felt Sense of Lemniscate

▶ Look at your right hand and move your arm in a figure-eight pattern, internally and externally rotating to form a figure eight.

▶ Notice that your hand moves your arm and as you make the figure-eight pattern larger.

▶ Allow your body to follow your hand; your hand and arm move your body from foot through spine to hand, as you weight-shift from side to side.

▶ You are spiraling in your body just by moving your hand—isn't that amazing?

Drawing Lemniscate Patterning

▶ Get a piece of paper, and draw a figure-eight pattern—from small to bigger—sensing the change from center to periphery.

▶ You may feel how relaxing this is as you flow in and out in your movement.

Now move into explorations and practices that emerge from and support the lemniscate and living bridge imagery discussed up to this point. The explorations also revolve around the physiology I just discussed and the practice of effort with ease. There are six explorations preceded by a preparation, which you might think of as set-up with awareness, which also bridges the theoretical and practical halves of this chapter.

EMBODIED PREPARATION FOR YOUR BREATHING SPINE

Sit comfortably on your sitting bones at the front edge of a chair, with your hips above your knees, sensing support in your feet, with your feet hip-width apart. Resting one hand on your low belly, place the other hand behind the base of your head at your occiput. Nod your head up and down, as in saying "yes," and notice if your head can nod freely on top of your neck, without your head and the base of your neck falling forward. **See Video 3.11 for deeper exploration.**

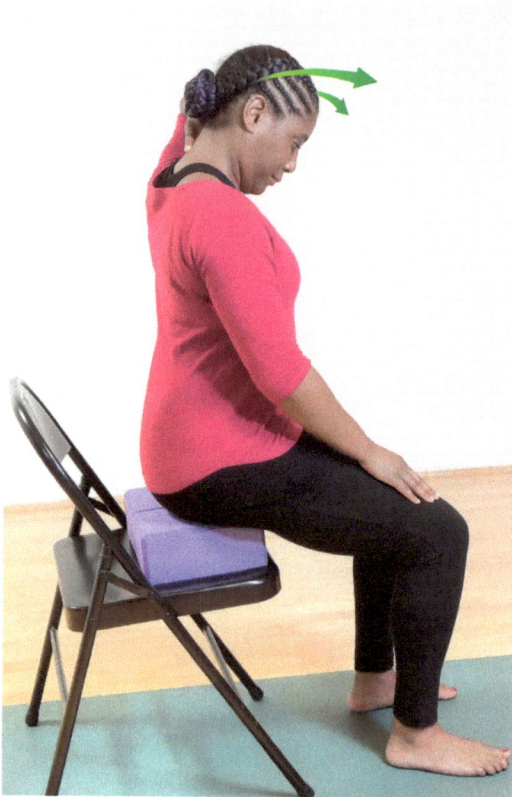

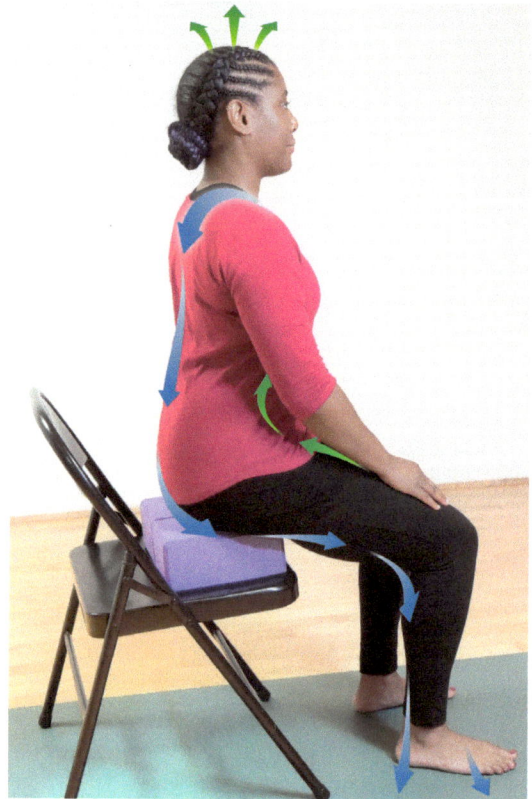

Figures 3.11A and 3.11B Awareness of head falling forward from C7, producing tension in jaw, tongue, face, and cranium

Your Practice for Breathing Spine: Exploring Breathwave

Remain seated with your hips above your knees, grounded in your sitting bones and feet. Notice the tilt of your pelvis—are you sitting on the front or back of your sitting bones? If you still feel tension in your back, lean forward from your sitting bones, and draw each sitting bone back, so as to transfer weight into your legs, onto the front of your sitting bones and feet, and then sit up with more ease from inner ear to sacrum.

We are attuning ourselves to the breathwave, which is the name often given to the fluid, naturally occurring rocking movement, synchronized by breath, that coordinates your body's motion between sphenoid (head) and sacrum (tail). To sense your breathwave, rest one hand at your solar plexus (in front of your diaphragm's roots/ crura) and your other hand on your low belly. **See Video 3.12 for deeper exploration.**

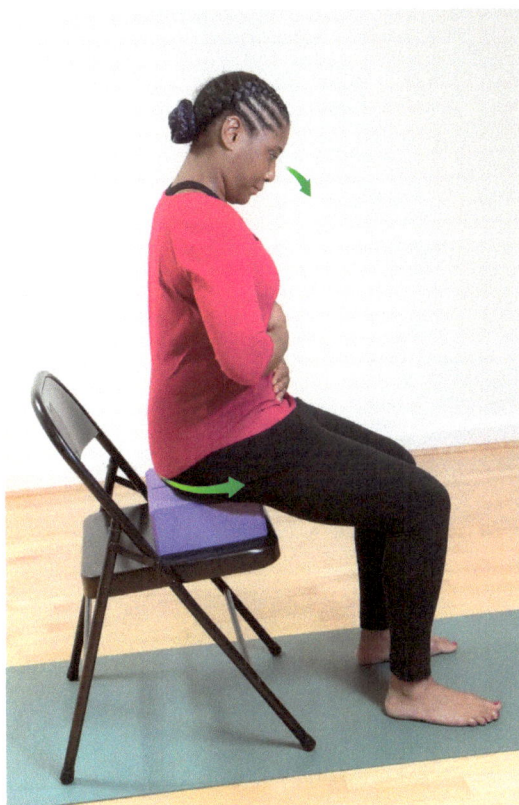

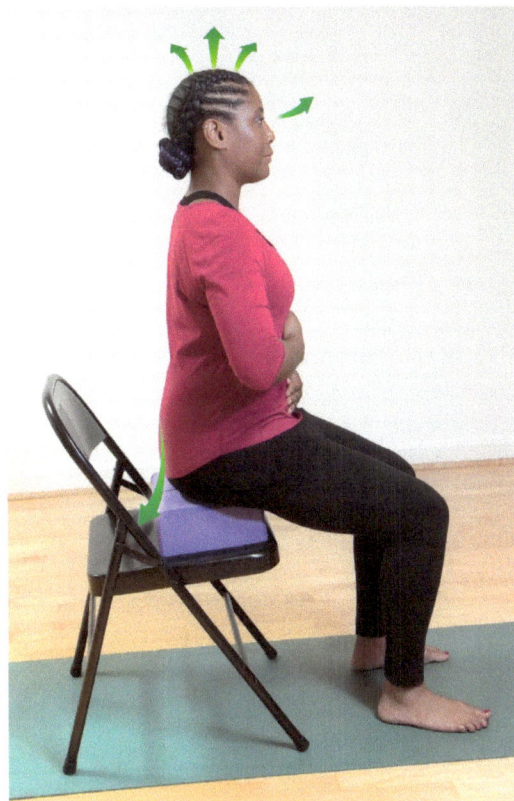

Figure 3.12A and 3.12B Sphenoid/inner ear to sacrum/tail—breathing spine "exploring breathwave"

Take your time and allow your breath and the gentle rocking motion through your sitting bones and feet to support your breathing spine. Exhale as you look down and curl your tail slightly (embryo shape); inhale as you look up and extend your tail. You may notice, after several breathwaves, a sigh, swallow, or yawn, which is your body's co-regulation of your autonomic nervous system through vagus nerve stimulation. If you would like to experience this breathwave in a more relaxed position, lie down in Constructive Rest Position, with your knees bent and feet in relationship with your sitting bones. See Golden Nugget Three: Cervical Pivot in Chapter 6 to deepen your relaxation from head to tail.

Your base of support, shared between your feet, pelvis, and spine's vertical orientation, creates a fluid massage along the full excursion of your spine, allowing the breathwave to massage your breathing internal organs and neuroendocrine glands. You may notice as you *do less* and *allow more* that the rhythm of your breath changes, becoming longer and deeper as you play with gravity. By slowing down, and discovering more fluid movement, you open a portal that is the foundation for any warm-up, workout, or traditional Pilates or yoga session.

WHY BREATHING THROUGH YOUR NOSE IS HEALTHIER

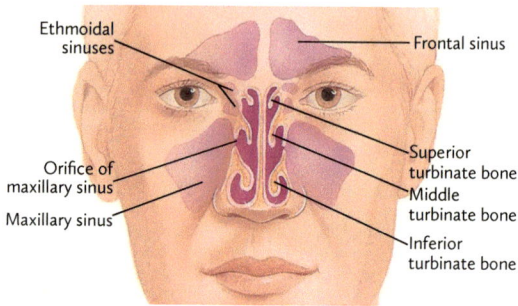

Figure 3.13 Paranasal sinuses

The air that enters your nose is swirled through your nasal turbinates, spiralic spongy bones that regulate the direction and velocity of the air to maximize exposure to a network of small arteries and veins and to the mucous blanket in order to warm, humidify, and sterilize the air before it is drawn into your lungs.

Nasal breathing is more than a good idea. It is the way your body wants to function by effectively using the air you breathe to feed your cells and tissues. Here are some benefits of nasal breathing:

- Encourages your tongue to rest on the roof of your mouth, which opens your airways.

- Filters out foreign particles (dust, allergens, pollen), preventing them from entering your lungs.

- Humidifies inhaled air by warming and moisturizing the air you breathe in, bringing your inhaled air to body temperature which makes it easier for your lungs to use.

- Directs your inhaled air into the lower lobes of your lungs where greatest oxygen and carbon dioxide exchange takes place.

- Produces nitric oxide in your nasal passages. Nitric oxide (NO) is beneficial to bacterial clearance and, as it is a vasodilator, lowers blood pressure, which helps to widen blood vessels and improve oxygen circulation in your body. NO also eases vascular tension in your head, neck, and thorax, and is recognized to be a key player in the process and essential for the development of the neurovascular response in the whole body.

- As the facial bones and teeth are forming, nasal breathing participates in the shaping of these and influences the placement of teeth and formation of the bite plate for better digestion.

Many people breathe mainly in the chest. This breath is performed largely by the expanding and lifting of the rib cage via the intercostal muscles and includes the clavicles in extreme states of air hunger. This action is more difficult than diaphragmatic breathing and requires more work and a higher heart rate to perform. Chest breathing fills the middle and upper portions of the lungs but doesn't efficiently engage the blood-rich lower lobes. Although it is easier to get large quantities of air in and out of the upper and middle lobes, the ample blood supply needed for a quality exchange, especially during oxygen-demanding exercise, is in the lower lobes. For chest breathing to supply enough oxygen, both breathing and heart rate must be faster (Douillard 2018, p.153).

When you breathe through your nose, air is channeled into the lower lobes and sacs of your lungs, where the greatest oxygen and blood exchange takes place. This deep inflation of the lower lobes of your lungs is a result of the omnidirectional energy facilitated by nasal breathing. As the lower portions of your lungs inflate, your back also expands, and your side body expands. Orientation with gravity is an active partner here, too, that supports a free head and neck. As your lower ribs and xiphoid melt down, as you exhale, your palate, respiratory diaphragm, and pelvic diaphragm can relax up, supported by your abdominal belly wall and crural midline from head to tail. The interplay of gravity and ground reaction force is present within the polarity motion of your breath, which is a lemniscate shaping of your body's biodynamic relationships. In this way, the activity of nasal breathing reminds us of the insight from the previous chapter on Core as Relationship which is a contextual shift from controlling your body to having a conversation with your body wisdom. **See Video 3.14 for deeper exploration**.

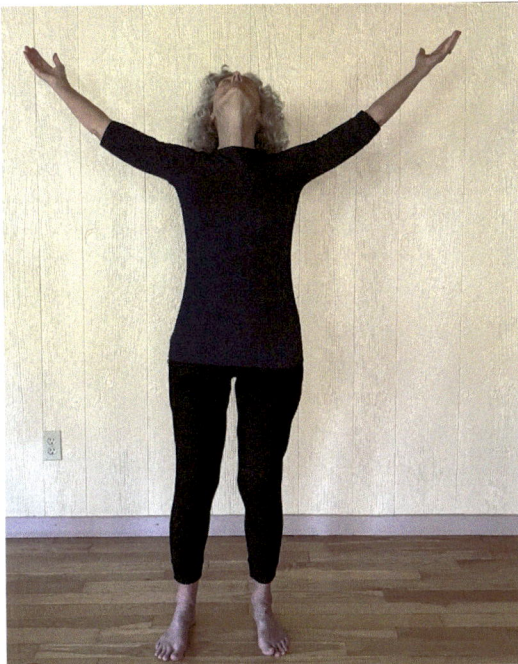

Figure 3.14 Lemniscate body with arms (internal-external) and legs (external-internal)

Regular mouth breathing actually triggers the body into emergency breathing. Mouth breathing can convince the body that there is a problem, which alerts the sympathetic nervous system and prepares the body to run or face danger. On the other hand, nasal breathing co-regulates the nervous system and circulation because carbon dioxide directly influences the toning of the vagus nerve by slowing the pulse and increasing oxygenation of the blood. This way of breathing alerts your parasympathetic nervous system, but alerts it in such a way as to work with your autonomic regulation to find balance.

When we change the pattern of our breathing, we change the pattern of what information is sent to our brain and how it responds to stimuli. The phrase "big breaths" almost always means big mouth breaths. These big breaths primarily activate the upper body. They release a lot of carbon dioxide, but, as a result, airways actually close up. Small nasal breaths, on the other hand, encourage your fascial matrix cellular body and breathing spine to breathe, which activates postural tone and supports your body's microfibril water matrix. What might at first feel like more resistance, because of the smaller aperture of the nostrils, rather than a large mouth opening, actually leads to more coherent support in the body, activating nitric oxide that, in turn, opens the airways, brings moisture to the tissues, and works in concert with the porosity of our living fascial matrix that supports whole-body awareness.

When we think of the healing bridge, notice how regular nasal breathing feels like roots growing in, through, and beyond my body, especially when the body is grounded through feet or sitting bones. Although regular mouth breathing might at times feel like a more controlled kind of breathing that helps when we are gasping for or are "out of" breath, it actually creates upper-body tension that stunts the growth of these roots. Regular mouth breathing is akin to growing a tree in a pot. Regular nasal breathing allows the roots to grow naturally and expand, eventually, out into the world beyond my body.

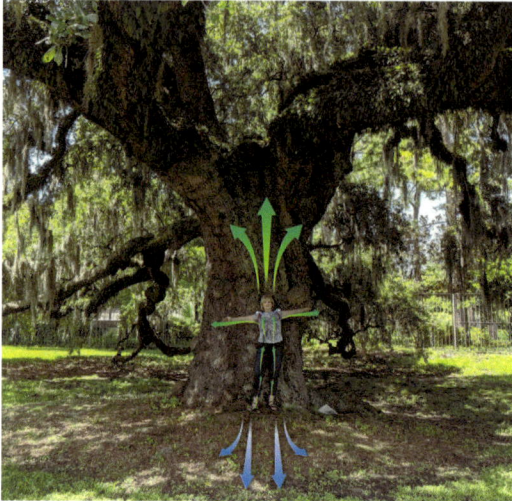

Figure 3.15 Live oak tree with full canopy and roots and person reaching and rooting

GRATITUDE TO MY SISTER PETA ANNE AND OUR FAVORITE MOTHER OAK IN CITY PARK, NEW ORLEANS

of CO_2 in the blood are low, the body cannot access the oxygen in the blood, which leads to poor body oxygenation. The practice of quieting and holding the breath allows CO_2 levels to build and increases overall body oxygenation. In 2017, a doctor at Subharti Medical College in India, Dr. Singh, who is also a yoga practitioner, wrote a detailed review of the benefits of carbon dioxide.

Dr. Singh, who has dedicated much time to researching how yoga works, discovered that increased levels of CO_2 stimulates the vagus nerve and slows the heart rate. He describes CO_2 as a natural sedative, soothing the irritability of the brain's conscious centers, promoting our ability to use logic, reason, and common sense. Without CO_2 we become anxious, depressed and angry. He goes on further to say that CO_2 is truly the breath of life. (McKeown 2021, p.17)

Regular nasal breathing bathes the pineal gland, which aids our ability to "see" beyond what the eyes see. When this bodily intuition is supported through breath, we honor the power of our embryonic beginnings, a power that is always flowing actively throughout our spine, from sphenoid to tail.

The following breath practices are ones I practice and teach as they are founded on strengthening our roots and building a healthy and functional breathing rhythm. In 1904, Danish physiologist Christian Bohr discovered the importance of carbon dioxide (CO_2) and how it supports the release of oxygen (O_2) from red blood cells into tissues and organs. Bohr discovered that CO_2 acts as a catalyst for hemoglobin to release O_2 for use in the body. When levels

In my Buteyko Practitioner Training with Patrick McKeown, I learned that for a person with a healthy breathing pattern, the breath hold after exhalation is about 40 seconds, which means that when inhaling through the nose, after the breath hold, you are breathing in a relaxed state. It has been shown that being able to hold the breath for at least 25 seconds allows one to be less symptomatic with conditions like asthma, chronic obstructive pulmonary disease (COPD), sleep apnea, hypervigilance, and more. My experience is that very few people have a breath hold of 40 seconds in the beginning, and that most of us would need to work up to this amount of time by cultivating a regular practice.

EXPLORATIONS FOR EMPOWERING THE BREATH AS A HEALING BRIDGE

Discovering Your BOLT Score (Body Oxygen Level Test)

The BOLT score is an awareness-building practice that you use to measure your breath hold time. It gives you a more accurate sense of how well your breath relates to your body's oxygen needs. A low BOLT score (0–25) indicates a low tolerance for CO_2, and a higher score (25–40)

indicates your body has a healthier oxygen/carbon dioxide ratio and your breathing, even under stress, will be slower, smoother, and deeper. **See Video 3.16 for full practice**.

Mini Pauses

This activity highlights a natural resistance *and* resilience formed through nasal breathing. This resistance may feel noticeable but should never feel threatening. It is caused by the purposeful build-up of CO_2. Throughout the activity, you will be playing with the sense that you *could* take in more breath, but you don't absolutely need to. It may seem as though you are feeling slightly breathless at first. You are beginning to discover what is just enough breath for your metabolic needs. **See Video 3.17 for full practice**.

Blocked Sinus Clearing

This is a practice which clears a blocked sinus through small breath holds and head nodding. **See Video 3.17 for full practice**.

I use these exercises to change your perspective about CO_2 in your body. Mini pauses help to build the proper ratio of CO_2, O_2, and nitrogen in your body. Once the ratio is established (and it will be slightly different for everyone), your airways find their optimal blossoming. Your capillary beds throughout your entire body are fed.

If you're comfortable building your breath hold capacity while sitting, then you can play with the deceptively complex task of breathing and moving with ease. Remember that you are inhaling and exhaling through your nose. **See Video 3.18 for full exploration**.

All of these explorations are an optimal way to enhance alveolar ventilation—the amount of oxygen that saturates the small air sacs of your lungs and capillary beds throughout your body. Since breathing through the mouth has a drying effect to your mouth and airways, and can lead to loss of essential bodily fluids, dehydration can occur without you even realizing it. Your body cannot function without an adequate supply of water, which also affects the slide and glide of internal organ function within your internal fascial matrix.

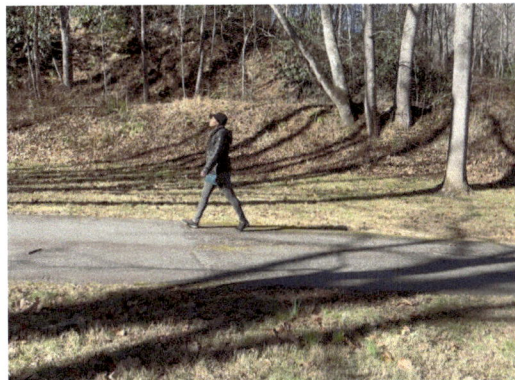

Figure 3.18 Nasal breathing while walking or exploring gentle movements

The way you breathe allows you to control your stress level, your emotional ecology, your physical and mental health, and your actions and behavior. This practice also introduces you to the sound and the power of your own voice. The following breath explorations are ones I practice in a variety of ways: in my daily practice, as the sounds not only oxygenate my entire cellular matrix, they also create an internal sonic massage from periphery to Meso midline. Sensing your internal midline is a major benefit of nasal breathing where you learn to bring your mind into the present moment, where it can rest in stillness and you can make clearer choices—called "being in the zone" in peak performance.

Counting Breath

The counting element of this exploration comes from Carl Stough's work, which he called Breathing Coordination, where he noted that everything is based on the *exhale*, and the *inhale* is a reflex. Counting Breath reinvigorates the elasticity of the diaphragm's ecological coordination in the body from pelvic diaphragm to palate—spiraling lemniscate breath. By naturally engaging the fascially supported abdominal muscles and internal organs to support the relaxation of the diaphragm on the exhale, you sense an inward and upward movement from pelvic diaphragm to palate. This, in turn, leads toward reestablishing the natural rhythm of each person's breath while releasing myofascial restrictions. **See Video 3.19 for full exploration**.

> **STORY:** A touching experience I had with my dad, who died of emphysema, was also a deep learning about how dysfunctional breathing changes the shape of our bones. As I supported my dad as he struggled with each breath, by placing my hands on either side of his ribs, massaging and gently breathing with him, I could feel that his lower ribs had distended into a *bell shape*, which prevented him from exhaling. In other words, the damage to his lungs and diaphragm was such that he couldn't exhale. His chest muscles were frozen and stiff, and his lower ribs couldn't move, because his diaphragm was atrophied, so he was prevented from receiving an inhale.

Humming Breath or Simple Bhramari (Bee Breath) Pranayama

Humming is another powerful practice which increases nitric oxide (NO) in the body. The chief benefit is improved vascular tone and alveolar ventilation, lowering blood pressure, which can help improve long-COVID symptoms. There is good research about the value of humming, and the many beneficial therapeutic effects.

Humming is a fluid-vibrational resonance of the extracellular matrix supporting lungs, throat, and capillaries through the production of nitric oxide. The resonance of the hum can travel throughout the entire body creating greater oxygenation.

The breath is transformed through these explorations so restrictions that are interfering with your natural breath rhythm can be addressed. With Counting Breath, the action of counting supports the movement of the pelvic and respiratory diaphragms, creating a deeper connection to your fluid midline. The result is that your elastic recoil breath and rib basket become stronger and more resilient. **See Video 3.20 for full exploration**.

As you breathe more naturally through your nose, the benefits are similar to those sensed through the previous explorations. The balance of O_2, CO_2, and NO sustained through a practice of nasal breathing will aid your body's metabolic needs more reliably than through regular mouth breathing.

Agni Sara

Agni (fire) Sara (essence) is a kriya yoga practice that is deeply transformational. This practice empowers abdominal "fire," balancing the spine's relationship with Down the Back (DTB) and Up the Front (UTF), toning neuroendocrine glands and chakras, bridging our relationship between matter and spirit, facilitating physical, mental, and emotional vitality and life.

Traditional Chinese Medicine (TCM) teaches that our life purpose is stored at birth in our kidneys as the root of life because they store our essence, and that expression is aligned with our heart's purpose. Before birth, our body receives nourishment through our umbilical cord, and after birth, this breathing center functions as our center for digestive fire. The Triple Warmer meridian, which is also aligned with our heart center and kidney essence, is fueled by our abdominal fire center. The Triple Warmer is the burner of respiration, digestion, and elimination. **See Video 3.21 for full exploration**.

Stand with feet slightly wider than hip-width apart, soft knees with hands on knees, upper body resting in hands and feet. Curl gently as sounding along spine from tail to solar plexus. Gently arch from solar plexus to tail.

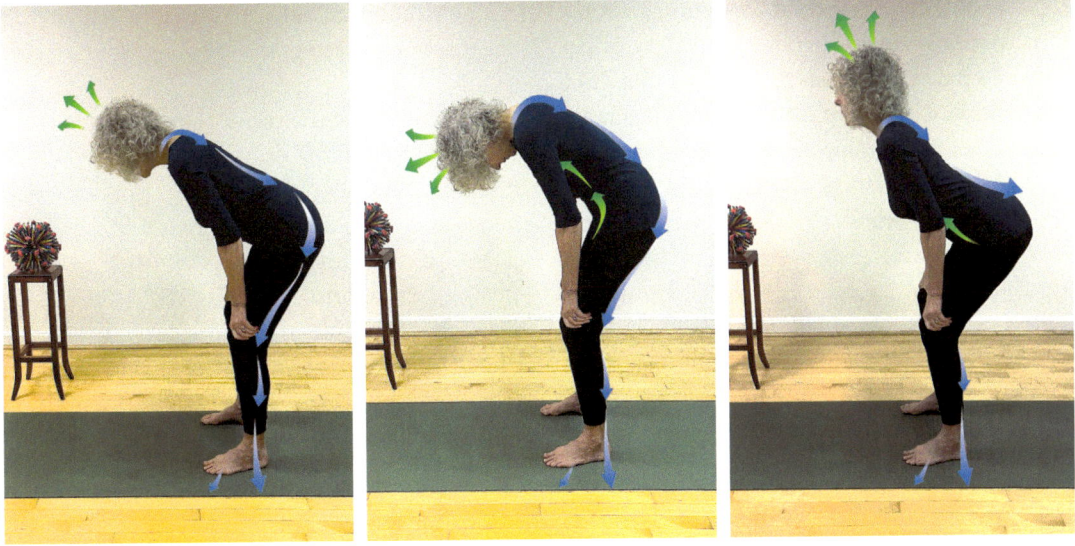

Figures 3.21A, 3.21B, and 3.21C Agni Sara

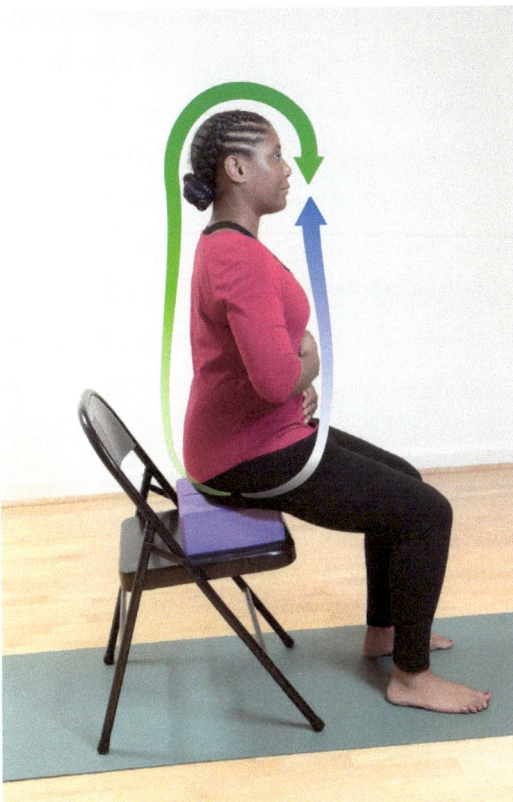

Figure 3.22 Central Channel—Governing and Conception Vessels—tongue at roof of mouth

It is important to emphasize the relationships enlivened through this kind of breathing practice. The physical, emotional, energetic, and psychological dimensions of the body are not separate. This breathing practice works from the principle that the whole person is composed of all these dimensions and that each dimension works in concert as we self-tune ourselves. Your body ecosystem as a whole is what you can access through the practice of Agni Sara, and is deeply nourished through this exploration.

You may have studied traditional Eastern movement forms like Qigong, Shiatsu, Do-In self-massage, and others. I am grateful to acupuncturist and osteopath Phillip Beach who utilizes this Eastern approach to create a deeper contextual awareness around the importance of self-tuning from an archetypal movement perspective, one that bridges our movement patterns with our rest patterns (Beach 2010). In *Moving Beyond Core*, we explore a world that teaches us a somatic approach to self-tuning our fascial matrix body by bridging our ability to sense our relationship between movement and rest, and cultivating support through our breathing spine in relationship with our environment.

In the following explorations, we explore the relationship between breath as a healing bridge between matter and spirit, through our fluid, fascial matrix body supporting our living architectural tension-compression body.

The traditional movements that we will begin exploring now, which are shown in Video 3.23, are ones that will:

- challenge awareness around relaxed breathing and help rehabilitate tension created by our right-angled chair sitting that doesn't support full excursion of our joint spaces and spinal elongation

- reverse the tendency to lack of movement from floor to standing in order to support venous return of blood circulation back to the heart as oscillator

- cultivate awareness around sensory deprivation of our feet that are often locked in shoes so we lose contact with our primal breathing relationship with earth's energy.

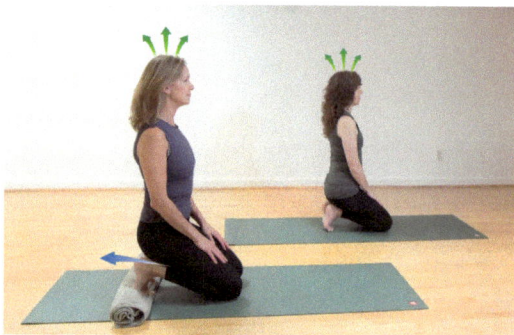

Figure 3.23A Toe sit

▶ This is a posture that many traditional cultures around the world use as a "resting" pose for sitting, cooking, eating, etc.

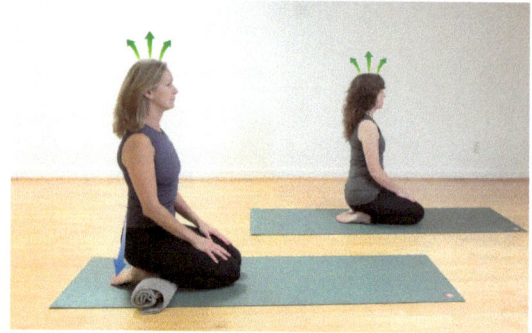

Figure 3.23B Hero

▶ This posture may be familiar as a meditation posture and is also one called "seiza" in Japanese culture. Even though I often sat in this pose over many years, it became more meaningful for me when I was gifted with participating in a traditional Japanese tea ceremony in Tokyo with hosting teachers.

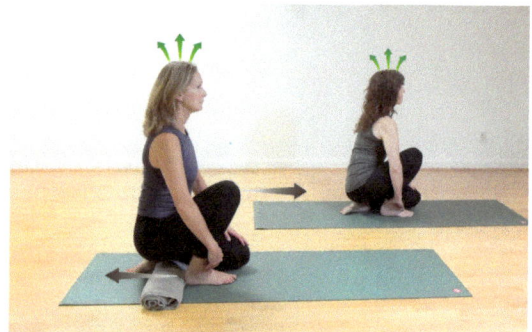

Figure 3.23C One-Leg Hero

▶ Still seated, one leg is in Hero and the other is in a squat position.

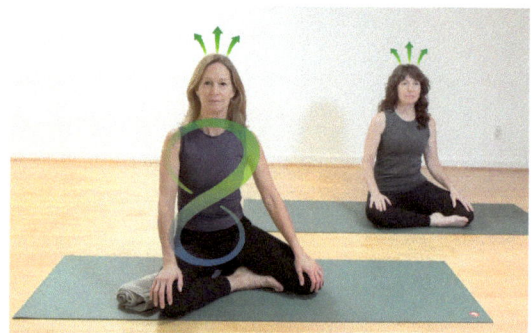

Figure 3.23D Z-sit—each side

- ▶ Sitting down in a Z position, which we use often in Rolf Structural Integration movement sessions to assess tension patterns and create awareness.
  - As you sit down, one leg is externally rotated and the other is internally rotated

transfer your weight through to your right hand and feet and rebound to come to standing.

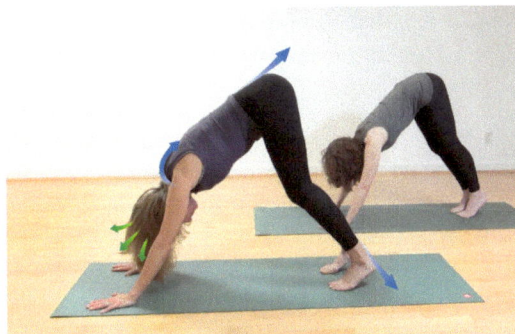

Figure 3.23E-2 Moving up

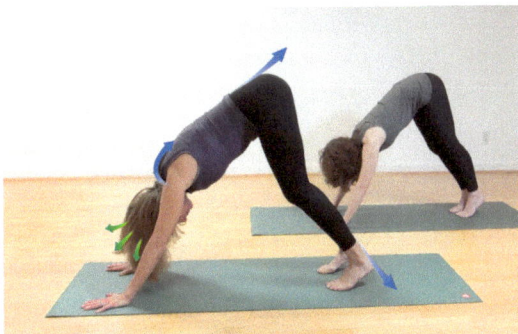

Figure 3.23E Begin in Downward Dog

- Rebound from sitting to standing up in Downward Dog with hands on floor.

- ▶ Play with standing up from sitting on each side with your spiraling, helical feet and rebound.

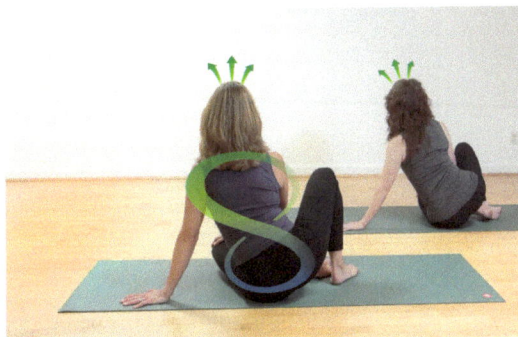

Figure 3.23E-3 Moving down

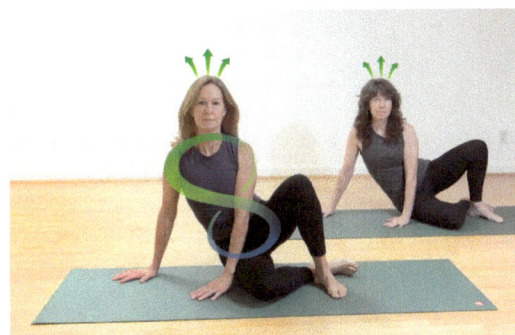

Figure 3.23E-1 Moving down

- Bend your knees and spiral down with your right hand support and release your right hip to the floor with bent knees.
- Play with this sit-to-stand spiraling movement 3–5 times in each direction.

- Starting position of Spiral Sitting on your left hip, bent knees, with your left hand on the floor, press into the floor with your left hand and spiral your hips up as you

THE INVITATION OF THE LIVING BRIDGE

This chapter shines a light on our most important function: the breath that breathes us. It invites you to consider breath as a living bridge of fluid relationships that spans the material and spiritual dimensions.

The practice of nasal breathing draws air into

your body, filling your lungs, enlivening your blood, and creating a deeper sense of presence through your fascial matrix body. Nasal breathing co-regulates your heart's support of your nervous system and leads to the establishment of a natural breathing pattern that further supports your body's ever-changing metabolic needs. At the same time, this natural breathing rhythm orients you to a relational patterning between gravity and spatial orientation that harnesses the mobius-like movement championed by researchers like Rohen and van der Wal. The elastic recoil of your natural breathing allows your conscious mind to sense the connection between the internal movement of breath and the relational connection of breath and the social and natural worlds in which you are embedded.

The essential activity facilitated through nasal breathing supported by the image of the living bridge is the co-regulation of the updated "new" view of your autonomic nervous system which, in turn, balances your heart rhythm and blood pressure through vagus nerve toning. Breath and blood flow together to massage your organs. Altogether, you center yourself this way. As the living bridge is connected to either side of a chasm through the root systems that have established themselves, your self is tethered to ground and sky, and this tethering provides a sense of centeredness. While the living bridge is sturdy and capable of holding weight, it is neither static nor immobile. The fluids in the capillaries of the roots collaborate with surrounding natural forces and allow the bridge to function in tandem with the surrounding world.

Once you orient with the living bridge of this breathing practice, many other practices are involved. Sound comes from breath vibrating your vocal cords. When you get comfortable with nasal breathing, you access the nitric oxide present in the nostrils. Nitric oxide dilates the blood vessels, thereby improving circulation and instituting a rhythmic breathing practice. In this way, you can begin to envision how conscious breath practices like these can mediate in your social world constructed through how we shape and express our sounding and speaking.

THE POWER OF SOUND

When I think of Stough's words, I also hear the words of my dear friend and mentor, Gael Rosewood, Advanced Rolfer and Continuum teacher. Many mentors have inspired me, and this quote about the deeply intrinsic value of sound sums up its value and importance to us at all levels of being:

> Sound has been used in many meditations over the centuries because it is one of the fastest ways to enrich an inner state of dynamic relaxation. [...] sound can be used as another form of movement as it helps us feel from the inside out as a sort of biofeedback to the system. We can feel the vibration of sound as it literally communicates through bone and tissue. When we become interested in the sensations and movement of sound, it has a way of organically opening and slowing breathing. As it goes with breath, so it goes with the nervous system. (Ohlgren and Litman 2008)

Sounding opened a primordial relationship between my pelvic diaphragm, respiratory diaphragm, and palate/throat. I was very silent as a child due to the fear I felt about my father's anger. Understanding the power of breath has been deeply nourishing and healing.

Sounds create "shapes" which support our shape-shifting body.

▸ To begin your practice, lie down on a soft mat. Then check in with your beginning baseline, where you sense breath in your body, the level of tension you may be holding on to, and what sensations or awarenesses show up before your practice, so you can see a comparison after your sounding and moving practice.

▸ There are so many sounds that are deeply resonant and create tissue change. Play with sounds that feel nourishing to you—for instance, the SSSSS sound can be a powerful fluid sound that creates internal lift for the pelvic diaphragm and domes of your body.

▸ Here, we will play with two sounds that Emilie Conrad introduced for lateral and midline support. Emilie felt that these two sounds (E and O) create a counterpoint for one another that decreases density and increases options.

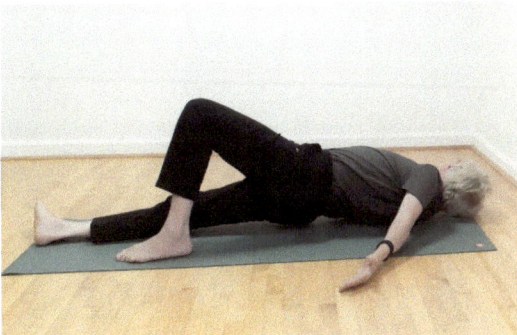

Figure 3.24A Exploring "E" sound

▸ "E" sounds create more of a lateral movement, like a smile.
  – You could explore rolling in a direction, pressing into the foot of your bent knee and rolling in the direction of your straight leg, sounding E-E-E, sensing your arms and legs responding to the vibratory resonance.
  – Upon completion of this phase of your practice, allow yourself to harvest the

benefits of what you have explored, which we call in Continuum "open attention"—this is where you have the opportunity to notice your intelligent body's response to your nourishing breath, sound, and movement. "Open attention acknowledges that the 'prime mover' is the innate intelligence of the organism, which when unencumbered will know exactly what to do" (Conrad 2007, p.336).

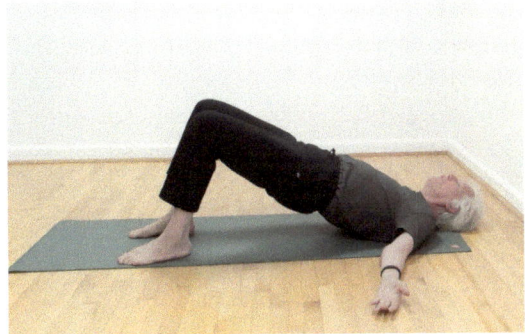

Figure 3.24B Exploring "O" sound

▸ When you are ready, move to exploring the "O" sound. "O" sound creates a tubular shape and can help to elongate or decompress an area of your body.

▸ You could explore a gentle midline curl between your head-to-tail, sounding "O-O-O" to support your midline curl as a wave-like motion.
  – Play with this wave motion and sounding, and notice where you can just allow your body to guide you, rather than forcing a movement.
  – Move to "open attention" and notice what you discover that might be new for you.

▸ This "E" and "O" sequence can be considered one round in your Continuum practice that would be a warm-up which would be ideally repeated two more times in order to optimize responsiveness. The second round opens your body to deeper explorations and is not the same body that began the exploration earlier. Breath, sound, and micromovement keep spiraling new information back into your shape-shifting organism, and your global body has the opportunity to become more informed, less dense, and increasingly receptive.

I have found that sounding or singing into areas of my body that are feeling distress through injury or illness can be a calming balm. What also becomes available is that in releasing tension, new opportunities come available that are unplanned, from my biointelligent body guiding me into adaptive movements that are deeply regenerative.

In the next chapter, I would like to explore with you how these activities need not equate to "doing things." Breathing as a living bridge transports you to a world of movement beyond doing.

Use the following QR code for all videos in this chapter:

REFERENCES

Beach, P. (2010) *Muscles and Meridians: The Manipulation of Shape*. Livingstone, NY: Churchill.

Conrad, E. (2007) *The Story of Continuum, the World-Renowned Self-Discovery and Movement Method*. Berkeley, CA: North Atlantic Books.

Douillard, J. (2018) *Body, Mind, and Sport: The Mind-Body Guide to Lifelong Health, Fitness, and Your Personal Best*. New York, NY: Harmony/Rodale.

Farhi, D. (1996) *The Breathing Book: Good Health and Vitality Through Essential Breath Work*. New York, NY: Holt Paperbacks.

Gintis, B. (2007) *Engaging the Movement of Life*. Berkeley, CA: North Atlantic Books.

Hunt, K. (2019) "India's Meghalaya 'living root bridges' get stronger as the trees grow." CNN. https://edition.cnn.com/style/article/living-bridges-india-scn/index.html

van der Kolk, B. (2015) *The Body Keeps the Score: Brain, Mind, and Body in the Healing of Trauma*. New York, NY: Penguin Books.

Litman, R. (2023) *The Breathable Body: Transforming Your World and Your Life, One Breath at a Time*. Carlsbad, CA: Hay House.

McKeown, P. (2015) *The Oxygen Advantage: Simple, Scientifically Proven Breathing Techniques to Help You Become Healthier, Slimmer, Faster, and Fitter*. New York, NY: William Morrow Paperbacks.

McKeown, P. (2021) *The Breathing Cure: Develop New Habits for a Healthier, Happier, and Longer Life*. New York, NY: Humanix Books.

Nestor, J. (2020) *Breath: The New Science of a Lost Art*. New York, NY: Riverhead Books.

Ohlgren, G. and Litman, R. (2008) "The Tao of Exercise and Self-Care." align.org. https://align.org/2008/01/02/exercise-breath

Ridley, C. (2006) *Stillness, Biodynamic Cranial Practice and the Evolution of Consciousness*. Berkeley, CA: North Atlantic Books.

Rothenberg, R. (2020) *Restoring Prana*. Philadelphia, PA: Singing Dragon.

Swami Rama, Ballentine, R., and Hymes, A. (2007) *The Science of Breath*. Honesdale, PA: Himalayan Institute Press.

Tracey, A. (2022) "Oxygen Advantage vs. Wim Hof: Is there a better way to breathe?" Bulldog Gear. https://bulldoggear.com/blogs/news/oxygen-advantage-vs-wim-hof-is-there-a-better-way-to-breathe?

Weil, A. (2006) "Breathing Basics: The How and the Why." Weil Nutrition Corner. www.drweil.com/health-wellness/body-mind-spirit/stress-anxiety/breathing-basics

Deep-Hearted Resources for Sounding and Singing

- Continuum Teachers Association: www.continuumteachers.com
- Susan Lincoln: www.susanlincoln.com/about-hilde-girls
- Jeremy Mossman: www.singingwithjmoss.com/bbvp
- Daniel Barber: www.danielbarber.com

CHAPTER 4

Movement Beyond Doing

In the previous chapters, we explored the importance of moving in resonance with our biointelligence, our awareness of bodies as deeply intelligent living processes, as beings that know innately how to self-heal, self-organize, and adapt. Doing this requires tuning into ourselves, sensing our internal vibrations and the ways we vibrate in resonance with our external environment. Advanced Rolf Structural Integration Practitioner Louis Schultz provides helpful language for understanding this tuning:

> When we talk about movement, we usually think of large gestures like walking, doing work, picking up the baby, washing the dishes, driving the car. Yet movement can be as subtle as slow breathing during sleep. A body never stops moving. Even the smallest movement creates a ripple throughout the entire organism. The tissue through which this ripple is transmitted is the connective tissue. When connective tissue is in tune, it is much like the cat gut on a properly tuned cello. It transmits movement. So, maybe we should say when we are properly "tuned," we hum to each person his or her characteristic tone. (Schultz and Feitis 1996, p.109)

This chapter looks at tuning, another way of doing, which is almost a non-doing. What I will call *movement beyond doing* unfolds from a recognition that there's a whole universe of movements that frequently go unacknowledged and are therefore undervalued. These are the subtle movements that we take for granted, but without which our dynamic selves would appear so much more rigid and constrained by binaries (such as right/wrong, healthy/sick). This chapter invites you to further develop an embodied personal practice through movement exploration to deepen awareness. I will explain how a deeper sense of movement beyond doing enlivens and transforms our teaching practice. This emphasis on "the teacher/practitioner" is important. I want to highlight the activity of listening in the studio or session space. This means listening to the Inner Guide, so we are tuning to the whole self of the person with whom we are collaborating.

Schultz's emphasis on subtle movement is important for attaining both of these goals because the category of "subtle" includes things like softening, internal orientation, interoceptive to exteroceptive awareness, noticing what is already happening that we don't have to "make happen." These and other awarenesses can be overlooked or ignored when we attempt to "do" exercise, "control" our breath, or "perfect" a posture. Achieving a deeper embodied personal practice requires learning to attend to these subtle movements. For this reason, both students and teachers of movement and bodywork are encouraged to increase their capacity to tune in to the subtle movements of themselves and others.

The ripple effect is equally important. For example, the action of softening the gaze requires subtle movements, one of which is the *pausing* of a certain activity—namely, you stop *staring* or *over-focusing* on something or someone in order to awaken to the perceptual field at the periphery of your vision. When you widen your gaze to peripheral vision, you directly experience and merge with spatial orientation, experiencing the act of looking, without labeling or objectifying. This perceptual shift orients you to sensing the two directions of your primordial midline through ground and space, and the living matrix of your fascial body's perineural nervous system, your *connective tissue consciousness*, which is responsible for wound healing and injury repair. This chapter looks at the fascial matrix. Our fascial matrix is like a musical instrument that is a network of pre-tension vibrating like a finely tuned instrument.

The fascial matrix:

informs cells and tissues of the movements, loads, compressions and tensions arising in different parts of the body. These signals join with those generated by other physiological processes, such as nervous signals, muscle potentials and sounds, and glandular secretory signals, to create a veritable symphony of oscillating electric fields that travel a certain distance through the living matrix. The cells and tissues then use this information to adjust their activities concerned with maintenance and nourishment. (Oschman 2003)

Once we understand movement beyond doing, it becomes possible to tap into that kind of awareness voluntarily. More than that, you begin to naturally include, on a conscious level, fascial matrix awareness in all of your movements.

Schultz refers to all of this activity—listening, open awareness, core coordination, and sensing into the fascial matrix—as tuning. This only tells part of the story. We certainly tune to ourselves by honoring our biointelligence, our ongoing dynamism that prepares us for life in the world. Beyond that, we also become tuned by the external environment and resonate *with* our external world. As I've discussed in previous chapters, our internal self is at all times in relationship with gravity, spatial orientation, and other external forces, as our body is a portal into presence that awakens us to our lived human experience. The bridge of the breath is a connective passage between our internal and external worlds, for example. When we breathe, we are also breathed, and thus our resonant inside and outside elemental body is tuned as we receive nourishment. At the same time, when we interact in harmony with other beings, we, in a sense, produce a chord sustained by our frequency and resonance. This is what Schultz, Emilie Conrad, and other somatic pioneers call our vibrational hum, in tune with the frequencies of the world within which we are embedded. *Tuning*, then, is something that happens internally and externally and also shows the ways in which our "selves" are always in contact with the outside world.

Tuning also names the way our fascial matrix channels the vibrations of our entire living architecture, as it surrounds, protects, and supports our bones, muscles, organs, blood vessels, nerves, and cells. Because our fascial matrix extends from the surface of our skin to the nucleus of every cell—essentially a porous membrane that connects the innermost and outermost parts of ourself—this living matrix is our body's internal communication web, and it exists from our earliest embryological beginnings. Without our fascial matrix, and its tensional-integrity relationship with the bioenergetics of our boney landscape, we would be unable to fold, unfold, rotate, sit, stand, walk, run, and move.

It is not possible to overstate the importance of listening and tuning through our fascial matrix, for it is this embodiment of ourselves that governs our quality of movement (especially as we age), our internal communication, our hydration, and our somatic consciousness. Later in this chapter, we will explore a few movements within our fascial matrix and its connection to our vibrational hum through familiar and novel explorations with an embodied lens. For now, it is important to emphasize that tuning ourselves means rediscovering our resonant relationship within the gravitational field through our spine's relationship between earth and sky, which reconnects us with whole-body breathing and peripheral vision, and increases vagal tone, our barometer of wellbeing.

For example, I hear a client say, "My back hurts." I tune to the tenor of those words, perhaps first by learning about which area of the back is holding the client's attention. I then tune into a wealth of unsaid information: what is the client's experience of walking—without judging, just witnessing and asking them to give feedback on what they notice as they sense their weight bearing into each foot, etc. The client can then settle into a collaborative session with me, noticing how or to what extent they are grounded/ungrounded; how they are relating to gravity in novel situations that are related to life skills, how they bend and extend their legs, in standing and walking, which can be a major problem in back pain. The client's sensorimotor awareness alters how they think about their back pain, through the body's language and experience. We inquire together into how their environmental set-up and habits at home, work, and play could be interfering with or limiting how they are using themselves, and we begin to unravel the context in which the back problem emerges.

Deep listening guides me to inquire with words and a gentle touch. Together, I listen through the movement evoked from the client's body wisdom. My main focus is supporting clients and mentoring teachers in remembering who they are through their body's innate blueprint of health. We all have habitual default patterns that can interfere with our biointelligence,

and we are constantly self-tuning and shaping ourselves.

The study of somatic, developmental, fascial matrix-informed awareness has contributed a powerful embodied lens to my mentoring of Pilates, yoga, and movement educators and bodyworkers of many disciplines. I have shifted my attention away from concerns of body image and attempts to gain control over posture and musculoskeletal movements. A somatic approach to movement and bodywork develops perceptual, kinesthetic, interoceptive, and proprioceptive awareness, with the vision of developing a sense of self that is empathetic and in relationship with all beings and the natural world.

What we eventually discover is that our ideal body is our *real body*. Through this lens, we give ourselves permission to step away from the emphasis on perfecting form and instead drop into an experience of sensation and support, from the body's perspective. This is a revolutionary approach of direct experience, in the moment, with your body's biointelligence directing how to move, so that movement is healing, empowering, and nourishing.

Scientist Mae-Wan Ho, who is best known for pioneering work on the physics of organisms and sustainable systems, affirms this by saying:

In the body nothing is in control, and yet everything is in control. Each part is as much in control as it is sensitive and responsive. Choreographer and dancer are one and the same. Global and local, whole and part, are indistinguishable. The living matrix network [i.e., the fascial matrix] is a molecular democracy of distributed control. More important than control is the source of the integration that gives rise to large-scale actions that are coordinated in a continuum from the macroscopic to the molecular. (Ho 1998, p.49)

Movement beyond doing requires dropping into

the meeting place between control and respon-siveness. It comes about once we stop trying to do movements perfectly and start listening to how our bodies respond to the forces that are shaping them. Once we find movement beyond doing so, we gain access to that "molecular democracy of distributed control." The challenge here is to tune to this democratic distribution consciously.

This embodied practice draws from the lessons of the body. The molecular democracy of distributed control expressed through the fascial matrix is an exemplary fluid dynamic that we can replicate in private sessions and group space. Here the practitioner learns from the student just as much as the student learns from the practitioner. Our bodies act with gravity and spatial orientation. The fluid field of gravitational forces acts through and extends our body's perceptual field. We would not ever undertake an exercise or movement exploration without considering the gravitational field and its relational effects. I never instruct students to control their abdomen to complete a movement sequence, which would be like driving a car with the parking brake on. I invite an exploration of Core as Relationship in order to help students and mentoring teachers/ practitioners to investigate the integrated relationships from foot to head and hand, which are awakened when the abdominals relate through movement, breath, and sound to our primordial midline. The Inner Guide, a major component of all movement and bodywork, is about *remembering*. Our bodies know how to self-heal, self-regulate, and adapt. When we compete with ourselves or strive to fix people, we can create unnecessary body tension and put our own body on hold, thereby interfering with our ability to serve. I often ask teachers to consider two life-altering questions: What is just enough effort for the movement? What can I let go of that I don't need to be doing? These questions bring us back around to the main focus of this chapter: movement beyond doing.

DEEPENING OUR SENSE OF MOVEMENT BEYOND DOING

When we try to complete a specific movement or initiate a sequence of movements, we may try to do it the *right way*. Doing often refers to the world of performance, achievement, effort, and hard work, and usually entails strain. There are times when doing is appropriate, such as taking action when someone is injured, or catching a flight on time. What is important to note is that in being overly focused on the end point of goals, we often give our health and wellbeing over to an outside entity and wait to be told what to do. By contrast, movement beyond doing is grounded in the world of orientation. This is a pre-verbal response directed by our fluid body which evolves prior to our nervous system. We discover where we are as babies, for example, by exploring our surroundings with peripheral vision, which develops prior to our central focus.

In other words, *who we are* is always linked to *where we are*. As adults, we can tap back into that early fluid knowledge by reawakening the ability to orient ourselves. Allowing ourselves to receive the various stimuli in our environment fosters a sense of curiosity, discovery, and groundedness. From that grounded and curious place, we move with ease and wonder what movement is occurring before we actively move. What is being called forth, even in apparent stillness? In what concert are we playing, even if we seem to be engaging in a task alone? How can our movements become responses to the other movements taking place within, around, and through us? The question ceases to be "How do we do this thing or achieve this goal?" and becomes "What might be interfering that I can become aware of and shift my perception which shifts my motor responses?"

Hubert Godard's notion of "pre-movement" drops us into this realm of movement beyond doing. Pre-movement is a perceptual shift that begins with questions. What is preparation for movement? What is it to consider that we move before we move and that the body prepares to do a movement by orienting itself? Before we execute a specific action, what happens when we connect to our location in the world? By sensing our relationship within the earth and the space around us, which softens our gaze, what information, nourishment, and energy do I find here? What is this way of being with myself that allows for a softening into and deeper presence within any given exploration? Is it possible that this way of being, this tuning, encourages a healing, relational response even before an action takes place?

With those questions in mind, try this:

▸ Stand to one side of a room and look across the room to a wall or a window.

▸ Select a point on which to focus your gaze.

▸ Walk across the room toward that point on which you are focused.

▸ As you walk, attend to your body. What do you notice in terms of tension in your eyes, jaw, tongue, throat, solar plexus, etc., that you might be holding? Also notice the force of your steps and the location of your center of gravity.

▸ When you reach the point of focus across the room, stop and see what sensations are present in your body.

Pause and now return to the place you first started. This time, let's explore the concept of pre-movement.

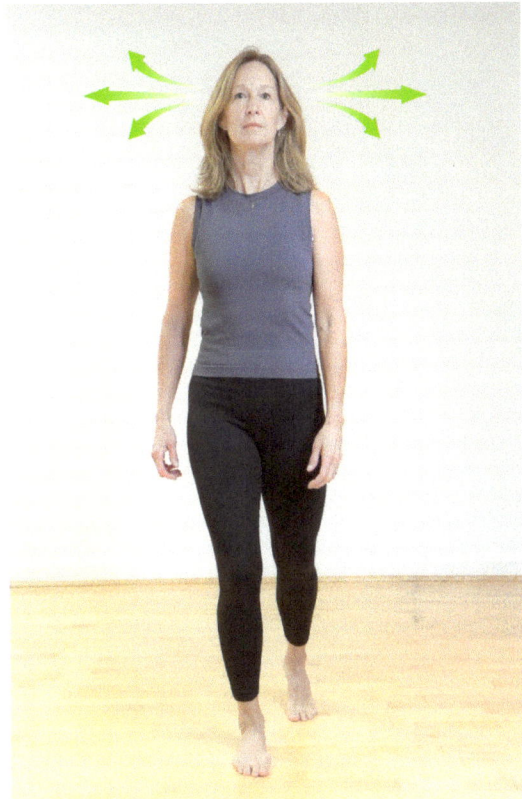

Figure 4.1 Peripheral vision

▸ As you look toward your point of focus, soften your gaze in order to awaken your relationship with the entire space of the room. In other words, as you gaze forward, can you also sense shapes, colors, etc. in your peripheral vision?

▸ Tune in to the relationship between your softening gaze and your jaw, tongue, throat, solar plexus, which can also soften. Now include your tail. Notice the fluid field of gravity's role in your tail's release, which allows your head to float and your feet to become more supportive of your whole body.

▸ Sense your feet. Feel into every part of your feet on the ground.

▸ Begin a subtle weight shift between your right and left foot. Acknowledge the fluidity of this movement, the way in which you can pour your weight from one foot into the other, supporting your gently swaying body.

▸ Eventually, take a step. To do so, come off the back foot and pour your weight into the front foot. Continue this pouring from foot to foot, as you sense walking.

▸ Walk with your soft focus, a sense of spaciousness and grounding. Walk in relationship with the space, including a point of focus.

▸ When you reach the other side of the room, stop. Pause. Notice what perceptual shift in awareness has awakened with this walking.

Think about the focus of your walking. We walk *in order to* get somewhere. However, a perceptual shift is a type of movement that we can drop into while walking through a forest or on the seashore, walking with a sense of presence. I find myself caught up in the first walking often, rushing somewhere, and my body wisdom wakes me up—"Wendy, you're doing it"—which shifts my awareness, slows me down, calms my breath, helps me to sense my feet and become more present while I am walking. The purpose of juxtaposing these two kinds of walking is not simply to exchange the first for the second. Rather, the exploration helps us bring attention to an automatic way of being, which creates more stress and strain. Remember that reuniting with connective tissue consciousness is your body-centered fascial matrix, and is a portal to presence. F.M. Alexander (the Alexander Technique) framed what I'm calling "movement-as-doing" as a function of unconscious habit. He discovered that his loss of voice as an actor was due to the closing of his throat caused by tension resulting from pulling his head back while efforting as

he spoke. By trying to speak as he thought he should (i.e., loudly), he ended up losing his voice. By reappraising his orientation through his feet (standing) and sitting bones (sitting), in relationship with the position of his head, he eventually discovered movement of ease that alleviated inappropriate tension, which changed his habitual perception of movement (and acting), and he found a new way of being as an actor and teacher.

Hubert Godard spoke to this shift in perception when he said, "A problem in movement may not be the result of faulty motor function, but of faulty perception" (Newton 1995, p.38).

STORY: A deep memory for me in studying with Hubert Godard was one of several weeklong immersions I attended in Canada on pre-movement and perceptual awareness. Following a movement exploration, we all walked around the room, sensing our peripheral vision. As Hubert walked toward me, his gaze and kinesthetic resonance was so softly focused and gentle that I felt held in the spatial awareness of his presence. His presence was receptive, and this receptivity was a direct result of his work with pre-movement. This experience changed my perception of myself, enabling me to create and hold space for others through my teaching. This sense memory remains with me to this day.

The "pre-movement" emphasized in walking consists of specific elements. We *locate* ourselves within a space, allowing for the possibility of 360-degree vision. Sensing through the side and back body helps to reduce visual tension from holding an erect posture with external muscular tension. Transferring energy from the abdomen to a peripheral, full-body gaze and connecting to ground through tail and feet releases tension, which, in turn, shifts our orientation to our intrinsic, gravity-based midline and fascial matrix. Releasing energy from external muscular holding and reorienting it into our fascial matrix midline support evokes our body's energetic Central Channel, giving a sense of coming home to ourselves. Through this homecoming, we connect with our ventral vagus nerve, or "soul nerve," which links breathing with vocalization and eye contact, based on signals from our intuitive gut microbiome.

Walking is not a simple action but a way we recalibrate our relationship with ourselves and our environment. Emphasizing the fluid nature of weight transfer in walking acknowledges that our internal systems are always moving and sharing spatial load within the gravitational field.

Pre-movement is the activation of our context for embodied movement in relationship with the world. We are in the space and the space is in us; we cannot know ourselves until we locate ourselves within the spatial context. Pre-movement is the foundation for movement beyond doing.

OUR RELATIONSHIP BETWEEN EARTH AND SKY

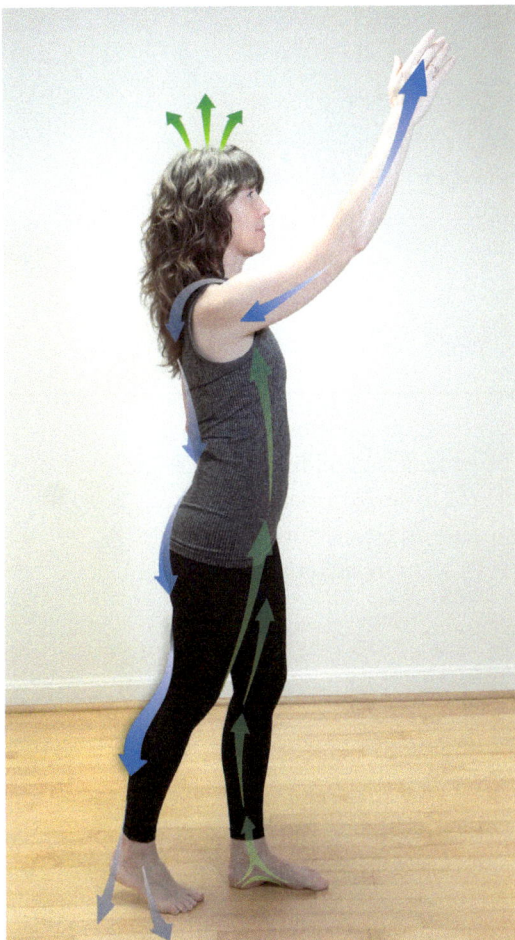

Figure 4.2 Lifting of arm and grounding of soleus

Hubert Godard calls this context activation *tonic*

function. This is the unconscious organization of tone in the body, expressed through our coherent relationship with earth and sky. We are oriented to either earth (grounding) or sky (spatial orientation), deeply conditioned by our earliest experiences of being held and touched, and by the landscapes (both natural and cultural) in which we find ourselves.

The word *tonic* connects to the intrinsic muscular support of our primordial midline structure and function. The fascial matrix that weaves through the intrinsic tonic muscles of your midline supports their ability to contract and release appropriately. Tonic function, ultimately, is our orientation, and that orientation (to grounding and spatial orientation) is pre-movement, which creates a free head and neck. To help you zoom in on an example of tonic function and pre-movement in action, consider this. As you lift your arm while standing, what muscle do you think activates first? Most people would say a shoulder muscle like the deltoid. In actuality, however, it is the soleus, the deepest of the calf muscles, which is in relationship with initiatory contractions in the muscles around your ankle joints. Awareness of the grounding pre-movement that supports the lifting of the arm awakens our sense of that midline tonic function, which, once awakened, helps expand our perception of a simple arm raise. When we raise our arm, the soleus responds to our relationship with gravity and spatial orientation, and that awareness evokes our grounding, extension, and reach. Remember that, as infants, we oriented in sitting prior to standing, so yielding to reach is an archetypal pattern that shapes the organization of our upper body and the position of the legs, and the positioning of our legs and pelvis is strongly influenced by the weight and position of the upper body. Consciously engaging with pre-movement throughout our lives helps us discover freer, more natural movements. Through this engagement, we access deeper strength, which leads us to become more receptive, compassionate, resilient, and adaptive.

A PERCEPTUAL WAY OF BEING IN THE WORLD

At stake here is the issue of a way of being in the world. As babies, we engage in primary developmental movements such as yielding, pushing, reaching, grasping, and pulling, developing our perceptual awareness. This foundational way of being supports our muscular suppleness and strength through gliding, spiralic movements. We develop ways of responding to and being strengthened by life's stressors through a broader movement palette that supports our behavior. By exploring our tensional-compression continuity within the fascial matrix and pre-movement through yielding as we play with gravity and spatial orientation, we learn to move with ease.

As babies, we are all born with flat feet. Through our gestural, spiralic movement patterning and appropriate tension and compression practiced on the floor through crawling, and then moving from sitting to standing and then walking, we develop the dynamic foundations of our fascial feet over our growing years. These foundations lead to the development of the primary and secondary curves of our fluid spine and our ability to come upright. The key to a dynamic, structural, and functional body is well-sprung arches developed through balanced tension and compression.

The way you inhabit your fascial feet through adolescence and adulthood is crucial to your whole-body development. It can serve to keep you connected to your innate biointelligence, which supports your ability to self-heal, self-regulate, and adapt.

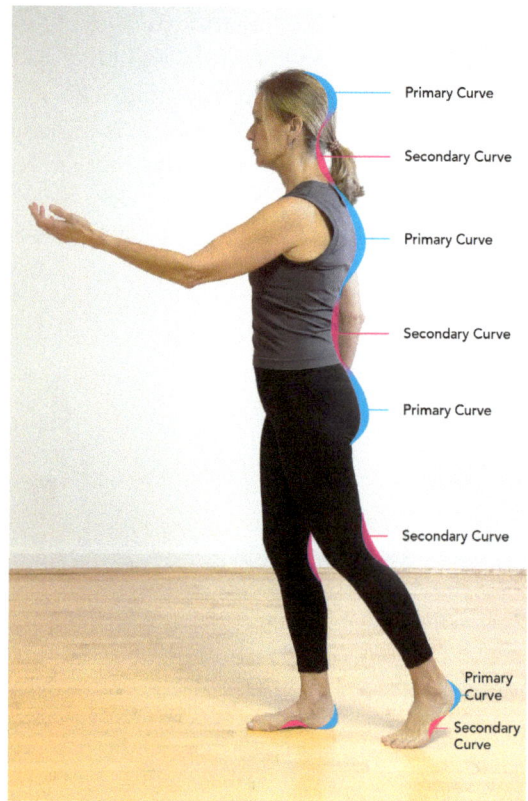

Figure 4.3 Primary and secondary curves of spine

Our fascial feet are proprioceptive organs through which the brain senses and maps the body. They form the foundation for the body's Domes of Uplift (inner ankles, pelvic diaphragm, respiratory diaphragm, thoracic inlet, palate/occiput, and cranium) and serve as the "true fulcrum or axis of your human body" (Sharkey 2021a). Conscious awareness of the interaction between these domes activates and enables uplift. Additionally, fascial feet facilitate a spiralic myo-fascial connection from the feet to the tongue. The health of the fascial feet is vital for the over-all dynamic health of the organism. Walking on uneven ground or rocky surfaces enhances pro-prioception. The fascial feet absorb knowledge from stress and transform it into growth.

As adults revisiting developmental, psycho-social, and fascial matrix-informed explorations, our bodies recall the knowledge of pre-move-ment, movement beyond doing, and effort with ease. As babies, learning to use both sides of our bodies develops communication between both brain hemispheres, transforming reflexive movements into integrated, graceful sequences. We also learn balance through vestibular aware-ness, detecting gravity and acceleration through our eyes and the three semicircular canals in our inner ears that lie on three axes: up and down, left and right, and forward and back (Blakeslee and Blakeslee 2007). This process enables us to progress from rolling to crawling, sitting, and standing, riding the wave of our emerging foot arches to whole-body core coordination.

> By much vigorous kicking and crying during the first months of its life, the baby develops those muscles which are needed to produce and stabilize the lumbar curve into its convex direction toward the front, to counteract the primary concavity of the thoracic curve. Not until this curve has been established is the baby able to hold its head up, to sit or stand alone... this lets me know that the cervical and lumbar curves, and thus the ability for self-support later on, come in response to the individual's own assertion of self as s/he makes desires or wants known in the world. (Todd 1991 [1943], p.94)

Developmental, Psychosocial Movements: Yielding to Gravity, Pushing to Reach; Rolling, Sitting, Standing

Grounding, centering, and uplift are ways that the body comes alive. The yield of the tail and feet and the reach of the head and hands cre-ate a new becoming. It is only later, through the trials of growing up, long-term sitting and screen watching, and socially informed disciplin-ing of our bodies, that this type of oneness with pre-movement and movement beyond doing becomes foreign to our natural selves. All of that knowledge is still embedded, and we can access it through simple movement explorations that communicate with the language of our bodies. **See Video 4.4 for full exploration.**

PRE-MOVEMENT IN PRACTICE

The next portion of this chapter is designed to help you raise conscious awareness of pre-movement through simple explorations and activities. I reg-ularly use all of these explorations in my personal practice. They evoke the living, emergent qualities of our movements. It isn't something to do; rather, it is a realm of awareness that helps us be present with our natural movement in relationship with the fluid intelligence of the natural world. This is *effort with ease*. All of these practices are grounded in accessing your primordial midline tonic func-tion's mobility and responsiveness through the *yield that underlies reach* within your breathing spine's relationship between earth and sky. This approach brings pre-movement into focus. "Yield that evokes reach" are fluid, ongoing mindfulness activities that support our embodied movements from foot to head and hand. This pre-movement makes possible a whole new world of movement. Activating awareness of this pre-movement and the possibilities of movement beyond doing cul-tivates a renewed attention to our innate postural tone. Frequently, we either collapse or artificially prop ourselves up. We collapse when we lose our uprightness by hunching forward—for example, when looking at a cell phone. We prop ourselves up by sitting or standing up with too much tension in our back, neck, shoulders, and knees, as if to show that we have "good" posture. Orientation within the gravitational field engages your body's innate awareness of tonic function through your spine's relationship between earth and sky, activating your body's fascial matrix that supports and embeds a deeper sense of whole-body movement, with core coordination and cultivating movement with ease.

To feel these ideas in action, let's re-experience the arm raise from above. This is a favorite partner exploration in my workshops and mentoring that is based on a traditional Aikido experiment known as the Unbendable Arm.

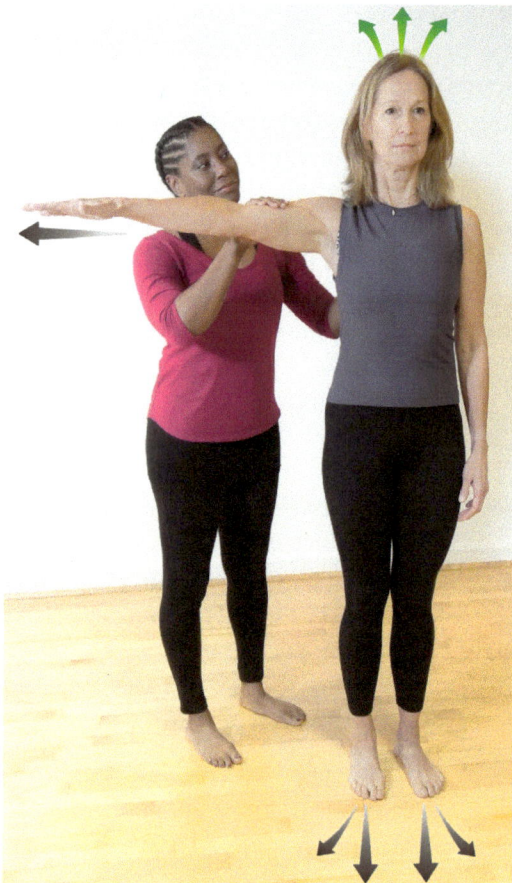

Figure 4.5 Unbendable Arm

With a partner, let's compare and contrast two types of arm raise. Choose one person to be A and the other to be B. In the first exploration, you will be sensing an energetic fascial matrix lift of your arm. In the second exploration you are lifting your arm through muscular scapular stabilization. **See Video 4.5 for full exploration.**

What you have just experienced is pre-movement through a perceptual shift in your relationship between earth and sky supporting the continuity of your fascial matrix in action. While it may seem that this partner activity is about arm raising, it is actually about something much richer. The sensory relationship between earth and sky of your "breathing spine" is a perceptual event which profoundly affects your motor patterns. "This example demonstrates, among other things, a phenomenon that we intuit: that perception is an action. Perception is a form of intentionality, a movement in a direction. To say it another way our perceptual state affects our motor patterns" (Newton 1995).

The arm-raising exploration is an extension of your body's fascial matrix in action, which is itself a manifestation of a deep process of nourishment that is key to your vital wellbeing. To focus on arm raising is to focus on your body's "doing." To soften into an awareness of the deep nourishment that comes from being supported by your pre-movement between earth and sky and the whole-body gestural support which lifts your arm is to enter the realm of *movement beyond doing*.

I have come to call this biointelligent, multi-dimensional, fluid approach to movement *movement as bodywork.*

Let's sense pre-movement again through the two directions of earth and sky. We will begin with a conversation between your inner ear/occiput, sacrum, and soft ankles/feet, as the mobility and responsiveness of your primordial midline through the support of pre-movement will be a good indicator of your body's ability to receive and adjust to new information, especially as you play with additional weight to increase gravity's support on your ankles, wrists, shoulders, or head. **See Video 4.6 for full exploration**.

so I added another 10lb sandbag to each shoulder. He became slightly interested, so I added another 10lb sandbag to each shoulder, so he now had 30lb on each shoulder. He smiled broadly and said, "Wow, my head just lengthened up—I feel great!"

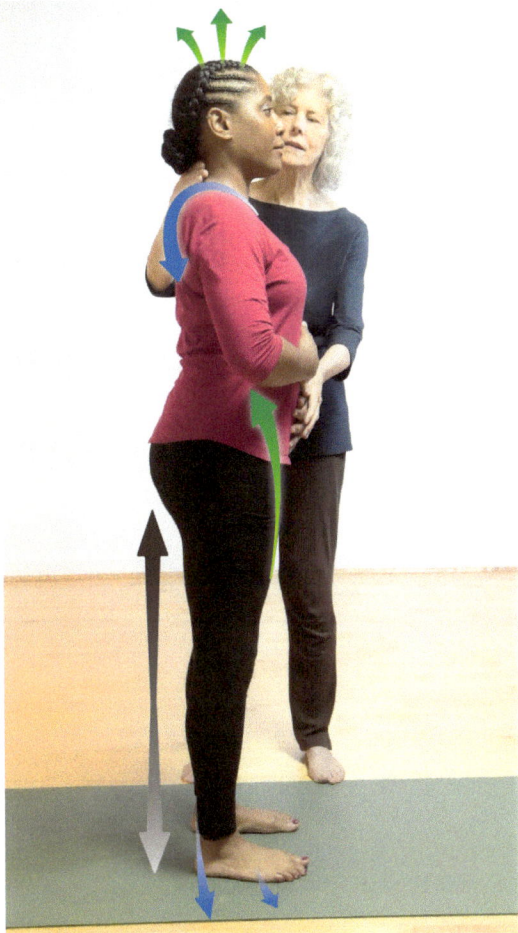

Figure 4.6 Pre-movement through the two directions of earth and sky

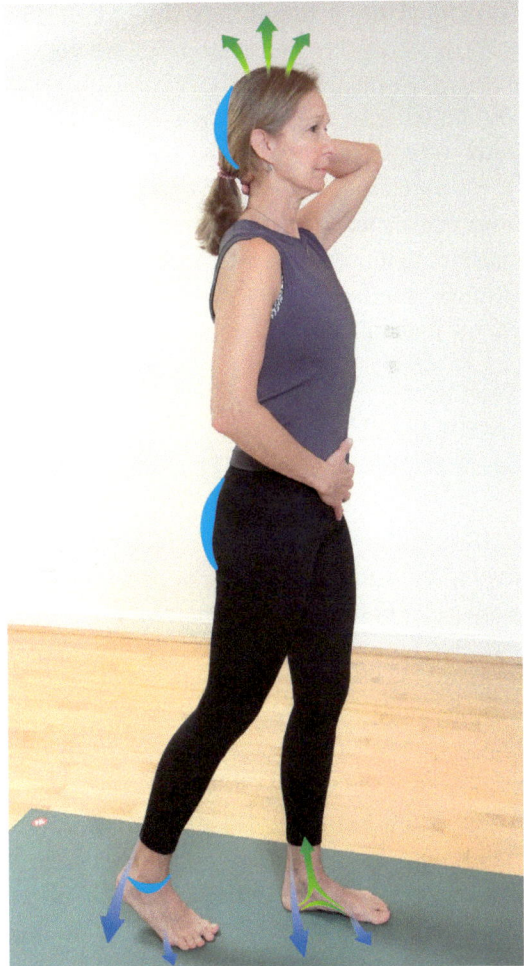

Figure 4.7 Occiput/sacrum/talus fluidic connection

STORY: A client was referred to me by a doctor following a surgery. He was used to lifting heavy weights as a workout. He was having difficulty releasing his shoulder tension, so I put a 10lb sandbag on each of his shoulders as he was standing. There was no real response,

Your sacrum has "weight" in standing, and your ischial tuberosities have "weight" in sitting, acting as counterweights to your head and pelvic diaphragm moving freely and finding uplift.

Relationship with a weighted sacrum evokes uplift through the front of your body from inner ankle to inner ear. Your tonic midline support engages as soon as there is a sensation of weight, provided that this sensation is not inhibited by excess tension. Holding *what is just enough* weight in your hands, or using a sense of weightedness on your ankles, wrists, head, shoulders, abdomen, etc., awakens a sense of grounding and uplift from inner ankle to inner ear and hand. This sensory, tonic function awareness can also be achieved through using sensory feedback props like Stretch-eze® and Tye4 whole-body bands, as you can see in Chapter 6.

In the embodied approach to movement and bodywork, your elbows and knees are "kinetic centers" that can amplify or inhibit movement through your hands and feet. As you move from center to periphery or periphery to center, they act as centers of communication through the portals of your feet and hands, from your midline to your environment and back again.

As Structural Integration bodywork pioneer Ida Rolf is attributed as saying: "When the body gets working appropriately, the force of gravity can flow through...then spontaneously, the body heals itself." In becoming a Structural Integration practitioner, what I experienced that she was referring to by that statement is that in whole-body movement, the shoulder and pelvic girdle become fully integrated into enlivened fascial matrix awareness from foot to head and hand. Inspired by this visionary perspective, we see "gravity as the therapist" and approach movement as an evolving, emerging conversation.

MOVEMENT EXPLORATIONS OF PRE-MOVEMENT AND MOVEMENT BEYOND DOING

A non-embodied, or even dis-embodied, approach to movement and bodywork treats people as a *thing to fix*. To mold the body to an idealized notion is to overlook the living process of the whole person.

There is a fundamental shift from seeing people as "broken" and needing to be fixed to being in collaboration with a client who is listening for guidance from their innate biointelligence to see what is needed. We are shifting from a judgmental position of right/wrong, to a collaborative relationship of noticing what is working and what is missing that we can provide.

Everything that follows is offered as a way to sense the embodied concept. To prepare for these movement explorations, we will deepen a foundational relationship within the gravitational field. We will call it Down the Back and Up the Front.

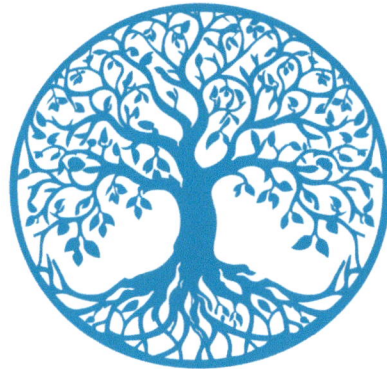

Figure 4.8 Celtic Tree of Life
GRATITUDE TO OMNITELIK

The Celtic Tree of Life symbolizes the axis mundi of the earth's center pole, uniting earth and sky. It is also a symbol of our primordial midline. This ancient image is a blueprint that helps us remember ourselves, restoring our connection to our living environment.

Down the Back (DTB) and Up the Front (UTF) are sensory images derived from first-person awareness of gravity and ground reaction force (GRF) which represent the embryonic, organizational intelligence of our midline's relationship between earth and sky. Just as the downward and upward energies of the tree roots and trunk produce the expansive, globe-like shape of the whole tree, the interplay of DTB and UTF produces an expansiveness through your spine's relationship with earth and sky and the gestural patterning of your peripheral limbs.

The flow between one's external and internal world is essentially seamless. It is the breath moving between our inhalation and exhalation. It is the movement between impression and expression, between "being" and "doing." It is an inquiry into the common-unity. It is a willingness to cultivate both an understanding and perception of the wholeness that lies beneath the surface of the illusion of separate individual parts. Whether we are speaking of a central core and midline, or spiraling flows of the torus resonating through the vastness, our moving, sensing, breathing bodies are in-formed and imprinted by the iterative patterns of vibratory intelligence which we call the geometric-energetic taxonomy. (Agneessens 2013)

The sensory image of DTB begins with a softening and widening of the clavicles that evokes a feeling of water falling Down the Back, toward your feet, and then circling the body to flow Up the Front from inner ankle to inner ear. The whole cycle is attuned to your body's pre-movement in relationship with the gravitational field.

The Fluid Interconnectedness of Down the Back and Up the Front

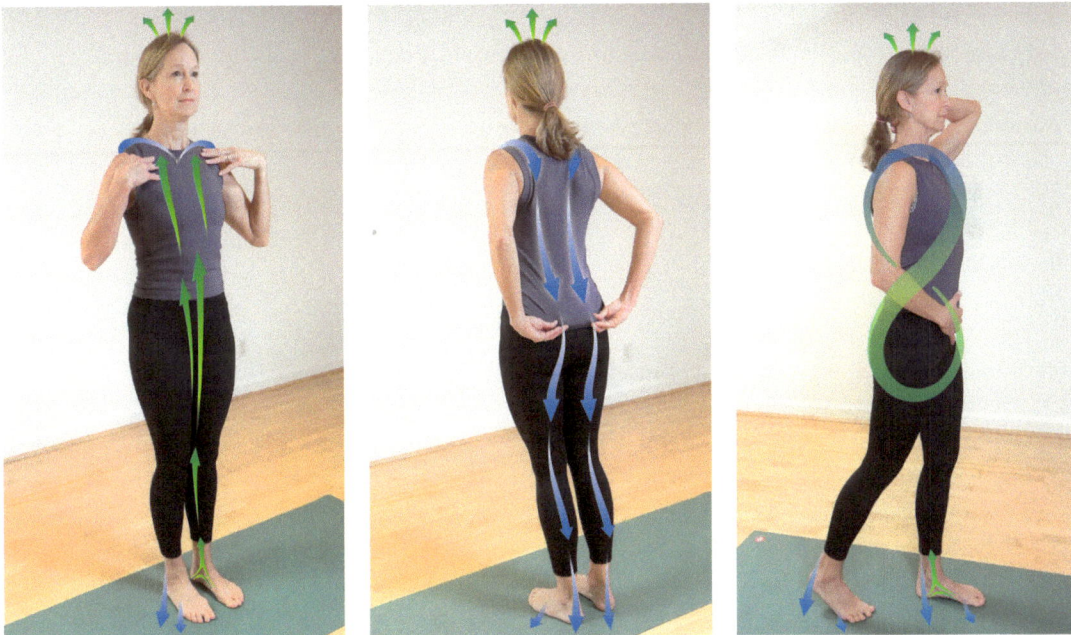

Figures 4.9A, 4.9B, and 4.9C Sensing with hands—your felt sense of Down the Back/Up the Front

Preparation for exploring DTB and UTF:

▸ Come to standing and place your hands on the top of your sternum, at your manubrium, where your shoulder girdle attaches to your rib basket.

▸ Notice that if your manubrium drops down, your shoulders and head will curl forward.

When this happens, you lose the feeling of water falling Down the Back. By activating and keeping active the DTB/UTF cycle, you continually sense your grounding and pre-movement yield to gravity, and find how to back yourself. As I mentioned in Chapter 1, "backing" refers to our embryonic backing into the womb and our ability to have our own back. Utilizing this imagery as an adult allows us to re-experience this embryonic self-organizing activity and sensation. For movement and bodywork educators, it's important to remember that we need to have our own backing before we can have someone else's back. **See Video 4.9 for full exploration**.

Down the Back—Compression Forces of Waterfall

▸ Standing up and starting from your manubrium, begin to trace your clavicles so you have a sense of them softening and widening, and trace over your shoulders to sense how that allows your shoulder blades to glide Down the Back.

▸ Pull your shirt down the back and imagine water rolling down your gliding shoulder blades along each side of your spine and back to your sitting bones and tailbone.

▸ Can you allow your front lower ribs and

xiphoid (end of sternum) to soften and not push or overarch forward?

▸ The waterfall continues down the backs of your legs to your feet, specifically the helical connections of the ball of the big toe, the ball of the little toe, and the inner and outer heel.

Up the Front—Tensile/Suspension Forces—Domes of Uplift

▸ UTF is generated/evoked from the internal lift starting with your inner ankles.

▸ Moving your hands along your midline, imagine an uplift from your inner ankles.

▸ Continue tracing up your inner legs, where your adductors innervate with your hamstrings* to connect to the front of your pelvic diaphragm—back of the leg to the front of the spine.

▸ Imagine each side of your low spine finding uplift (pull up your waistband to sense your low belly suspenders), along each side of your mid and upper spine, through your respiratory diaphragm and thoracic inlet (widening clavicles and open armpits), and continuing all the way up through to your inner ears, palate, and cranium.

---

* Remember the embryonic helical internal movement of hamstrings spiraling from front to back of leg, where they connect fascially through the inner thigh and front of the pelvic diaphragm to the front of the spine.

Like the Celtic Tree, we are omnidirectional beings, orienting within the gravitational field. Finding your grounding and backing by sensing the waterfall DTB with breath evokes the internal lift of the "low belly suspenders" UTF, which in our embodied approach we call "shoulder blades to internal belly" (SBIB)—a felt sense of your elastic recoil fascial matrix breath support. For Pilates practitioners, this awareness provides an embodied approach to what is often referred to as the *Pilates Powerhouse*. **See Video 4.10A to deepen exploration. See Video 4.10B to explore the elastic recoil fascial matrix breath on the Pilates Cadillac with Push Thru Bar and Guide as partner**.

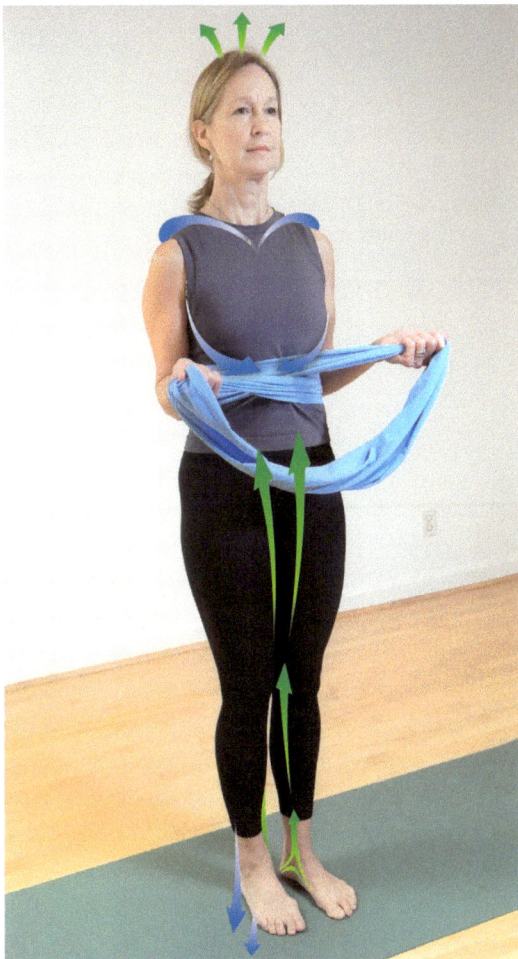

Figure 4.10 Elastic recoil fascial matrix breath

If you feel like nothing is happening or you aren't "doing something," that's the point. There is a non-action linked to movement beyond doing

and supported by pre-movement taking place within the fascial matrix. You are allowing your body and breath to respond naturally to your exhale and inhale. You are seeking to sense the subtle movements taking place, without interfering with excessive muscular tension.

Additionally, the language and orienting intelligence of DTB and UTF help you sense your body's metabolic need in any activity through relationship with your shape-shifting, elastic fascial matrix breath. Sensing this need helps you to avoid overriding your body's capacity (e.g., "over-stretching or over-stabilizing"—forcing a movement) and, instead, to honor your interoceptive awareness of an ongoing conversation with your body's core connections.

As you explore the following awareness-enhancing movements in this chapter, there will be suggestions to notice embodied distinctions which will deepen your kinesthetic awareness and ability to respond to your body's needs. For instance, as we explore our spiralic nature through movement, we are reminded by osteopath Phillip Beach that

mammalian limbs are seen as power amplifiers of helical biodynamics: the upper limbs amplify the body's ability to twist the torso from the suboccipital complex to the waist, whereas the lower limbs empower the caudal body to twist from the pelvic floor up. (Beach 2010, p.15)

- Freedom for your head, neck, shoulders, and upper spine.

- Embodied organization for all Upper Core movements.

- Remember that arms and legs amplify (increase) or inhibit (decrease) movement potential.

- Notice that your arms move from your

kinetic center of your elbows in two directions:

– your upper arms root through your shoulder girdle to your Breathing Spine and your sacrum (Down the Back).

• **See Video 4.11 for deeper exploration**.

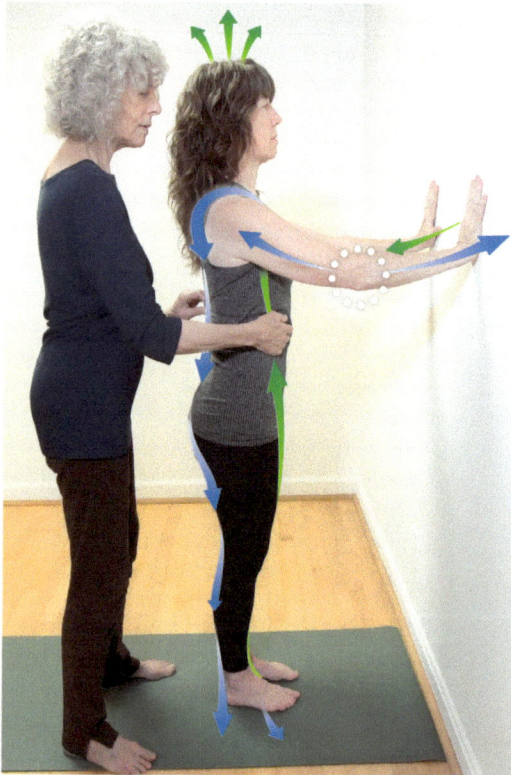

Figure 4.11 Rooting and reaching of arms from kinetic centers at elbows

If standing and reaching to the wall front or side bothers your shoulder, you can also lie on the floor on your back, with bent knees, with a rock or small weight in each hand that is reaching toward the ceiling—then soften and straighten your arms from a heavy shoulder blade and notice how your elbows can be soft and your hands can reach (going away from you), as your upper arms can root toward your shoulder blade, spine, sacrum, and feet (connecting with yourself).

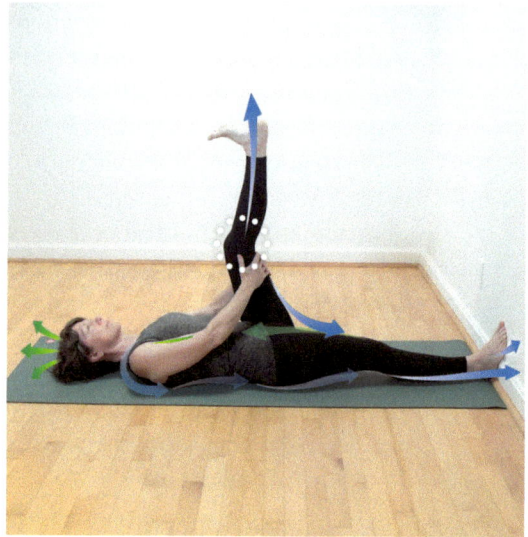

Figure 4.12 Rooting and reaching of legs from kinetic centers at knees—freedom for your feet, ankles, hips, sacrum, low back, and mid-spine

• Embodied organization for all Lower Core movements.

• Remember that arms and legs amplify (increase) or inhibit (decrease) movement potential.

• Notice that your upper thigh moves from your kinetic centers at your knees in two directions:

– Your upper thigh roots from the spiral of your hamstrings innervating *through* the front of your pelvic diaphragm to the crura/roots of your diaphragm and Breathing Spine to your inner ear (Up the Front).

• Notice set-up for Pilates Leg Circles at wall—with Rooting (upper leg to breathing spine) and Reaching (lower leg and foot to wall or space around you).

• **See Video 4.12 for deeper exploration**.

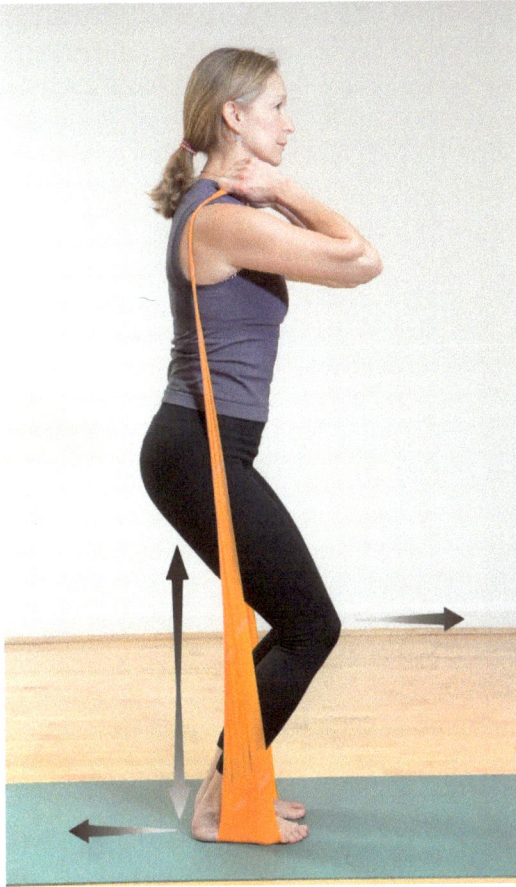

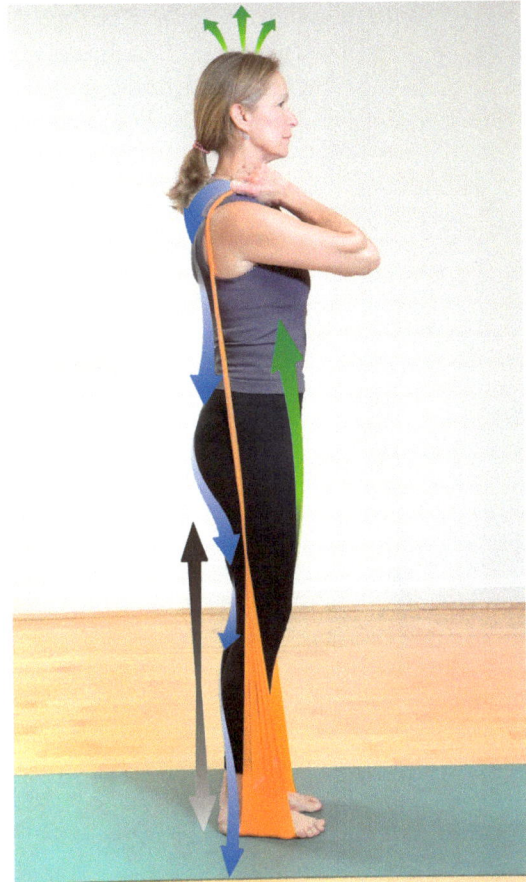

Figures 4.13A and 4.13B Sitting bones to heels connection

- Notice that your body *knows* an innate relationship between your sitting bones and heels.

  - This fascial matrix awareness—same side or opposite sitting bone to opposite heel—creates a spring-like awareness in how you soften and straighten your ankles, knees, and hip coordination to your breathing spine in standing, sitting, walking, running, etc.

  - Standing up, can you straighten your knees, without hyperextending, and notice a felt sense connection with your feet? Isn't it interesting that you

don't fall down as you soften your knees? There is a spring-like action happening throughout your fascial matrix body that supports softening and straightening your legs.

DTB and UTF are embodied connections, where your innate relationship between earth and sky supports information coming in through your lower hindbrain to support frontal lobe insights.

As Bonnie Bainbridge Cohen shares, "When we open the back of the brain to receive new information and allow it to absorb forward to the front of the brain, we can expand our ability to organize and make choices that lead to new behavior" (Bainbridge Cohen 2023).

Body intelligence is thus evoked from sensory

receptivity in the extremities and vectors of directionality through hands, feet, head, and tail. As Kevin Frank and Caryn McHose share: "To bring alive the experience of one's hands and feet creates integration as hand contact and foot contact is linked to eccentric movement in the spine" (Frank and McHose 2020, pp.8–10).

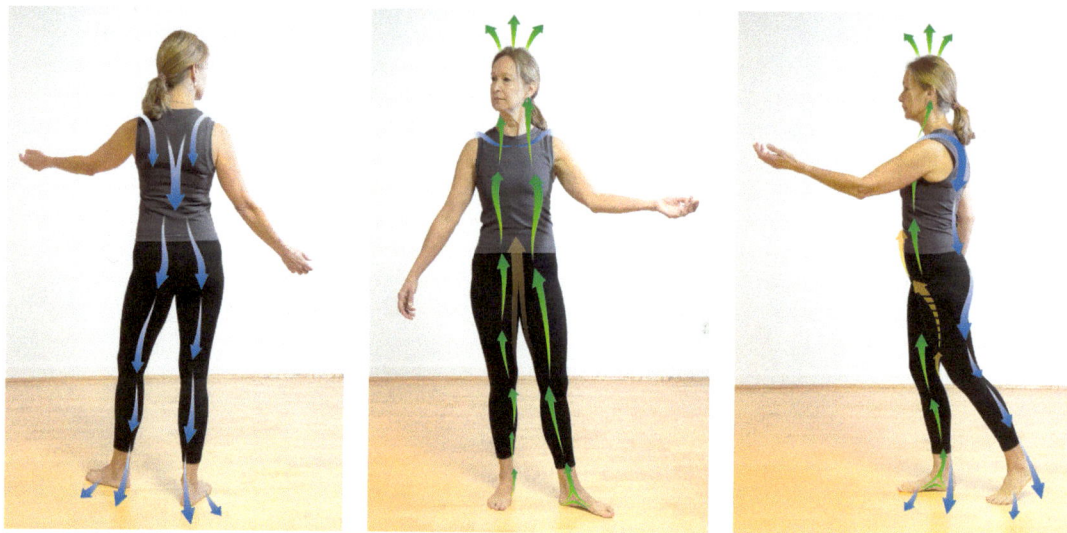

Figures 4.14A, 4.14B, and 4.14C Down the Back and Up the Front—how grounding evokes uplift

Notice that as you explore the following novel fascial matrix-informed movements, you are sensing how your body is a shape-shifting, fluid emergent field, curling, arching, spiraling in response to sensory feedback. This way of being with yourself is like having a conversation with your body and listening for guidance, which is *energizing rather than exercising.*

As we explore movement in all directions, through the vectors of our feet, hands, head, and tail, we are exploring our body's length, depth, and width, which Irmgard Bartenieff and her teacher, Rudolph Laban, cross-cultural scholars and pioneers in the field of dance/ movement therapy, called our "kinesphere." Their visions offered new perceptions of ourselves, in relationship with our world, which they felt would enhance all our lives (Bartenieff 1983, p.v).

These movements prepare us to practice a more fluid, embryonic, fascial matrix-informed approach to traditional Pilates, yoga, and other movement and bodywork disciplines (see embodied biotensegrity, Pilates, and yoga movement flow sessions in Chapter 7). As you engage with the novel movement explorations below, it will be helpful to keep this awareness of the fluid, embryonic, fascial matrix-informed approach in mind. Before you are supported by your legs, for example, you are supported by your breathing spine, so the relationship between your sacrum and your occiput is one your body knows from your embryonic beginnings. When you allow weight to release through your sacrum in sitting or standing, ground reaction force or uplift will be evoked from the inner ankles of your feet (standing) or sitting bones (sitting), along the front of your pelvic diaphragm and spine to each inner ear to awaken and restore your primordial midline lift or extension in any direction. This is felt as your familiar "center of gravity." All of these connections and lines of embodied communication are active before we do any given movement. We orient to this concert of activity and carry knowledge produced through this activity into our movements.

Additionally, along with our well-known lower center of gravity, around L3, studying with Hubert Godard opened another awareness—there is an upper center of gravity within our body. This moving center around the fourth thoracic vertebra derives from the rooting of your arms to your mid-spine, heart center, and is felt as a softening and widening of your clavicles, chest, and back and uplift through your occiput, and results in organization and freedom of movement in your neck in relationship with your head and arms. This center of gravity is often lost in the compressive postures of sitting too much or the collapsed, flexed posture in aging, where we lose uplift and internal support for our hands to function in everyday activities of daily living.

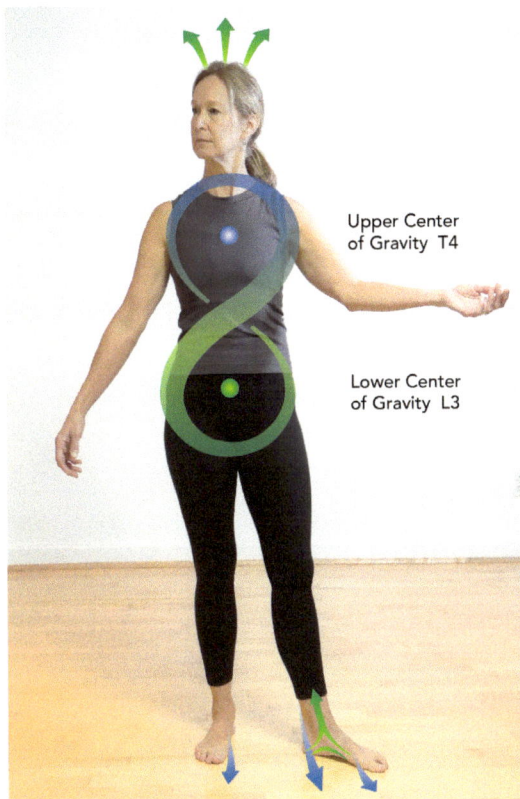

Figure 4.15 Lemniscate body with upper and lower center of gravity

Upper Center of Gravity T4

Lower Center of Gravity L3

Remember that in our embodied approach to movement and bodywork, your elbows and knees are "kinetic centers" that can amplify or inhibit movement through the helical movements of your hands and feet. When you can access your spine's relationship between earth and sky, with freedom in your occiput and sacrum, your neck and jaw can be free and your arms can hang freely, ready for gestural actions of reaching/receiving or taking/pushing away. As you move from center to periphery or periphery to center, your elbows and knees act as centers of communication through your fascial matrix, from your midline to your environment and your environment to your midline, unless that movement is blocked.

For bodyworkers, this is also essential for therapeutic work. It is crucial to be able to access your own breathing spine's tonic function, with your center of movement open, with a free neck, and with weight in your own sacrum, so you can find freedom in your elbows and knees, enabling you to "touch" a client from whole person to whole person. From this place, you don't put them "on hold" as Judith Aston so astutely said many years ago.

Whether you are a new student to embodied movement or a seasoned practitioner, preparing to engage in any movement activity, therapeutic hands-on sessions, or exercise, you benefit from consciously evoking the interdependence of your upper and lower centers of gravity so as to address the tendency to lose one of your spine's primal relationships between earth and sky by *collapsing* (lack of energy) or *propping* (too much energy). When we collapse, we lose the balance of grounding and uplift through our roots, and when we prop, we use too much energy to sit, stand, touch a client therapeutically, etc. *What is just enough effort for the movement* is our mantra, which evokes your fascial matrix spine's fluid, wave-like polarity of Down the Back and Up the Front, preventing chronic spinal cord and nerve compression that happens from habitual forward head positioning and eye strain. Bodyworkers will also notice that Down the Back and Up the Front prevents chronic strain through shoulders, neck, and arms that leads to early retirement due to arthritic joints.

EXPLORING YOUR LIVING ARCHITECTURE

Up to this point in the chapter, I have primarily utilized narrative—interspersed with demonstration through guided activity—to explain and describe the notion of movement beyond doing and its partner, pre-movement. Everything that follows from this point is offered as a guided movement exploration with which you can sense your body's experience of these same ideas. If you want to skip ahead to the next chapter, now is a great time to do that. If you'd like to deepen your embodied knowledge of movement beyond doing, proceed to the movement explorations below.

To summarize the major takeaway of "movement beyond doing," the over-exertion caused by trying to muscle through any given movement or exercise has the unintended side-effect of silencing an entire world of embodied, fascial matrix movement.

FROM ISOLATED MUSCLES TO FASCIAL MATRIX AWARENESS

Sensing your *fluid spine awareness* changes your way of being with yourself from one of muscular holding and controlling yourself to a fluid connection with your fascial matrix's support from foot to head and hand. This change is important because it helps to unravel long-held tension and trauma patterns held in the tissue. The unraveling begins with a yield to gravity and regulates the triune nervous system (sympathetic, parasympathetic, social), thereby preparing the body for deeper connection with ourselves and one another. To imagine this fluid connection, let's look at how your head balances on the *rockers/fulcrum* of your skull (occipital condyles at atlas) and how this support relates to the (talus/calcaneus) *rockers/fulcrum* of your lower leg and feet. This relationship is one your body knows from an "orienting" place, when your sacrum/tail are released and just enough effort for the movement engages UTF from your feet and/or sitting bones, through the front of your pelvic diaphragm to your inner ears. **See Video 4.16 for full exploration**.

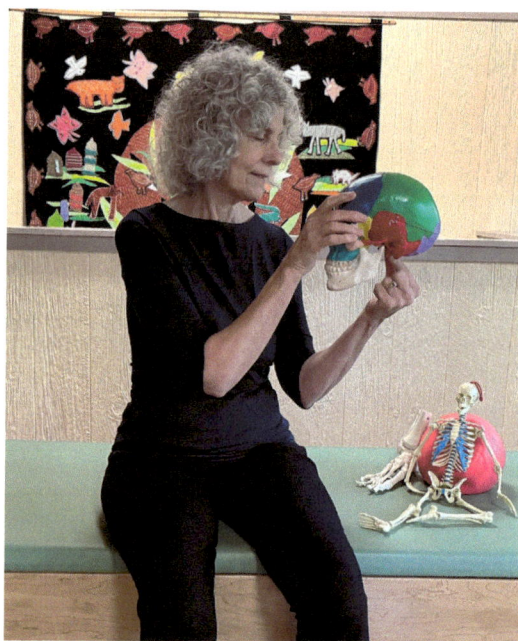

Figure 4.16 Relationship of sphenoid/inner ear to sacrum/tail to talus—how the "rockers" of the skull and foot talk to one another

Lower Center of Gravity Awareness—Lower Core

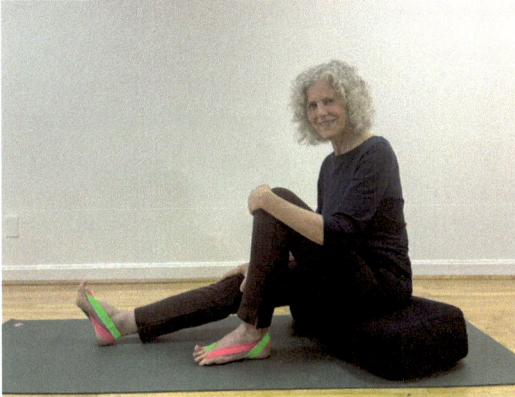

Figure 4.17 Your fascial feet—doming your emergent inner ankle uplift

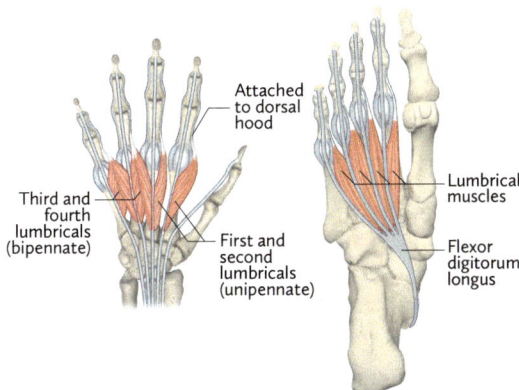

Figure 4.17A Interosseous and lumbrical suction-cup muscles

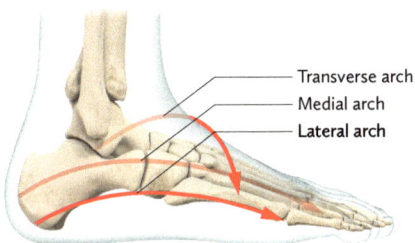

Figure 4.17B Domes—transverse, medial, lateral arches of feet

▸ Standing up or sitting on your sitting bones, you are *doming* your foot, drawing your heel toward the balls of your toes, while keeping your toes long.

▸ You are engaging the fascial matrix that supports the smallest muscles of your feet, the lumbricals and interosseous—your suction-cup support.

▸ You are also engaging your living architecture's three arches which are the scaffolding for your fascial foot's *domes* and build whole-body fascial matrix support:
  – medial longitudinal arch
  – lateral longitudinal arch
  – transverse arch.

▸ See Video 4.17 for deeper exploration.

Sensing the Helix of Your Feet to Whole-Body Awareness

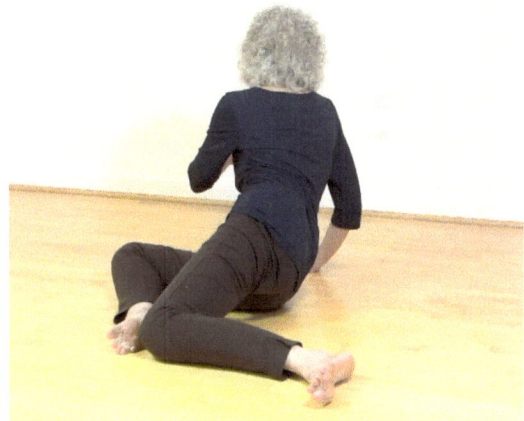

Figure 4.18 Sensing the helix of your feet to spiraling whole-body awareness

Your fascial matrix body moves through gestural patterning from your earliest embryonic beginnings. Here we are exploring our helical nature from foot to head and hand. You can explore humming, SSSSS, counting, or any sound you are drawn to on your exhale to sense your fascial matrix breath supporting your spiralic nature. **See Video 4.18 for deeper exploration.**

Sensing Domes of Uplift at Wall

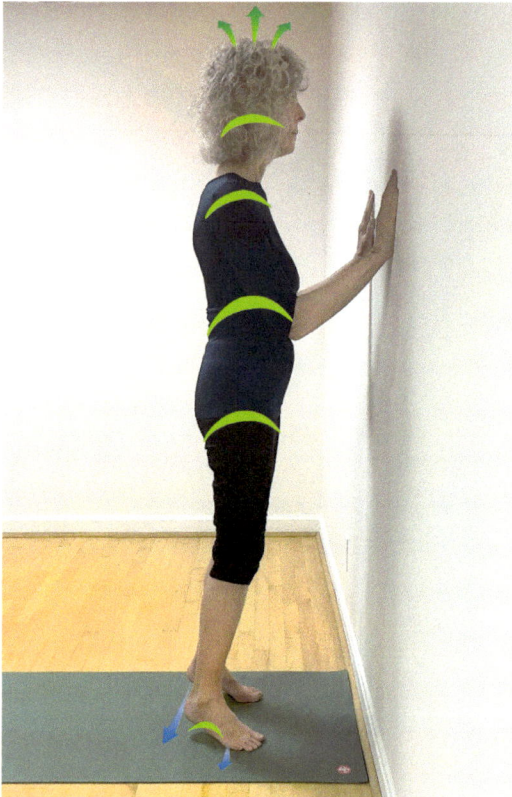

Figure 4.19 Sensing Domes of Uplift at wall

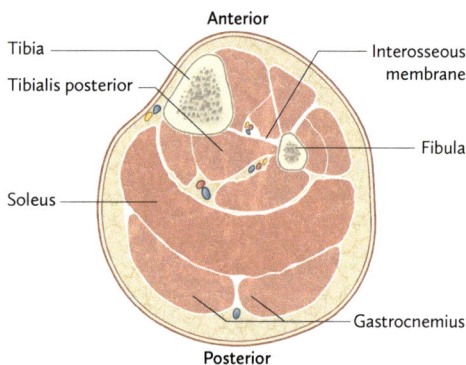

Figure 4.20 Internal calf showing Domes of Uplift of tibialis posterior, interosseous membrane, etc.

From this awareness of opening your suction-cup domes in the previous two explorations, I have found it important to notice the interdependent relationships between the muscles and fascial matrix that support the interior calf from the dome of the foot to the inner ears. In particular, the tibialis posterior (TP), whose function is to hold up the arch and support the foot in walking. The TP adjoins the interosseous membrane that spans the tibia and fibula, which I have experienced as "fascial listening pegs" that support the fascial foot softening and widening to meet the energizing exchange between gravity (grounding) and ground reaction force (uplift) (Sharkey 2021b).

In this exploration while standing in front of a wall, with your hands lightly touching the wall, you will be noticing how to compare and contrast the difference between:

▶ *External* control, marked by:

  – gripping and tightening of your gastrocnemius calf muscles (external calf muscles) to lift your heels in order to float onto the balls of your feet, which, in turn, tightens your knees and buttocks and restricts your hips.

  – As a result, you need to "work hard" to feel your suspension onto the balls of your feet.

▶ And *Internal* support, which is:

  – an embodied approach to the same movement facilitated through the pre-movement of relaxing your tail, sensing heavy heels, and gently floating forward onto the balls of your feet.

  – Internal support allows your internal calf

to draw support from your Domes of Uplift from inner ankles to inner ears— your inner ankles, pelvic diaphragm, respiratory diaphragm, thoracic inlet, palate, cranium, and palms of your hands.

▶ **See Video 4.19 for deeper exploration.**

Footwork at the Wall

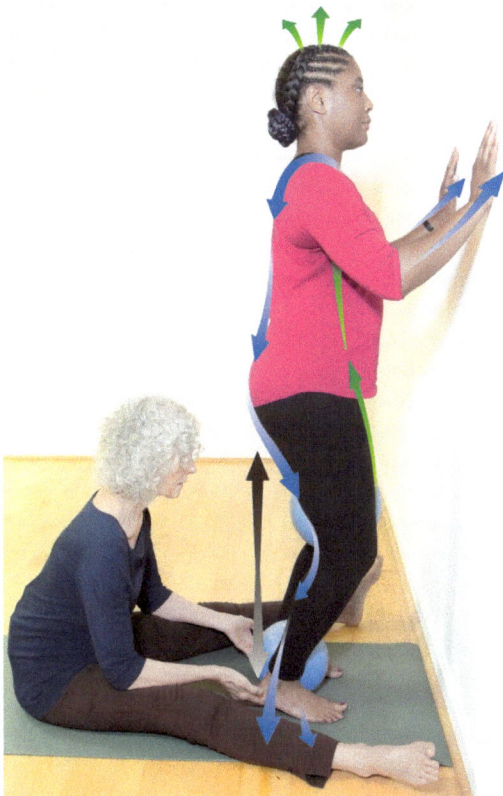

Figure 4.21 Footwork at the wall

Building on the awareness of "Sensing the Domes of Uplift at the Wall," this exploration is especially helpful for Pilates students and practitioners who are often cued to "squeeze your midline with heels together, toes apart, and inner thighs glued," which often results in sacroiliac, hip, and back pain. By engaging *what's just enough effort* to meet the floor, ball, or wall, you sense

pre-movement of yield to gravity through the grounding of your feet as you soften your knees and ankles to support the polarity of your sitting bones to heels. Heels and hips release back as your knees soften forward over your forefoot. This action evokes internal uplift through your Domes of Uplift, as you straighten your legs through the support of DTB and UTF.

These sequences recalibrate your *primordial midline* support from foot to sacrum to head, DTB and UTF. We are constantly shape-shifting as we move gesturally within the rooting and reaching nature of our hands and feet, supporting our biointelligent body on our soul journey. See Video 4.21 for deeper exploration.

Squat Holding Weights in Hands

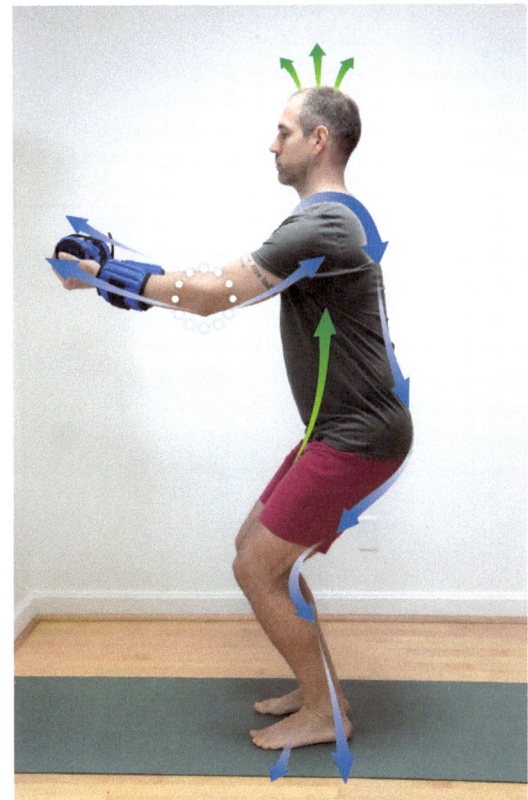

Figure 4.22 Squat holding weights in hands

Holding a weight or stable base of support gives you a sense of reaching through your lower arm while rooting through your upper arm to your waterfall Down the Back into your feet. Can you relax your neck and ankles? **See Video 4.22 for deeper exploration.**

▸ See Golden Nugget Six: Embodied Squatting at the Kitchen Sink in Chapter 6.

▸ How does this awareness allow you to lift weight with gravity's support (through your feet)—with less back and neck tension?

Remembering that rocks are the *bones of the earth*, our bones know this supportive relationship.

If you have shoulder tension on one side, start with the side that is more comfortable. The arm with less or no tension will experience the lifting first, and the knowledge gained from that side of the body can support the shoulder that is compromised on the other side. **See Video 4.23 for deeper exploration.**

Upper Center of Gravity Awareness—Upper Core

Wall Push-Up Progressing to Plank

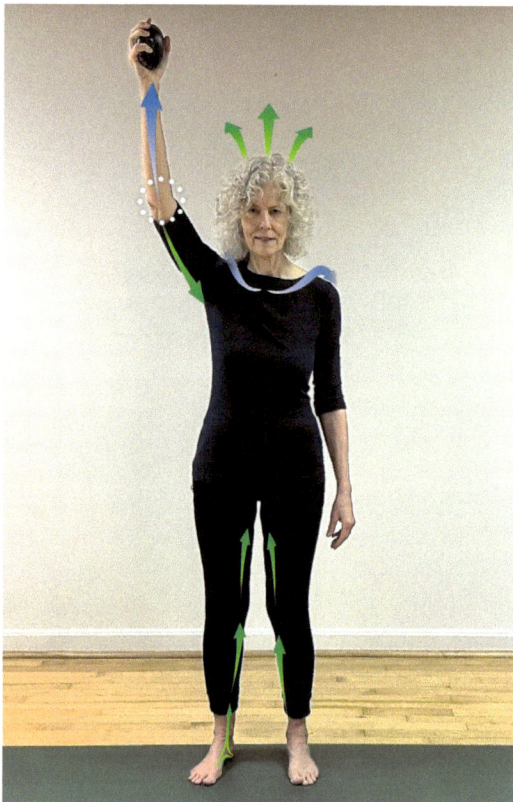

Figure 4.23 Lifting a rock or small weight from DTB and UTF

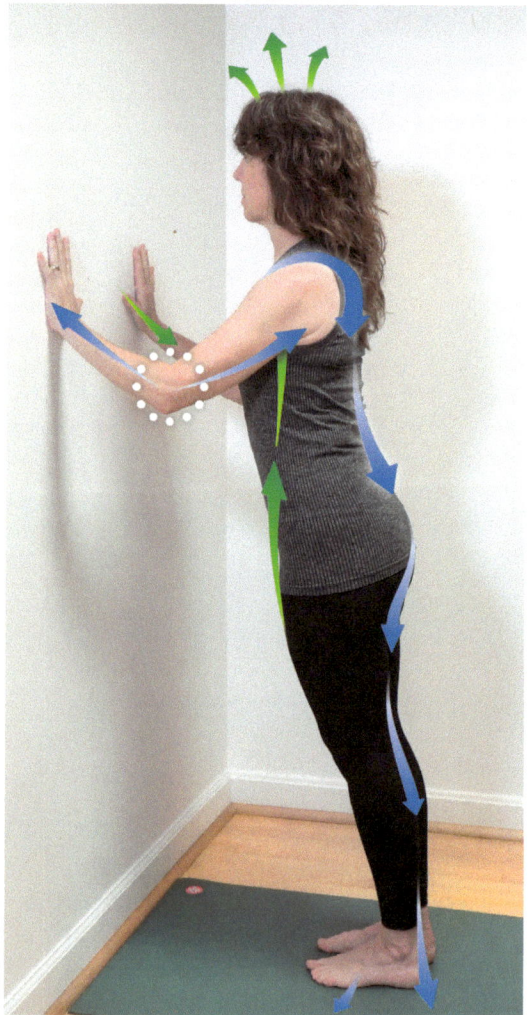

Figure 4.24 Wall push-up to full plank

With the next sequence, remember the awareness of elbows and knees as "kinetic listening centers," which help to modulate, in this movement, how to soften and straighten your arms and legs in order to make whole-person contact with your environment or another person. Additionally, in our embodied fascial matrix approach to movement, there is a relational rooting of your arms through your shoulder girdle, and your legs through your pelvic girdle to your breathing spine, and a grounding support from foot to head. Noticing *what's just enough* while softening and straightening your elbows gives you the elastic feeling of biotensegrity. See Video 4.24 for deeper exploration.

Important for movement and bodywork educators: When we check in on our own holding patterns before making contact with a client, by softening our eyes and finding our pre-movement awareness, we allow them to be fully present, rather than "putting them on hold" by our own tension pattern.

Similar to Embodied Squatting at the Kitchen Sink (see Golden Nugget Six in Chapter 6), the exploration is beyond the activity itself. In other words, the named push-up isn't the end of the activity; rather, it is a way of being within the gravitational field that is nourishing and strengthening and relates to all movement. That relational rooting with ourselves and our environment is the activity that gives us perceptual awareness of the pre-movement of tonic awareness.

The Power of Hanging from Hands and Feet

We meet and interact with the world through the core coordination of our fascial matrix between our hands and feet and our breathing spine. Consider an aging posture, where the upper body is curved forward, which weakens the hands, yet the hands can often become weak even in a younger person due to an over-sitting, collapsed posture. Let's create awareness around the higher position of the hands in senior walkers to support Upper Core orientation through inner ear uplift and greater health into end of life.

Feet that never touch the irregularities of the ground or stay locked in shoes lose their aliveness and helical nature. Our choices of movement through our feet and hands stimulate portals through our fascial matrix via mechanotransduction which signals our body to adapt to any situation. Lack of movement creates weaker bones; quality of movement such as *hanging* creates robust, strong bones:

> Mechanotransduction refers to the process by which the body converts mechanical loading into cellular responses. These cellular responses, in turn, promote structural change. A classic example of mechanotransduction in action is bone adapting to load. A small, relatively weak bone can become larger and stronger in response to the appropriate load through the process of mechanotransduction. (Khan and Scott 2009)

Here are some powerful ways to enliven your relationship with your hands and feet and their relationship with your breathing spine.

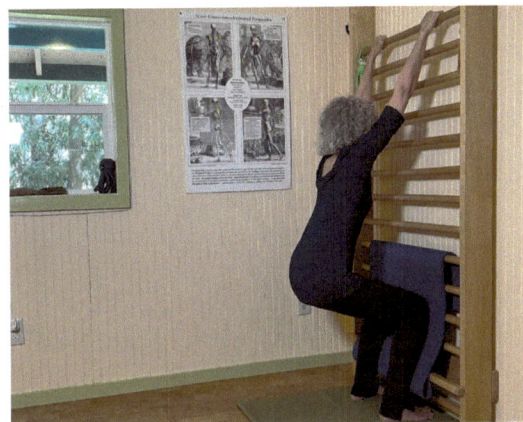

Figure 4.25 Transformational shape-shifting for healthy shoulders

About ten years ago I discovered the work of orthopedic surgeon John Kirsch, which transformed my understanding of how gravity can heal shoulder pain. He spoke about the "forgotten joint" in the shoulder that he discovered and called the *acromiohumeral joint*, and noted that so much attention is paid to the glenohumeral joint, with little attention paid to what allows full excursion of the humeral head without impinging the rotator cuff.

> This joint is engaged and visible while hanging from an overhead support or bar. When engaged, the humerus (upper arm bone) leans on the acromion, bending this structure, providing more room beneath the acromion. This leads to healing subacromial impingement syndrome, frozen shoulder and rotator cuff tear symptoms. (Kirsch 2019, p.77)

This awareness speaks to the principle of "Wolff's Law," a theory developed by German anatomist and surgeon Julius Wolff, which states that "bone in a healthy animal will adapt to the loads under which it is placed. If loading on a particular bone increases, the bone will remodel itself over time to become stronger to resist that sort of loading" (Wikipedia contributors).

See Video 4.25A for deeper exploration of Power of Hanging from the Hands. See also Videos 4.25B and 4.25C which show the Power of Hanging from the Feet.

The Power of Throwing— Core as Relationship

This distinction helps to self-correct the effects of repetitive strain injury in one-sided sports such as golf and tennis. See Video 4.26 for full practice.

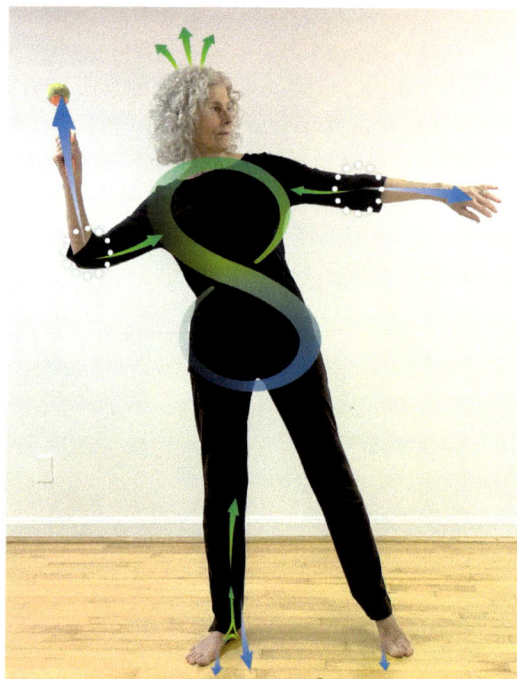

Figure 4.26 The power of throwing— Core as Relationship

STORY: I developed a new appreciation for the regenerative power of throwing one and a half years ago. I developed a severe microbiome issue and had diarrhea, which continued every day for almost a year—I couldn't stabilize my microbiome. My body normally readjusts so easily, so this was very difficult. Then about a year later, I felt a deep pain in my right hip, so went in to have it checked out with an x-ray and MRI. I was told I had osteoarthritis.

Just two years earlier, I had a bone density test and was told that, for my age, 74 at the time, I had mild osteopenia. Apparently, the dehydration during the year of diarrhea caused bone loss.

So I begin upping my hydration program and movements that feel regenerative to my body. Throwing has been a powerful balm which has surprised me in many ways. I had natural rotation, stored energy, and upper-body velocity when throwing on my right side; however, throwing on my left side was difficult—the ball just plopped in front of me. So I studied the patterning of my right side throwing from foot to head and hand, and began to match the gesture of the throw with the rotation, wind-up, and weight transfer to throw on my left, and slowly, just like moving my computer mouse to my left hand, my body adapted. It was remarkable as the force transferred from foot to hand became stronger. Now my throw on my left side is as strong and distanced as my right, as I throw the ball for Jockamo, our seven-year-old furry friend. And I'm strengthening and remodeling my fascial matrix body from all the deep listening and spiralic whole-body movements.

Lying Spiral with Wall

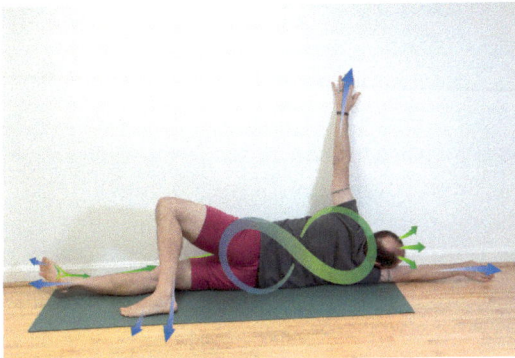

Figure 4.27 Lying spiral with wall

This is a powerful recalibration of your fascial matrix from foot to head and hand, which unravels fascial restrictions and provides a clear felt sense of grounding, centering, and uplift.

This simple yet profound act of rolling is a reset for our fascial matrix perineural nervous system which supports our central nervous system. When we sense our weight shift from one foot to the opposite hip, we awaken a cascade of myofascial releases from foot to head and hand. Remember to take your time and notice that each side of your body has its own intelligence, timing, and needs.

This self-corrects the effects of repetitive strain injury in one-sided sports such as golf and tennis. See Video 4.27 for deeper exploration.

Bridge with Domes of Feet at the Wall

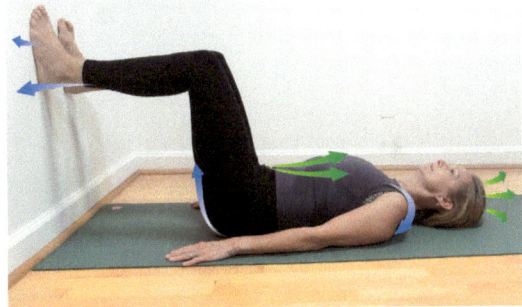

Figure 4.28 Bridge with domes of feet at the wall

Sense your Central and Upper Core from Lower Core awareness. Sense grounding into your feet (DTB) to evoke uplift along the front of your pelvic diaphragm and breathing spine (UTF).

You may notice that as you experiment with various breath patterns and as your spinal curl continues to your midback, your arms want to participate in the expression of the movement. If one side feels less fluid, be mindful of allowing that arm to lead the movement of your arm range, rather than the more mobile side pushing the more tense side to go beyond what feels supported by grounding, centering, and uplift—that way, you will support whole-organism change. When we listen to our bodies and learn, we are guided to heal long-standing trauma patterns stored in deep places. See Video 4.28 for deeper exploration.

Going deeper:

- Place a sandbag across your low belly to support the softening and widening of your low back and belly wall to allow your tail to curl from fascial flossing awareness.

- Place a sandbag along your sternum from manubrium to xiphoid to sense the softening and widening of your sternum and chest, releasing your arms and neck.

- Place a sandbag across each clavicle to sense the softening and widening of your clavicles, allowing your chest to soften as your tail and breathing spine curl.

Embodied Upper Body Curl to Lift Head

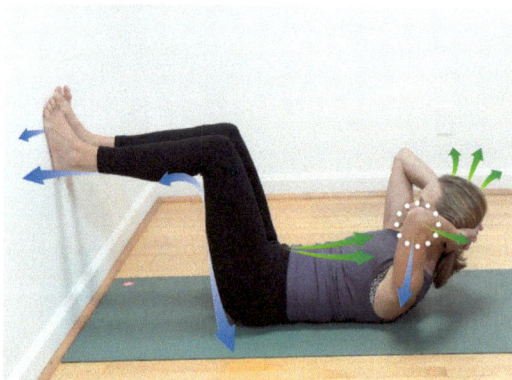

Figure 4.29 Embodied upper body curl to lift head

Explore a transition to sensing gravity's support to curl your head and upper body from a whole-body awareness. Notice how the lift of your head/inner ear (UTF) happens from the reach/pressing into your feet (DTB). Play with your feet on the wall for the Pilates Matwork, yoga, etc., using weights in your hands/wrists or on your ankles, to gain more rooting and reaching through your upper body as your shoulder blades waterfall DTB to your sacrum and feet. **See Video 4.29A for deeper exploration. See Video 4.29B to explore the process of curling**

forward to Teaser on the Pilates Cadillac with the Push Thru Bar.

Domes of Hands Touching Wall—Embodied Lower Body Curl from Sacrum/Tail

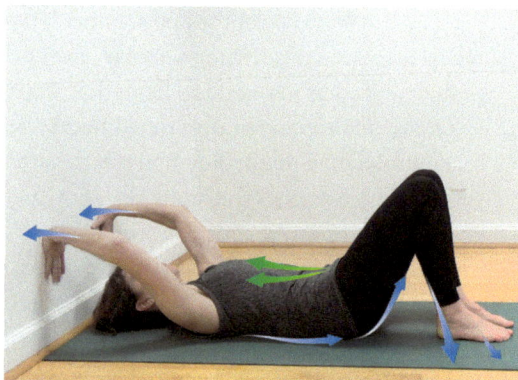

Figure 4.30 Domes of hands touching wall— embodied lower body curl from sacrum/tail

Sense your Central and Lower Core from Upper Core awareness. Notice if you can sense that feeling of DTB from your *doming* hands touching the wall, waterfalling through your shoulder blades, sitting bones, and sacrum/tailbone all the way to your feet. **See Video 4.30 for deeper exploration.**

Embodied Exploration for Leg Extension—Hands on Wall

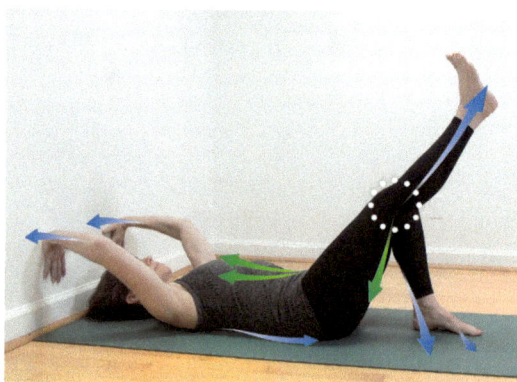

Figure 4.31 Embodied leg extension—hands on wall

Your *doming* hands are touching the wall, supported by your waterfall; both knees are bent and feet flat on the floor. Notice how the pre-movement of pressing gently into your hands supports reaching your leg away from you toward the floor, and then press into your hands and opposite foot to lift the extended leg over your hip, and notice how that can progress to a low bridge with leg extended. This is a set-up for Pilates Shoulder Bridge with Kicks. **See Video 4.31 for deeper exploration.**

RE-IMAGINING GROUNDING, CENTERING, AND UPLIFT

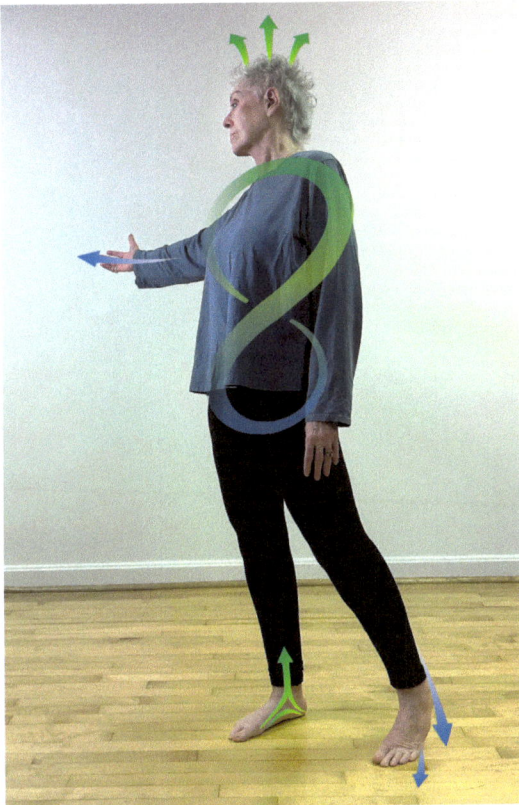

Figure 4.32 The pre-movement fluid fields of grounding, centering, and uplift

body. What we're most interested in is the context and pre-movement that supports a deeper fascial matrix support for sitting, standing, and breathing. When we open to the supportive fluid fields that are acting upon us and through us (gravity, ground reaction force, breath, and sound), we feel more spacious, receptive, and resonant with our surroundings. See Video 4.32 for deeper exploration.

▸ Helps to self-correct the effects of repetitive strain injury in one-sided sports such as golf and tennis.

▸ Sitting: Point and flex your feet and ankles to encourage the soleus pump of your lymph and blood support from Lower Core to Central and Upper Cores.

▸ Sitting or standing: Play with the push/pull movement of your arms—pushing one hand away and pulling the other toward you, noticing the relationship with your breathing spine (pelvic diaphragm to palate) with soft head and eyes.

This practice invites us to sense our relationship with the vitality of earth and sky, *wu wei* effortless doing, allowing yourself to be supported by DTB and UTF. The primary action here, while sitting or standing, is to exhale to connect/*yield* with the earth, and then just "allow" your inhale to draw energy up through your feet into your

Our fluids (e.g., cerebrospinal, cardiovascular, lymphatic) are responsive to gravity, breath, sound, and movement, not unlike the way the tides are affected by the moon. Once pre-movement is activated, the spine transforms, at least in my mind, to a fluid "breathing spine," which is marked by a conscious meeting of our fluid supports, both within and outside of our bodies. When pre-movement awareness is cultivated and our attention has shifted from "doing" to movement beyond doing, we are able to maintain attention for long periods. This attention cultivates a deeper connection to the present moment. And this connection helps foster more open engagement with other beings and with the living environment.

As babies, we cultivate postural tone through the process of pushing, pulling, reaching, rocking, rolling over, and moving between crawling, sitting, standing, and walking. We are in self-discovery mode, yet there is a tendency to lose this sense of self-discovery as we grow, by over-focusing on external needs and desires. We can become spectators in our own lives. By sensing our pre-movement to the floor/ground, we cultivate our relationship with the earth's support. By sensing soft eyes, we reawaken our relationship with our spatial orientation and expand our perceptual field. Together, this relationship with earth and sky through spatial orientation opens us to sense and support another's pre-movement. Instead of simply standing *in order to* get up or sitting *in order to* rest, this exploration brings us into a regenerative awareness of Core as Relationship, an empathetic way of observing our own and one another's movement awareness, as explored in Chapter 2.

Long Sitting

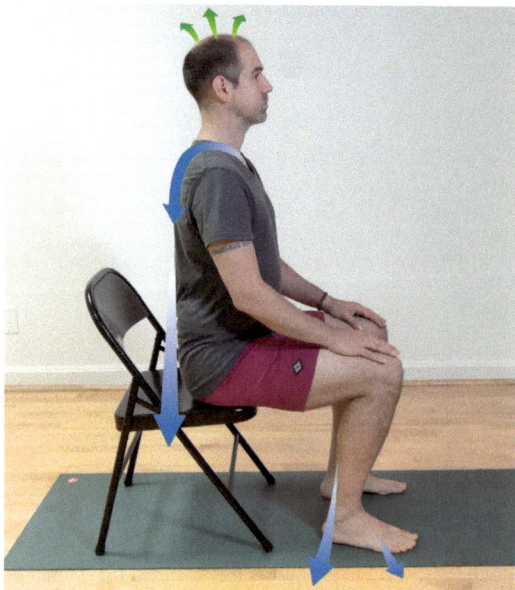

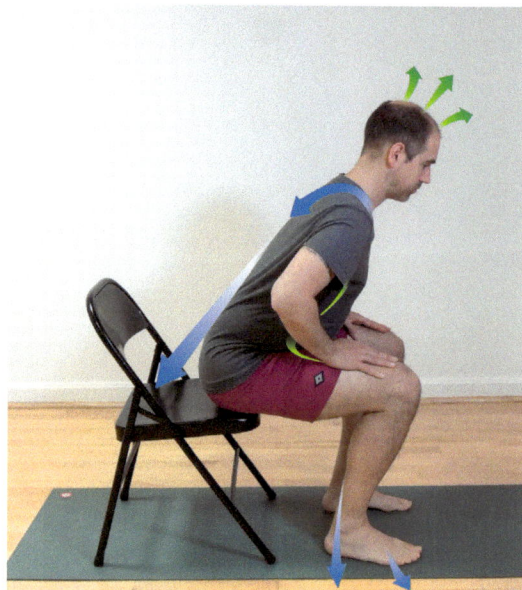

Figures 4.33A and 4.33B Long sitting

Moving from a compressive sitting posture to an enlivening, refreshing toning posture, you are *reorienting with gravity* and improving the circulation of blood to the brainstem, which also improves the function of the ventral branch of the vagus nerve. This Long Sitting Practice resets your sitting awareness with more full-body breathing by activating internal lift from the yield of grounding through your feet. When you lean forward out of your hips, your body thinks you are going to stand up, and so it lengthens in preparation for standing. But then you sense weight into your feet and, with the support of breath, pour that spinal lengthening back into the postural tone of sitting upright, with the two directions of your spine now supported by grounding and uplift (through the front of the pelvic diaphragm—Down the Back and Up the Front). As a direct result of resetting your sitting posture, range of motion for your neck and shoulders is likely to increase.

An insight that arises here is that, in our busy day-to-day lives, we have cultivated a sitting-as-doing that brings excessive tension into this most common of physical states due to a tendency to collapse and then self-correct by propping ourselves up. By engaging in Long Sitting and activating the pre-movement tonic function of sitting, we gently challenge the habitual form of collapse and propping while sitting that we acquire through work (at a desk or in front of a computer), reading, writing, etc. When we take regular breaks during sitting at a computer at work, on a project, etc., we reset to the primal movement of sitting with *gravity as a partner* that gets overwritten by tension, breath-holding habits, and modern social life. **See Video 4.33 for deeper exploration.**

NOTE TO SELF: Reset my sitting position and soft gaze regularly while driving, working, reading, etc. to refresh and enliven my breathing spine and peripheral vision!

Long Sitting Breathwave with Spiral and Vector Reach

Your initial movement in this exploration is to sense your sitting "breathwave"—the gentle movement of your sacrum and tail articulating with your occiput/sphenoid. This is a very gentle movement where there is initially very little movement of the pelvis—more of an up-and-down movement through your midline, rather than forward and back. You will be articulating in front and behind your sitting bones, and your peripheral vision will support your exploration of spacious and grounded movement.

▸ Sit on the front of your chair, hips above knees, noticing that you can sit in front of your sitting bones as in Long Sitting which relaxes your back and allows gravity to support your uplift.

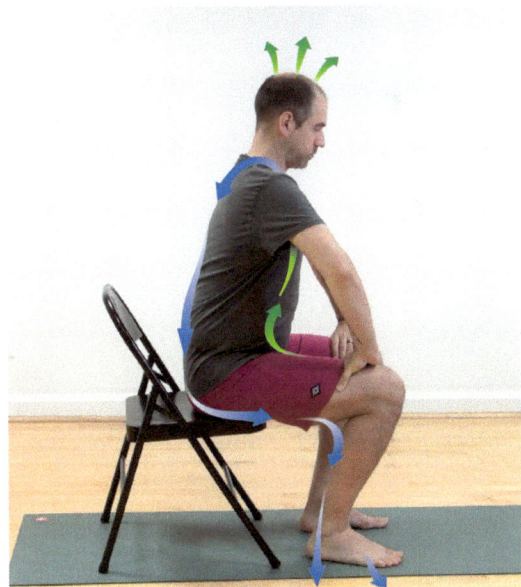

Figure 4.34A Sensing Head to Tail

▸ Place your hands on the tops of your knees with thumbs touching outer knee and fingers on inner knee so your back feels wide.

Did you find leading with your tail to be a bit disorienting? That will change as you practice—which creates a deeper sense of grounding rootedness that evokes uplift in your body. **See Video 4.34 for full exploration.**

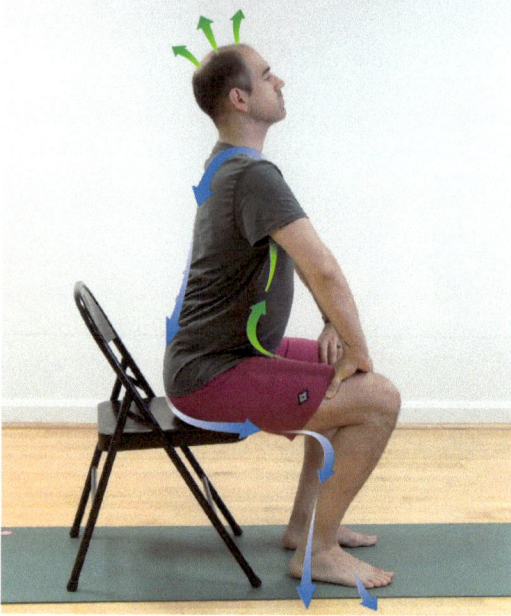

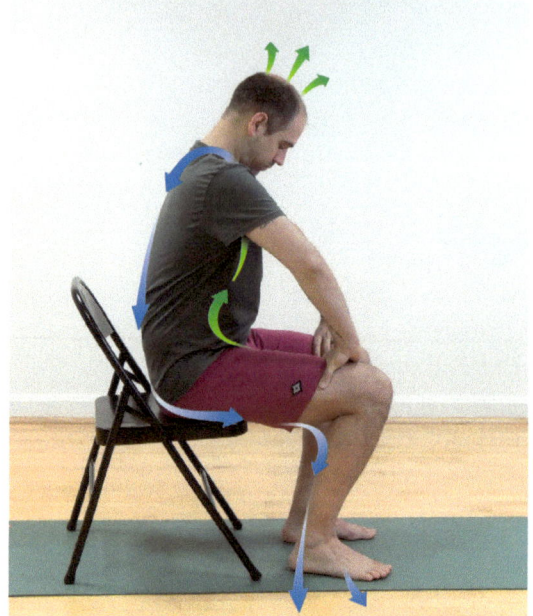

Figures 4.34B and 4.34C Playing with arch and curl

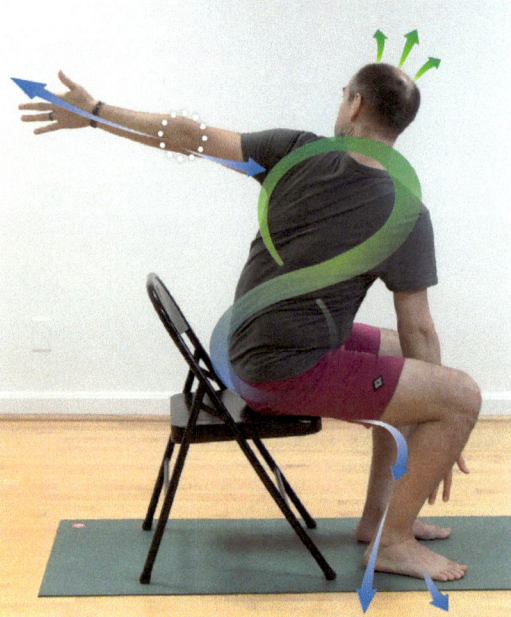

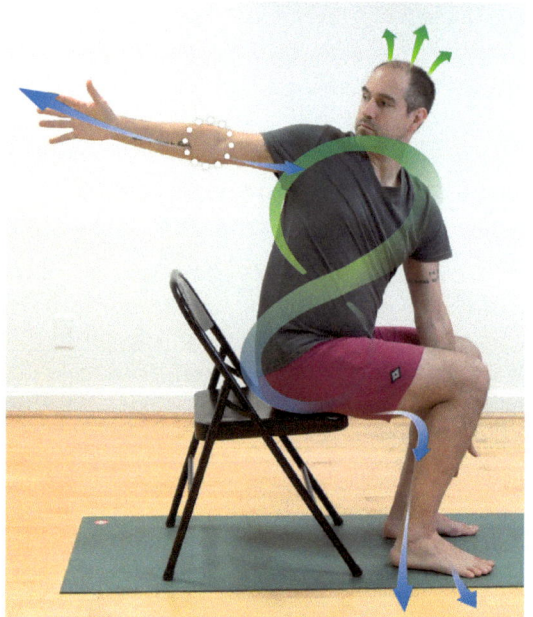

Figures 4.34D and 4.34E Spiraling to reach

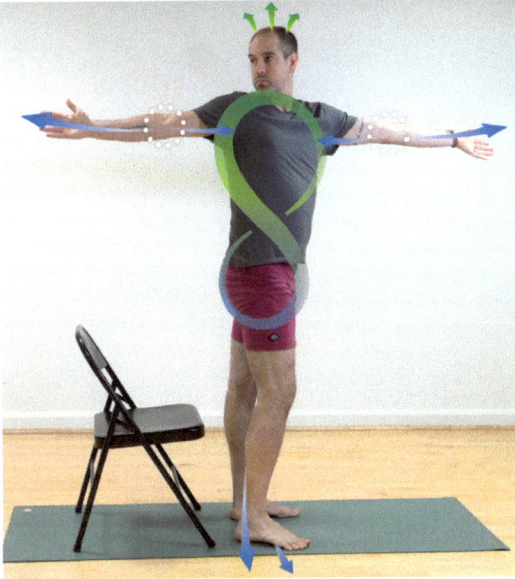

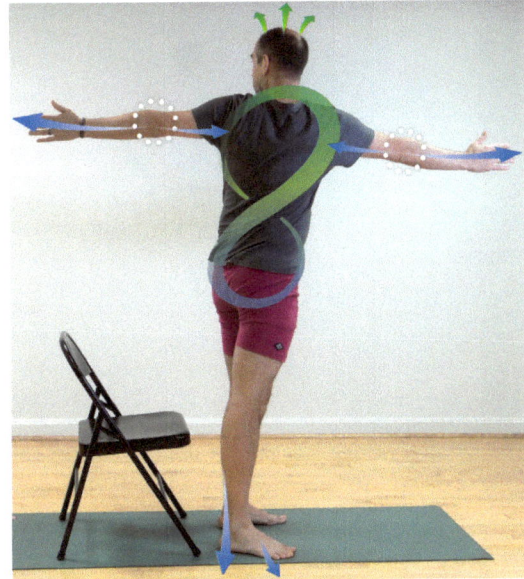

Figures 4.34F and 4.34G Spiraling to standing and sitting

Long Sitting into Standing and Walking

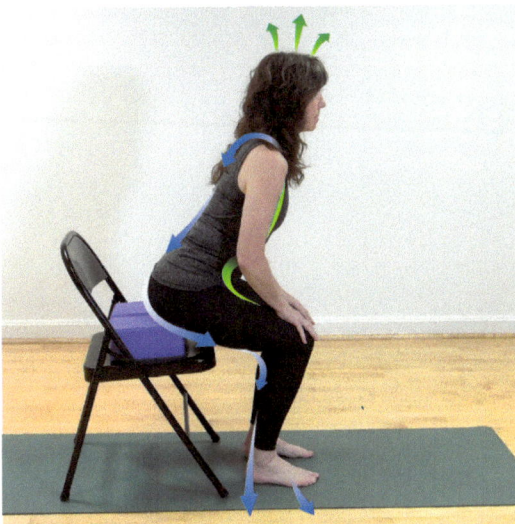

Figure 4.35 Long sitting into standing and walking

This time, repeat the forward motion from Long Sitting, but continue on to standing. Allowing your tail to release, pour your weight into your feet as though you're preparing to stand. As your sphenoid/inner ear floats up, your back can lengthen and widen as you press gently into your feet and come to standing. Once standing, carry that fluid momentum into walking. As you walk, notice how your interoceptive and proprioceptive awareness and social engagement blossom. **See Video 4.35 for full exploration.**

Lunge Facing Wall

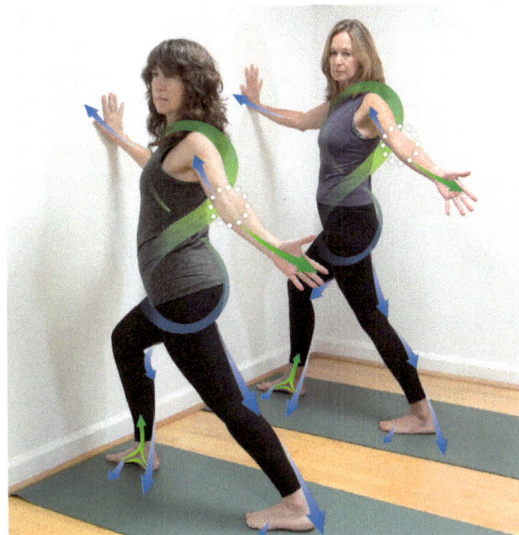

Figure 4.36 Lunge facing wall—inner and outer spirals

With a hand on a wall in front of you, straighten your elbows only as much as you are able to maintain your *waterfall Down the Back* support from hands to shoulder blades. Find a simple lunge by bending your right knee forward, foot facing forward, extending the left leg behind, allowing your pelvis to be suspended between the movement of your bending knee and front foot, sensing your back foot (very important foundational awareness for your yoga practice and teaching to not square and stabilize the pelvis as this shear pattern creates hip and sacroiliac problems).

You might add humming or counting on your exhale and/or deepening the movement with a lemniscate, figure-eight movement of your arm as you spiral in each direction. **See Video 4.36 for deeper exploration.**

Bent Knee Roll Down

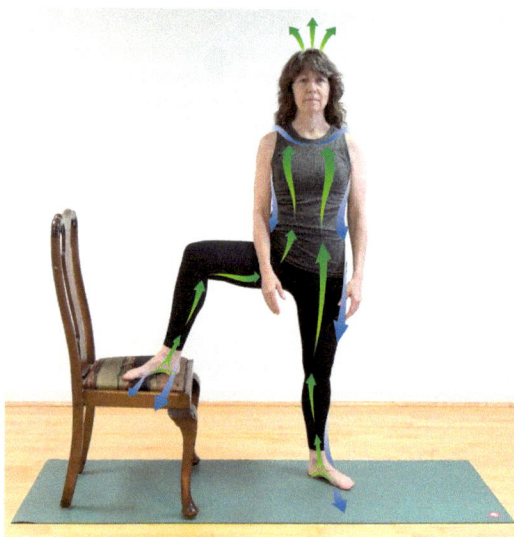

Figure 4.37 Bent knee roll down

Stand facing a chair and then turn to the left so that the chair is on your right side. Make sure the chair is on a sticky mat or placed next to a wall so that it doesn't move.

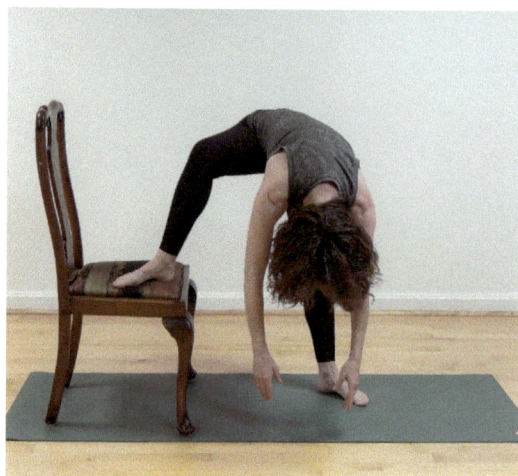

Figure 4.37A Finding your hover

▸ Place your right foot on the chair, with your left foot about hip-distance apart or with enough room to let you comfortably curl your upper body down toward the floor. Curl down and allow your arms, spine, and head to hang.

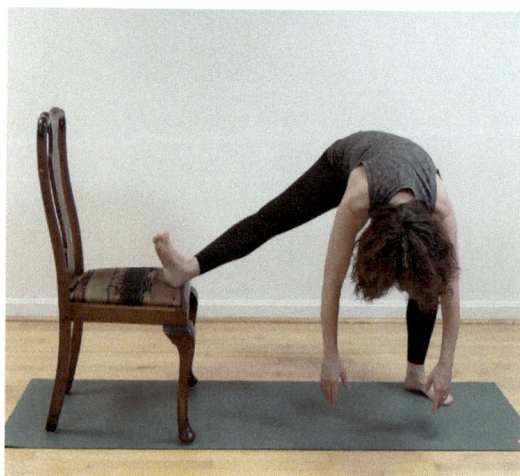

Figure 4.37B Extending leg to spine

▸ Staying rounded over, gently widen your standing leg from your bent knee leg (by pivoting heel, toe, heel, toe). Your right leg will slowly straighten with your foot on the chair.

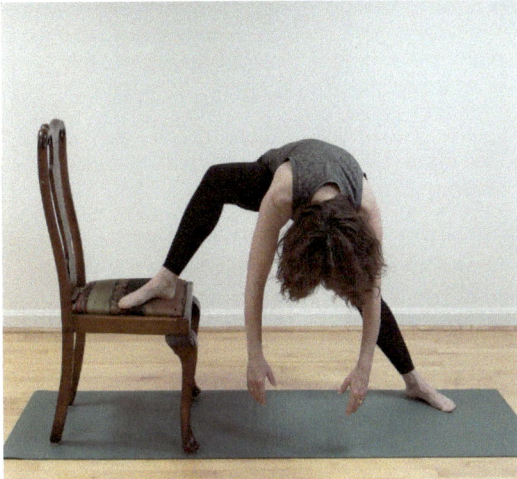

Figure 4.37C Moving toward bent leg foot

▶ Bend your right leg as you weight-shift toward that foot on the chair.

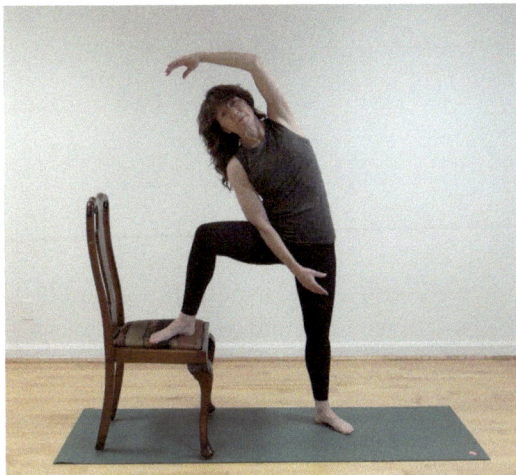

Figure 4.37D Rolling up to sidebend

▶ Sidebend over as you soften your standing knee.

Listening to our ongoing interoceptive awareness from pre-movement support changes the way we approach formal exercise and activities of daily living. The next chapter, Communicating from Our Way of Being, explains why this type of heightened awareness matters. The chapter speaks to how renewed attention to our innate embodied knowledge, combined with awareness of the external relationships in which we are embedded, changes our understanding of our porous self, our connection with other people, and our ways of communicating between self and other beings. **See Video 4.37 for full explorations**.

Use the following QR code for all videos in this chapter:

REFERENCES

Agneessens, C. (2013) "Carol Agneessens—flowing wholeness." Street Smart Craniosacral. https://blog.cranioschool.com/carol-agneesens-flowing-wholeness

Bainbridge Cohen, B. (2023) "Receiving information through sensory nerves and motor nerves." Body-Mind Centering. www.bodymindcentering.com/receiving-information-through-sensory-nerves-and-motor-nerves

Bartenieff, I. (1983) *Body Movement, Coping with the Environment*. New York, NY: Gordon and Breach Science Publishers.

Beach, P. (2010) *Muscles and Meridians: The Manipulation of Shape*. Livingstone, NY: Churchill.

Blakeslee, M. and Blakeslee, S. (2007) *The Body Has a Mind of Its Own*. New York, NY: Random House.

Frank, K. and McHose, C. (2020) "Peripheral stability through the lens of Rolf Movement." *DIRI* 48, 1 (March), 8–10.

Ho, M.-W. (1998) "Organism and Psyche in a Participatory Universe." In D. Loye (ed.) *The Evolutionary Outrider. The Impact of the Human Agent on Evolution, Essays in Honour of Ervin Laszlo*, pp.49–65. Westport, CT: Praeger.

Khan, K.M. and Scott, A. (2009) "Mechanotherapy: How physical therapists' prescription of exercise promotes tissue repair." *British Journal of Sports Medicine 43*, 4, 247–252. https://doi.org/10.1136/bjsm.2008.054239

Kirsch, J. (2019) *Shoulder Pain? The Solution & Prevention: Fifth Edition, Revised & Expanded*. New York, NY: Bookstand Publishing.

Newton, A. (1995) "Basic concepts in the theory of Hubert Godard." *Rolf Lines 23*, 32–43.

Oschman, J. (2003) *Energy Medicine in Therapeutics and Human Performance*. Oxford: Butterworth-Heinemann.

Schultz, R.L. and Feitis, R. (1996) *The Endless Web: Fascial Anatomy and Physical Reality*. Berkeley, CA: North Atlantic Books.

Sharkey, J. (2021a) "John Sharkey—Tuning the fascia net." YouTube. www.youtube.com/watch?v=DvDEMDVxcCl

Sharkey, J. (2021b) "The Fascial Foot." The Fascia Hub. https://thefasciahub.com/blog/the-fascial-foot-2

Todd, M. (1991 [1943]) *The Thinking Body: A Study of Balancing Forces of Dynamic Man*. Princeton, NJ: Princeton Books.

Wikipedia contributors (n.d.) "Wolff's law." Wikipedia: The Free Encyclopedia. https://en.wikipedia.org/w/index.php?title=Wolff%27s_law&oldid=1189218004

CHAPTER 5

Communicating from Our Way of Being

The first four chapters of *Moving Beyond Core* focus on lifelong learners, those devoted to exploring movement and bodywork beyond techniques like Pilates or yoga. Those chapters emphasize cultivating an understanding of the Inner Guide, Core as Relationship, Breath as a Healing Bridge, and Movement Beyond Doing, and fostering a holistic connection with the natural living world. This chapter shifts slightly, targeting both students and educators of this biointelligent perspective, exploring how to teach and partner with others to plant seeds for a better world. It emphasizes that transformational teaching stems from our way of being, and includes verbal and non-verbal communication.

Educators of biointelligent ways of being need to consider not only what they communicate but also how they go about it. Effective teaching requires clear and vivid communication, but it also asks educators to connect with their inner selves, finding and expressing their emergent voices. This is modeling authenticity.

In the 1980s, I experienced the transformative power of language, communication, and self-expression through participation in transformational programs. These programs deeply impacted me on all levels, allowing me to forgive and transform my relationship with my father before his death, and to gain confidence in my ability to make a difference and to contribute to the world. They highlighted the difference between informational learning (downloading information) and transformational learning, which involves holding space, listening, and speaking from a deeper awareness and commitment.

> **STORY:** I was leading a workshop a few years ago, and a practitioner was having difficulty with breathing while lying on her back. I asked if she would mind if I placed my hands on her to follow her breath pattern, and placed a small pillow under her head and a pillow under her thighs so she could let go and allow gravity to support her. She was used to controlling her breath and was holding a lot of tension in her face, neck, shoulders, and belly through concern that she wasn't "doing it right." Without telling her to do anything, I just began very gently rocking her, moving both of my hands on either side of her ribs and gently tracing her softening and widening her clavicles as her breath found new pathways. Very slowly, her midline breath wave began to emerge and she began to sob. We all held space for her to take the time she needed. Finally, she looked at me and said, "That was amazing—I feel so free."

My participation in the process was informed by my pre-movement awareness, which allowed me to hold space from my Inner Guide. This approach cultivated the grounding and space for this practitioner to remember she was a living process who knew how to self-heal. By meeting her where she was and gently pulsing her body, moving with her breathing spine's metabolic need, her body began to unwind the tension that had been held inside for years. Holding space is about Wholehearted Deep Listening that allows someone to feel their wholeness, which, in turn, allows their body to access their biological blueprint of health, their shape-shifting ecology body.

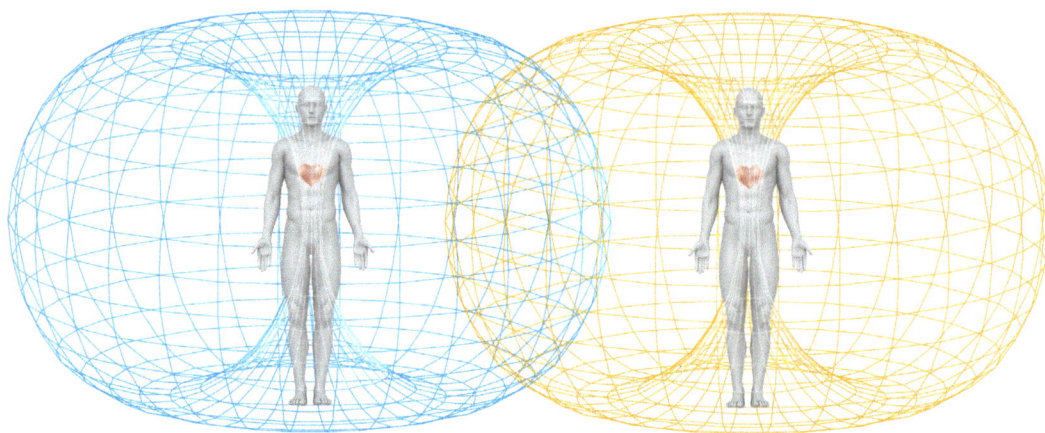

Figure 5.1 Toroidal field of heart-to-heart communication
IMAGE COURTESY OF THE HEARTMATH® INSTITUTE—www.heartmath.org

Letting go of the notion of fixing someone means trusting our heart to communicate with another's heart. In terms of the literal dimension of the heart in *Wholehearted Deep Listening*, there is good research being conducted at HeartMath Research Center, which tells us that the heart is the most powerful source of electromagnetic energy in the human body and that the magnetic fields produced by the heart are involved in energetic communication. Your heart's electrical field is approximately 60 times greater in amplitude than the electrical activity created in your brain and is an important carrier of information. Your heart sends more communication to your brain than your brain sends information to your heart, and your thoughts and emotions affect your heart's magnetic field, which energetically affects other beings in your environment, whether you are conscious of it or not. Wholehearted Deep Listening proceeds from this trust.

I've had many heart-to-heart communication experiences in my life. Being coached by dedicated mentors and participating in transformational programs gave me my own wholehearted experiences with transformational learning.

My experiences within transformational programs taught me so much about *speaking and listening* communication. Here, in *Moving Beyond Core*, I also focus on another type of communication, one which utilizes a way of being. This means communication can take place without words and where we communicate through sensing the world through the vibrancy of living tissue from fascial matrix to fascial matrix. This communication takes place through holding space and often through the way we touch, through our hearts and hands, and through the way we receive touch as empathetic beings. All of this unites the structural, connective, and energetic dimensions of the body.

SHIFTING MY WAY OF BEING

When I first began teaching, my focus was on having the answer to every question a client might ask, so I placed a lot of pressure on myself to be an expert. I scoured books and took many courses to fill the bottomless pit of *not being enough*. I was immersed in informational learning. Over time, I became more and more curious about our self-healing ability and had a breakthrough when I read Ida Rolf, who said that gravity is the therapist and that our orientation in the gravitational field changes our physiology, psychology, and behavior. I realized that the role of expert that I was striving to play was actually inhibiting my partnering with gravity and other beings. When I let go into gravity's support, I also let go of that false notion of posturing expertise and discovered a collaborative approach, which empowered clients to be the "expert" in their own body.

The breakthrough lay in discovering that gravity, that force that is always pulling us down, and that I had been fighting or collapsing into for years, had a partner—ground reaction force—spatial orientation. I shared about my physical experience in Chapter 2, but here I want to emphasize the importance of developing a befriending relationship with gravity. Using more effort than needed to move around in life—resisting gravity—becomes exhausting, physically, mentally, emotionally, and spiritually. My perceptions about myself, my job, my husband, etc. were often focused on what was wrong that needed to be fixed (another type of resisting). It was only when I befriended or accepted or yielded to gravity and awakened my peripheral attitude (peripheral vision as a body-wide perceptual communication)—and, likewise, to the perceived challenges in my life—that I began to see the world and myself anew. I didn't have to resist because there was a vital resilience within me, an innate constitutive order, always working together with gravity and also the challenges that I faced.

As I became aware of sensing my body as a living process, a whole new world opened—the natural world and my embedded relationship within it came alive. I hadn't realized how much I perceived nature as "out there" and had the belief that my brain controlled my speaking and listening. Sensing the earth beneath my feet and awakening to breath as a primal relationship between earth and sky opened me to a whole-hearted awareness and bathed my tissues with a loving touch that wakes me up when I lose focus, and continues to deepen every day.

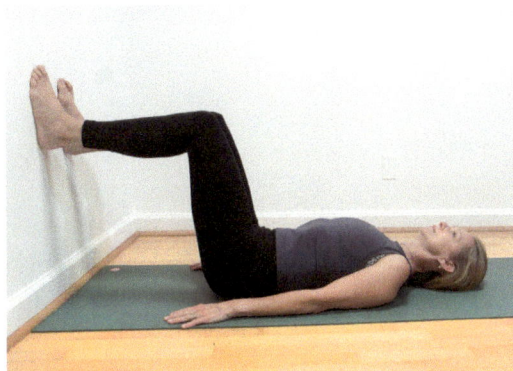

Figure 5.2 Finding your backing with feet on wall

I also discovered how to meet myself through listening and speaking from my body's perspective and finding and embodying my own *backing*, which is a felt sense, a physiological activity. Even though I had a rich meditation practice, there was a place of not letting go that I found in backing myself, as if my spirit could rest into the here and now on earth. As I mentioned in Chapter 4, we can't have someone else's back till we have our own back. That backing happened through studying transformational learning and rich somatic practices where I found my authentic, emergent voice and let go into sensing a direct experience of gravity as my partner. What opened was a deeper voice from a place of vision where

I felt my connection within the matrix of our global community and lifeforce of the cosmos. **See Video 5.2 for full exploration**.

Another life-altering discovery was that *perception shapes our reality*. The story I had been living was that life is difficult and I didn't have the proper education to really thrive. What I learned was that I was living a "story" from my past that had nothing to do with the present and future. Too often, we forget that we are the author of our own storybook. My perception completely shifted when I learned that this was just the fearful, small-minded, automatic listening and the speaking part of my brain, looking for what is *wrong*. To change my life, I changed my story. With that change of story came a major change in perception and my way of being.

> **STORY:** There is an old story about how our attention and intention affect our energy level: There were three masons who were laying brick. A man walks up and asks each of them the same question—What are you doing? The first mason says, "I'm laying brick—what do you think I'm doing?" The second mason wipes his brow and says, "I'm making a living." The third mason looks up with light in his eyes and says, "I'm building a cathedral!"
>
> The moral of the story is that the third mason allows the aspiration of the finished cathedral to shape the care with which he places each brick, and by allowing that larger vision to guide his daily work, his way of being is transformed.

This visionary foundation is what enables us to get back on track when we fall off—this is the soil we are cultivating in our lives that grows us as wholehearted beings. For instance, here are a few of my affirmations:

- I am a life partner who feeds my husband Michael's spirit, passion, and purpose.

- I am a global citizen who lives life passionately and respectfully so that all beings flourish.

- I am committed to a global shift from a reductionist, body-as-machine approach to ourselves, to a whole-organism, body-as-a-living-process approach, through the language, fluid resonance, and brilliant guidance of our embodied wisdom.

- I care for my body, mind, and spirit as my best friend.

This is a life-shifting practice which underpins my year-long mentoring program.

There are two main ways to alter life: one is change and the other is transformation. Change is an alteration in some aspect of your reality, which happens through informational learning. You change the circumstances in your life—new job, get more information, move, buy new clothes, change the shape of your body. The effects of change are short-lived—a fundamental shift in our way of being as a lived experience is missing.

Transformational learning, by contrast, is an alteration of your *perception of reality*. When you alter your perception of your reality, you create a new relationship with yourself and your circumstances. For instance, rather than altering the circumstances, you can make a conscious choice to shift the way you think about and respond to someone or some situation. In order to transform any situation, what is needed is a new relationship with what we are calling the *Gift of Communication*. With this, we examine how we relate to ourselves and others, how we meet the other person, and by noticing how we are communicating a sense of connection and trust. The transformation here is one that moves away from a narrow focus on *what* is communicated toward a broader focus on how my way of being influences *how* I communicate.

HOW COMMUNICATION ALTERS OUR WAY OF BEING

STORY: Several years ago, a client was referred to me by a doctor who was concerned that she was so afraid of moving due to the pain she was experiencing from the many surgeries she had undergone over decades. As we sat down for me to ask her about her medical record and hear where she was at this time, she began describing everything that was "wrong" with her. After a time, I asked if I might ask a question. We paused and I asked her, "How did you get here to the studio?" She looked surprised and said, "Well, I drove and walked in." I said, "Yes! So there is a lot that is working well in your body to get you here! And that is your innate biointelligence that we will be working to support in our sessions together." She looked at me with such a sweet expression, and I knew that our hearts had connected in a trusting relationship—it was such a beautiful moment!

This client's session began by meeting her where she was and by introducing myself as a welcoming presence who was deeply listening. Once she voiced her worry about losing her mobility, I spoke to her Inner Guide from my Inner Guide, assuring her that we are not objects to be trained and fixed, and that our sessions would build on her inner resilience in ways that would surprise her. In our first session, she was amazed at how her biointelligent body moved. She became curious. That curiosity helped her feel supported in the gravitational field. Out of that place, her sitting, standing, and walking felt more internally supported and fluid. She felt much less pain and was empowered at the end of our session by her ability to help herself by calling upon her innate self-knowledge. I was inspired to hear her exclaim how committed she was to continue sessions.

This client experienced a transformational shift away from the belief that she was broken and unable to help herself, because we were speaking to her Inner Guide, the fascial matrix communication network that is self-healing and adaptive. This paradigm shifts away from fixing toward self-curiosity and exploration, putting her in touch with her biological blueprint of health that is her transformational birthright.

The flow of energy in this client's session between us was exchanged on bridges of connection. These bridges are how we connect on Core-to-Core teaching—whole fascial matrix to whole fascial matrix. Calibrating, empathy, and rapport create these powerful bridges. These three dynamics produce awareness, connection, and resonance. They are ways of being which help you to reach out and make contact. All three are about stepping out of our world as the expert ready to fix and entering into someone else's world to collaborate through a powerful flow of energy.

Communication is fundamental to our humanity and is the greatest resource we possess. Every stage of our evolution has relied on communication to expand our ability to think, create, and make meaning. I have found that communication is the means through which cooperation takes place, community is formed, and lives are fulfilled. It is how we live our soul journey.

If you closely watch people in heartful communication, you see an exchange of energy—a give and take, breathing out and in. In a sense, we are held within the pre-tensed network of the biotensegrity of life. There is a tensional integrity that feeds the exchange. When you speak, and even when you are attending bodily without speaking, you are projecting, sending your energy into the world. When you listen, you are receiving, picking up, and allowing in another's energy. This energy is the heart of what I am calling *Wholehearted Speaking and Deep Listening*. It is made up of sound waves, moods, intentions, perceptions, and beliefs. You are literally creating a flow of information and feelings from one person to another—fascial matrix to fascial matrix. *You are exchanging who you are with others.*

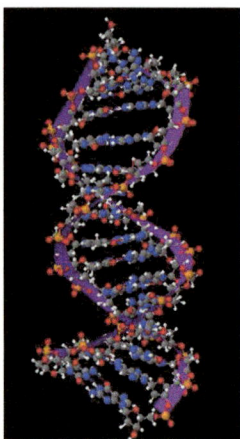

Figure 5.3 DNA sequencing
GENEIOUS BASIC 4.0.2, CC BY-SA 3.0. https://commons.wikimedia.org/w/index.php?curid=5056868, VIA WIKIMEDIA COMMONS

We are energetic, bioelectric beings who communicate non-verbally through our cells and fascial matrix to the multi-universe. When we create space for another person, or client, we are held in this luminous spatial orientation that is our shared social nervous system.

Observing two people in conversation, begin noticing how the speaking and listening affects each of them. There is also a non-verbal communication happening through our vibratory fascial matrix bodies that sets up a spatial way of being before the verbal communication occurs. I call this presencing. Presencing, listening, and speaking are channels for our thoughts, feelings, and commitments, all of which are forms of energy. When we are in tune with the spirit of an exchange between ourselves and others, we begin to feel the embodied dance that communication is. When we attend purposefully to this dance, we tune into who others are and what they are communicating with their full selves. It is the space of that dance where embodied communication happens and can be perceived as either positive or negative.

Although we don't like to admit it, all of us have experience with negative communication exchanges. In those exchanges, there is a whole-hearted (contributing) side, but it is challenged by a self-serving (judgmental) side. When we let our guard down or when we aren't aware of this judgmental side, conversations can become awkward, stilted, or even disempowering. These conversations usually thrive on old, habitual patterns and perceptions. Becoming aware of the dynamics of this negative exchange, however, leads to a shift through which judgment gives way to respect for the other person. This respect usually comes from first befriending yourself, and from there, negative communication patterns give birth to new, positive, empowering exchanges.

STORY: I met a neighbor at a local gathering and she mentioned that she was very limited in her movement. She shared that she had stage 4 bone cancer and was "terrified" to move because she was told she could fracture her bones very easily. I invited her to come in for a very gentle session at no charge that would help her have ease in her activities of daily living. She was grateful for the support, and when we met, it was surprising to her how much effort she noticed that she was using in sitting, standing, walking, and supporting her upper body in motion. As I supported her movement with embodied touch, she could feel more ease. She also shared how much her fear of moving in her body was affecting her relationships, and was surprised how much our embodied approach felt so therapeutic and was freeing long-held tension patterns in her body. She rediscovered how to access her pre-movement awareness, and her relationship with gravity shifted from a compressive one to finding lightness and fun in movement. What was most powerful for her, though, was that we addressed her *fear* of moving. She learned how to use gravity as a partner and discovered a wholehearted approach to herself, which will ripple into her relationships. She saw that her movement awareness could come from a place of grounding, centering, and uplift by listening for her Inner Guide to guide her. Seeing the smile on her face at the end of our session was a priceless gift.

WIDENING THE CIRCLE OF RELATIONSHIP

We have many different aspects of our character. Our wholehearted side is generous, caring, pro-active, and considerate. It has strong values, listens closely, and wants everybody to win. It is our best nature. We are acting from this side when we are centered, compassionate, and in touch with a larger vision that will hold the conversation to support all parties involved in a win/win.

Our small-minded side is petty, selfish, uncaring, demeaning of ourselves and others, cold, and reactive. It behaves in ways that are inconsistent with our values and tends to come from win/lose, an ego-based place. When we are having a good day, when things are going our way and our needs are being met, it's easy to be our best or wholehearted self. We narrow our relatedness to the small-minded side when things aren't going the way we want them to go.

We can bring these ideas into the arena of movement or bodywork by considering the following. I've had many teachers tell me that, at some point in their lives, they were told, "You don't have the right body for Pilates (or yoga)."

Claims like this come from a dogmatic position that ends up measuring (and judging) an individual student against some imagined ideal. At worst, this type of judgment can be denigrating and cause great amounts of shame. Even when expressed with less venom, dogmatic judgment still shuts down the two-way flow of communication between teacher and student. Whenever our words or touch or presence shuts down communication in that way, we aren't creating space for wholehearted communication. The remedy for closed communication is speaking, listening, and touching from a place of safety and support in which our teaching guides and honors our students' Inner Guide.

We can create a safe and supportive space for our students only once we have found our own backing and support. To do this, we access the *powerful bridges of Calibrating, Empathy, and Rapport* so as to connect with the wholeness of who we are and bridge the world of our client. By entering their world from a place of *Wholehearted Speaking and Deep Listening*, we create a flow of energy exchange that impacts our social nervous system and enables wholehearted connection.

PRACTICAL APPLICATIONS FOR TRANSFORMATIONAL TEACHING

- *Calibrating, Empathy, and Rapport:* These elements create bridges of connection in communication. By calibrating our responses, showing empathy, and building rapport, we facilitate deeper understanding and mutual respect.

- *Wholehearted Speaking and Deep Listening:* This approach involves fully engaging with others through mindful, empathetic, and responsive communication. It emphasizes the importance of being present and genuinely connecting with others.

- *Empowering Clients:* In teaching or therapeutic settings, shifting the focus from fixing problems to fostering curiosity and self-exploration can empower individuals. This approach taps into their innate resilience and self-healing capabilities.

- *Transformational Learning:* Encouraging a shift in perception and relationship with oneself and circumstances involves creating a space for reflection, self-discovery, and the development of new, empowering communication patterns.

- *Respect and Self-Befriending:* Developing respect for others starts with befriending oneself. This self-awareness and self-acceptance create a foundation for positive, empowering interactions with others.

By integrating these concepts and practices, educators and practitioners can foster environments that support transformational learning and meaningful, empathetic communication. This holistic approach not only enhances individual growth but also strengthens the interconnectedness of our shared human experience.

WHOLEHEARTED DEEP LISTENING

STORY: In a private session with a seasoned practitioner, I asked her to walk back and forth in order to assess how walking occurred for her. In order to witness her walking, I first sensed my own pre-movement awareness with peripheral vision and then asked her to share with me what she was noticing as she weight-shifted from her left to her right foot and back again. What was interesting? What might be calling for her attention? As she walked toward me the third time, she began to tear up and shared that it was so powerful for her not to be judged. She was so used to being told what was wrong (with her body) that she had learned to carry a heaviness within. When I assessed her walking by collaborating with her own direct experience of her body in motion, something shifted. This wholehearted collaboration enabled her to feel seen, and a lightness radiated from within. She stopped judging herself and became first curious and then excited to learn more so that she could bring this approach to her clients.

What I find so powerful in this non-judgmental way of assessing and teaching is how freeing it is, especially for seasoned practitioners of movement and bodywork who are often used to external validation and correction. To address problems from a collaborative perspective, for example, to how the global fascial matrix body supports problems, leads to an empowering form of teaching. The client/practitioner I reference in this story gained interoceptive awareness through our empowering communication and was able to articulate what she was noticing by letting go of the judging voice and relaxing into a new way of being with herself. To bring forward the language of the previous chapter, this client was used to *doing* walking, based on many interpretations of the "right" way to walk. In our session, she found the permission to discover a relational way of being with herself within her environment and settled into "effort with ease." She let go of her overriding desire to be perfect and saw, at the same time, the value in helping her own clients in a similar way. When we settle into a place of curiosity, rather than trying to correct ourselves, we open to our biointelligent reservoir, release habitual tension in our spiralic fascial matrix, and gain the ability to naturally access the shape-shifting support of grounding, centering, and uplift.

From the practitioner/guide perspective of this session, by setting myself up with pre-movement awareness and peripheral vision, the tone of the session became one of collaboration and non-judgment, which shaped the client's sense of safety, support, and receptivity. That type of environment can only be created by my fostering a deep communication with my Inner Guide who is, at all times, seeking to communicate with another's Inner Guide. Again, I call this communication Wholehearted or Deep Listening and Speaking.

To listen to the Inner Guide is to listen deeply. Unfortunately, we rarely hear what others are really saying to us because we are mostly listening to our *little voice*—the one in our internal dialogue that sows self-doubt and that is talking to us all day long. Listening to this little voice has, for many of us, become automatic. This little voice is often talking to ourselves even when someone else is talking to us, and because this internal dialogue is also by nature self-centered and judgmental, it often obscures what others are trying to communicate.

The internal dialogue with the little voice cannot be simply switched off. It is hardwired into our brain's functioning. We can, however, learn to reduce the internal dialogue's volume. By learning Deep Listening, we can train the mind to listen for the spirit or *wholehearted commitment* of what someone is telling us. When we listen for a wholehearted commitment, we are listening *for* what the person values and what moves them deeply. I have found that a client's request to be more flexible, stronger, relaxed, etc. is usually driven by a much deeper desire to be in relationship with the fullness of life. So, just stretching some muscle group never truly addresses what is needed—whole-body integration, connection, and core coordination. When the act of listening becomes a conscious inquiry into the spirit of whatever message you are receiving, the internal dialogue with the little voice loses its power and strength. In its place arises a new communication

with the self that, in turn, transforms how we communicate with others.

The client I shared about a moment ago who had negative thoughts about herself got in touch with her wholehearted commitment and ability to help herself through our collaborative conversation which inspired her to perceive herself newly through her biointelligent wisdom. I have noticed that in order to engage in Wholehearted Listening, I must consciously shift both my *attention* and *intention* in a conversation in order to create a space where safety, support, and self-expression are foregrounded and valued. First, I must shift the focus of my attention away from my own world and toward that of the other person's world. Then I shift the intention of my focus away from the voice of the "expert" toward the voice of one who envisions and creates a space designed to benefit both parties—a collaborative conversation.

With Deep Listening, you receive, register, and echo what is going on with that person. For instance, if a friend or client confides in you about feeling disconnected from their body, you have the opportunity to just hear what they are saying and have them feel heard. Witnessing someone's upset can be a healing gift. Then pay attention to what that person's deeper commitment might be in the conversation, rather than just giving advice or trying to fix. When you listen with the intention that your friend or client will experience a feeling of support and self-expression, being met where they are can awaken a space of resolution and curiosity about the next steps to take. All your questions and comments revolve around that supportive intention, so that something new might be birthed over time out of the space of empathy, commitment, and relationship.

I have experienced that by making this shift in orientation from myself to others, I have almost immediately begun to see and hear things in conversations with mentoring teachers and clients that were previously inaccessible to me. It is said that energy flows where attention goes. The power of Deep Listening is that it creates a kind of force field that attracts more of whatever its attention focuses on, which in turn helps you to manifest the attention and intention for any conversation.

Wholehearted Listening is an act of generosity. You are seeking the authentic nature of the person speaking, instead of settling for only the most obvious meaning in their words. That authentic nature exists for everyone, all the time, even when it is not apparent. A person may have low self-esteem, but that is not the totality of who that person is. What I have noticed is that if I become receptive and open to the unexpected outcomes of my encounters with others, I will recognize the heartfelt commitment behind what the person is saying, and then the conversation can become more authentic and empowering, and both of us learn and grow in the process.

Responding to this client by finding my own centering and grounding through pre-movement awareness allowed me to hold her in the potent space of her biointelligent awareness, which enabled her to enter a new self-healing possibility. Remember that your fascial matrix is a fluid, fiber-optic electrical network that communicates like a finely tuned musical instrument to other social beings, and so listening closely in this way through Deep Listening has the potential to be a transformative physical and interpersonal action. Within the spatial orientation of Deep Listening, any conversation becomes more mindful and meaningful to you and to the person with whom you are speaking. That is the magic of Wholehearted Listening through the pre-tensed fascial matrix—it is multi-dimensional and omnidirectional. We are listening to our biointelligent Inner Guide, and deep healing on many levels happens in the process. This is an embodied listening.

AUTOMATIC LISTENING AND WHOLEHEARTED LISTENING

Wholehearted Listening has an opposite—what I call "Automatic Listening." To demonstrate the difference between the two, consider a situation in which a Pilates teacher introduces a student to the Footwork on the Reformer.

Teaching Through Automatic Listening

- Client is told to put a prescribed spring weight on, without noticing or being supported in discovering what works best for their body and movement needs.

- Client is given cues as to how to move by the "expert" who is teaching, and is not asked if that makes sense to them.

- An opportunity may never be considered: By teaching the "perfect form" of the exercise only one way, am I devaluing the client's curiosity of exploring *their experience* of that form and whether or not it is meeting their body's needs at that time?

- A not uncommon result is that the client feels like they're doing things the *right* way (to please the teacher).

If a session leads to the actions outlined in that bulleted list, the teacher is likely relying on Automatic Listening. The client, on the other hand, misses the opportunity to develop interoceptive listening awareness, through which they would begin to sense how to help themselves, rather than just perform exercises.

Teaching Through Wholehearted Listening

- Client is asked what spring weight allows them to feel their whole body from foot to head when they straighten their legs.

- Client is engaged as a collaborative partner with the person teaching the session, so cues are used to deepen the client's interoceptive awareness. Even a great cue that may work for one person might not work for another, so the teacher does not think, "This client just doesn't get my great cue," but, rather, adjusts the language, touch, image, or demonstration of the cue. Cueing can be transformational when the practitioner/guide is being present with what each client needs and supports their shape-shifting nature.

- Client and practitioner/guide are in resonance and can move through a rhythmical flow of movements with a sense of collaboration and playful elasticity.

- Client is treated as a deeply intelligent living process who knows how to self-heal, self-organize, and adapt.

- Since each person is unique, each session is unique. A practitioner/guide may feel like they've experienced a new approach to a familiar technique, as if for the first time, because of their deep listening to the unique feedback of an individual client within a session.

Guided by Wholehearted Listening, the client is treated as an active participant in the exploration of Footwork, with the intention of having the client step off the Reformer and be more aware in their body in walking and every other activity of daily living. Wholehearted Listening is a potent space that a practitioner gifts to their client, within which clients and students can access a way of being in life that empowers their ability to help themselves. This level of learning cannot be unlearned as it is in dialogue with the biointelligent awareness of the client. This space of Deep Listening is only possible when the practitioner has a befriending relationship with themselves prior to meeting the client or student.

As we are exploring, the act of listening is related to both verbal and non-verbal communication. Someone sends out vibrations through the air with their voice, your ears pick up these sounds, your fascial matrix body senses whole-body communication (your innate biotensegrity body connected through a tension-compression relationship internally and externally, from cellular nucleus to cosmos), and your bodymind translates the communication into something meaningful. In English, we pack all of this into the word "listening." It is interesting to turn for a moment to Chinese where the symbol for listening contains reminders of the whole-body collaboration involved in this seemingly simple and passive act. Note that, in that symbol, "listening" doesn't exist without collaboration between mind, ears, eyes, undivided attention, and, of course, heart.

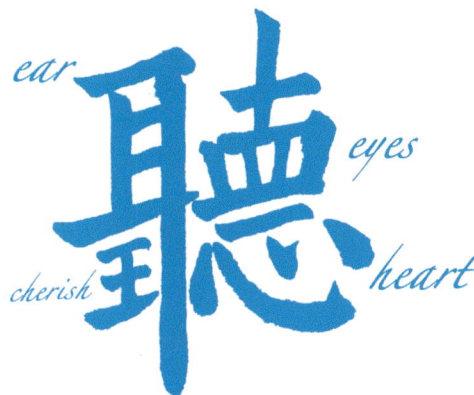

Figure 5.4 Listening from the whole body
CHINESE SCRIPT: www.skillpacks.com/chinese-character-listening-5day-plan

Deep Listening is a more complex exchange that is taking place in the teaching–learning relationship. There are two main ways of listening—Automatic Listening and Wholehearted Listening.

The most important aspect of listening is your focus of *attention* and *intention*. Being aware of these two basics can transform your listening ability. Listening is a force field that attracts whatever it focuses its attention on. My early life was dominated by the internal dialogue going on in my head all day long. I had low self-esteem and felt I wasn't smart enough, which colored my perception about my ability to live fully and caused me to be mistrustful of other people—this is Automatic Listening. Through participating in transformation programs, I began to see these perceptions as "story boxes" that determined who I was, how I felt, and the actions I took in life. I also realized that I had everyone and everything in my life in some sort of "story box"—stuck in past-based thinking.

As I was coached to see that these stories were mostly perceptions that I had shaped into reality, I had the ability to alter them. This stroke of insight, that reality and perception get collapsed into "the truth" by Automatic Listening, was a defining moment in my life. What I realized was that I had a perception of what happened, and that is "my truth" rather than "the truth."

My attention to being able to shift my awareness was then focused on a second life-altering lesson—that the quality of my life and my peace of mind are more determined by my mental attitude than my physical circumstances.

What I have discovered is that the Automatic Listening internal dialogue:

- tends to be me-focused—not open to new ways of thinking or collaboration

- is judgmental—always seeing the flaws in others and ourselves

- goes for win/lose—resists the search for middle ground

- decides and judges everything on the basis of the past.

An exercise that I explore with mentoring practitioners illuminates the direct experience of this kind of negative listening:

- Each partner chooses to be A or B.

- Partner A (speaker) is instructed to speak to partner B for two minutes about something that A is passionate and excited about.

- Partner B (listener) is instructed to behave in a self-focused, Automatic Listening way and think distracted, negative thoughts about A, such as "This person is boring," "This person doesn't know what they are talking about," "This person doesn't really matter."

- Partner A as the speaker becomes totally deflated very rapidly, even though they know that B has been instructed to be a poor listener. Afterwards, A reports that they lost their train of thought and began stumbling in their speaking, even though they knew their subject matter very well. They lost confidence in the topics they were so passionate about. Then they began to lose confidence in *themselves*. Within two minutes of being exposed to Automatic Listening, they became someone who doesn't matter, with nothing of interest to say!

In Wholehearted Listening, attention and intention are actually co-created by both parties within the conversation. A listener may set an intention before the dialogue begins, such as "I will meet this person where they are, and something beneficial will come from this encounter." As the dialogue commences, precisely what this intention means will become clear. Intention is co-created through the content of the speaker and the constantly refined listening of the receiver.

To listen on this level, you become aware of your negative listening filters and return to your wholehearted commitment to be generous and have the other person be empowered. To do this, the focus of attention shifts from your world to their world, and your intention shifts from benefiting just you to benefiting both of you. The second you shift away from Automatic Listening, the whole energy of the conversation changes, and you then begin to see and hear new things. You are now attending to the speaker and what is really going on with them. You are looking for their wholehearted commitment. This is the level of listening where you can begin to pick up messages in their speaking—facts, feelings, and wholehearted commitments or values.

The philosophy active in this scenario translates seamlessly into the teaching sessions within movement and bodywork.

This shift from Automatic to Wholehearted Listening is an act of generosity. Instead of seeing only one aspect of your partner or student, you are looking for their wholehearted nature. Suddenly, what they are saying, or how they are saying it, takes on a whole different meaning. You will begin to understand what they are really trying to say and what they need. When you alter your listening in the middle of a conversation, you can feel the transformation. It becomes a more empowering environment.

STORY: My father was a very abused child and became an abuser. I had written off our relationship until I participated in transformational work. In one program, a man who was a recovering alcoholic stood up and began sharing. At that moment, my father came to mind, which surprised me. What was even more shocking was that his very difficult, sad life flashed before my eyes, and unbelievably, I saw his pain and sadness in ways I never could before. I also saw how hard he had worked to be a good father, and that was the first time I had ever realized that. My heart opened to him, and I decided to write him a letter. Then I decided to take it to him. I hadn't seen him in quite a while, and when he, surprised, opened the door, I said, "I have something for you." We sat on the sofa, and I gave him the letter where I told him things he did not believe about himself—that I loved him and was proud of him and knew he had done his best job as my dad. I can still feel the incredible heart space open now that opened then. He started crying, put his hand on my knee, and said, "You have no idea what this means to me." I immediately touched his hand, and our hearts touched. What was also incredible about this experience was how this action changed my dad—he became more receptive, loving, and vulnerable to his daughters and my mom, and we had some beautiful conversations before he died.

What is most important here is the *healing story* that was birthed as I re-examined my life's experience through the lens of compassion, which gave new meaning to old pain and wounds.

WHOLEHEARTED LISTENING AND SPEAKING WITH INTENTION

This is the other end of the spectrum. It is an act of co-creation. You begin to use your listening and speaking in a conscious way to shape and co-create reality. Like the "knife of the carver," your words give birth to whatever you say. As in Wholehearted Listening, what is important is to focus your attention and intention. The focus of attention is on the other person, and your intention is that your listening and speaking is wholehearted. It creates a totally different dynamic, a dance of creation and possibility. In Wholehearted Listening and Speaking with Intention, collaborative conversations begin to happen naturally.

Moving Beyond Core, up until this point, has provided a roadmap for how we sense this for ourselves. We awaken to the wisdom of our Inner Guide by bridging biomechanical approaches to our bodies with relational and biointelligent ways of movement through fascial matrix awareness. We befriend our breath as a bridge connecting matter and spirit. We look beyond "doing" to the realm of *effort with ease*. And then, at that point, after becoming fully aware of our pre-movement and ongoing relationships with our spatial surroundings, we are ready to meet a client.

For those of us who are also bodyworkers, whose ways of touching are equally as important as our ways of speaking, it is exciting to consider how that is a form of communication:

When we touch the surface, we stir the depths. (Juhan 2003, p.43)

There is a picture from an article, years ago, called "The Rescuing Hug." The article details the first week of life of a set of twins. Each were in their respective incubators, and one was not expected to live. A hospital nurse fought against hospital rules and placed the babies in one incubator. When they were placed together, the healthier of the two threw an arm over her sister in an endearing embrace. The smaller baby's heart rate stabilized and her temperature rose to normal.

The process at work in this story is co-regulation, where the healthier twin effectively communicated its vibrancy to its sibling. As practitioners, we can challenge ourselves to allow each word we speak and our entire way of being

in our sessions and workshops to touch our students and clients in a way not unlike the way this sibling touches her twin.

Touch, which we will remember is our first sense to develop in the womb, awakens an entire way of being for the client, for the teacher, and for the collaboration between both parties. Touch from fascial matrix to fascial matrix evokes a space of transformation which takes place in each collaborative session.

For instance, here is a testimonial from a gentleman who attended a one-hour presentation I offered at a weekend retreat:

I found your invitations to explore my relationship with gravity to be gentle, accessible, and profound. With your enthusiastic guidance, I could feel what you were explaining in my own body. That is a type of learning that cannot be unlearned. From the brief exercises that we were guided through, I came away with a whole new sense of my relationship with gravity and the earth's support. I feel it now as I sit at my computer, the gentle lifting of the edge of my desk supporting my palms...the firm encouragement of my chair...and the floor beneath my feet. There is a grounded-ness which is absurdly freeing. As though having my roots firmly planted allows my branches to reach out and wave with abandon. I like it!

My words touched this client as he shared: "I could *feel* what you were explaining in my own body." The meaning of my words (the intention I wanted to impart to him as a student) only became clear as the meaning came alive for him within his own body. My words were landing through *touch*. His listening was embodied. Together we collaborated and met in that space where meaning is evoked, which in his particular case was a felt sense of his biotensegrity body—his tension-compression continuity, and fascial communication.

BODY IMAGE AND BODY SCHEMA

When you work with instructors of dance, yoga, tai chi, Pilates, Alexander Technique, Feldenkrais or dozens of other kinds of movement training, you are basically working on *body schema* awareness. These methods teach you to purposefully attend to the many core elements of your schema as a means of self-exploration. (Blakeslee and Blakeslee 2007, p.37)

Let's examine the dueling body maps that are constantly at play in our lives and which deeply affect us: body image and body schema. *Body schema* is your internal conversation, a felt sense of your body based on physical properties and perceptions. *Body image* is a retroactively applied map of your own body designed by others—for example, media, family members, stories we hear.

Let's look at a great story that Oprah Winfrey shared about her lion-hearted battle with yo-yo dieting. She shared that for 20 years she lived her life unconsciously, feeling out of control, ashamed, lonely, and filled with self-loathing. Because she was afraid to confront her traumatic past, she ate compulsively just to dull the pain. Finally, she decided to take control of her life and, with hard work and determination, took on a physical conditioning and food awareness program that changed her life. What is not so well known is that her transformation can also be described as a story of dueling body maps, of how she used one body map (body schema) to remodel a second body map (body image). In other words, she had applied an image of her body to herself and her sense of identity, even though that image was not created by her or for her benefit. The fit was always uneasy, and the struggle against it perpetuated disordered eating. Only when she stopped obeying the command of the external image and started befriending herself through optimal (physical and emotional) nutrition and movement was she able to create a new body schema for her identity, a new model from which a new self-created body image could emerge.

I call that transformation the process of *your ideal body becoming your real body*.

What I have discovered and noticed in 40 years of studies and my own personal practice with pioneers of somatic arts and sciences, breath, bodywork, embryology, and energy medicine is that when we learn to listen and be guided by our body wisdom, in relationship with gravity and spatial orientation, body schema begins to support, feed, and transform our body image. We learn to embody our true selves.

When we discover the inherent wisdom and intelligence within every organ and cell of our body and our body-wide fascial matrix by allowing ourselves to rediscover how, for example, to *rest down* and find our backing, we connect with the natural healing energy of the earth, and realign with our primal nature and relationship within the matrix of the natural world. This is the first step toward empowering our body schema to actively shape our identity of self.

Body Schema

You have sensors all over your body surface that are responsive to tender caresses, pressure, pain, heat, or cold. Your body is also endowed with specialized receptors that detect tiny movements—through muscle fibers, bones, joint spaces, and throughout your fascial matrix, especially feet and hands. Whenever these sensors undergo changes through movement, which are first organized through your primary touch map, they signal your brain to update your sense of where you are in space and how your body is configured at the time. The weight of your body and its postures are calculated by these sensors in what is called "proprioception"—meaning perception of one's own (place, position). Your body schema is a physiological construct. Your bodymind creates it from the interaction of touch, vision, proprioception, balance, and hearing. It even extends out into the space around your body. For instance, when a golfer addresses a ball on the green before putting, that club becomes part of that golfer's body and allows them to scan their surroundings, adjusting in micromovements for how far, fast, and delicately to putt the ball toward the hole.

There are two other sensors within your body's felt sense, or body schema, that operate on a subconsciousness level: one reads signals from inside your body, and the other reads signals from your inner ear to assist you with a sense of balance. Balance is achieved by integrating your inner ear "vestibular system," three little canals, tiny stones, and hairs inside your inner ear that specialize in detecting gravity and acceleration on three axes—up and down, left and right, forward and back.

Balance does not happen just in your head; vestibular signals are intimately tied to touch. Nothing stabilizes your balance better than contact with your environment. Balance is dynamic, and gravity is constant—we are recalibrating all the time.

The soles of your feet have touch receptors that send signals to your brain when you stand and put pressure on the ground, making them essential resources in the production of body schema. Signals conducted through the feet connect with higher brain maps and vestibular, visual, and other touch information to keep you balanced and adaptive. These foot signals can dull with aging and health issues that affect blood flow, but also by not using your feet, which is why walking on stones or barefoot on uneven ground can keep your vestibular system in tune.

Body Image

Like your body schema, body image has its basis in the way your body maps itself.

Table 5.1 Quick reference for body image and body schema

Body image—our external conversation	Body schema—our internal conversation
• This is where we "put on the mask" from *learned* attitudes about our body, and create "storyboxes" about ourselves and others • It is *personal* and patterned by our history, life circumstances, and development through imitation of others, which can result in positive or negative experiences • It is a potential filter through which "coordination" often has to pass, and can interfere with natural movement, because we want to "look good" to the teacher, rather than become more aware of what is presently happening or needed • It is oriented with what others think of us or tell us to do • It is guided by over-recruitment of muscles to act in an idealized way • It is oriented with a biomechanical notion of the body as an object to be trained and fixed—a doing-it-the-right-way approach to movement	• This is *our felt sense* based on our body wisdom and relationship with gravity • It is *not personal* and does not differentiate "body" from the space around the body • It is oriented with the development of our inner ear/vestibular awareness and a sense of *grounded presence* • It doesn't "think" about a particular muscle, like the psoas or fascia, as being the most important. It "knows" the body as a complex palette of whole-body movements, gestures, and behaviors • It is oriented with a biointelligent biotensegrity—with a body as a living process that learns through curiosity, exploration, adaptation, and discovery movement approach

Your body schema is based on how your brain perceives touch, vision, proprioception, balance, and hearing, and how that awareness extends out to the space around your body. Your body image, on the other hand, includes the beliefs you have about your body. These beliefs are produced by the cells in your brain and body, cells that also create, store, and update information that shapes your expectations about how the world operates.

While the body schema is largely a function of body parts in motion, your body image draws on a larger web involving your library of personal experiences and memories. Your family, peers, and culture provide the content, and you provide the interpretation.

If you lose weight and still feel overweight, it may be due to a mismatch between your body image and body schema.

Moving Beyond Core is a way of being with ourselves that brings us back to favoring our body schema by sensing whole-body relationships in novel ways. When we allow our body schema to shape our sense of self, we can heal traumas and discover a more authentic way of being with ourselves within the gravitational field.

As educators of movement and/or bodywork, we live in a world that is saturated with images of "ideal" bodies, so it is not surprising that so many people struggle with self-esteem and body image issues. We have the opportunity through Wholehearted Deep Listening and Speaking, however, to create a new story. I know that when we truly befriend and value ourselves, we wake up to a loving way of being of gratitude and acceptance that feeds our wholeheartedness. This way of being enables us to create spaces of safety, support, and loving kindness for ourselves, clients, and mentoring teachers.

EMBODIED PARTNERING WITH ANOTHER PERSON (A COLLABORATIVE CONVERSATION)

Partnering with a client or colleague is a very potent experience that can be transformational. We have the opportunity to truly "meet" one another through an embodied sense of touch, from cellular awareness to fascial matrix resonance, communicating "what is just enough effort" to evoke an embodied awareness that is loving presence. I call this approach "Core to Core" or "whole-person to whole-person" touch. This embodied touch enables the client to cultivate and grow their relationship with their own Inner Guide. This way of approaching touch has a co-regulatory, therapeutic effect.

As we are a porous self, in relationship with gravity, ourselves, one another, and our environment, we have the opportunity to experience the exquisite dance of self with other—meeting ourselves and being met—Core as Relationship.

Gravity Press Embodied Assessment with Partner as Guide

This is a powerful orienting experience for the client to become their own Inner Guide. The guide first establishes their own pre-movement awareness with peripheral vision and sensing their feet—as we explored in Chapter 4. There is a pre-test and post-test for the client to notice that, in the course of the exploration with their Guide, their experience of being in their body, in standing balance, evokes their own bio-intelligent wisdom. **See Video 5.5 for deeper exploration.**

▸ Developing Lower Core awareness—pre-test.

▸ Client sensing how their pelvis relates to their whole foot.

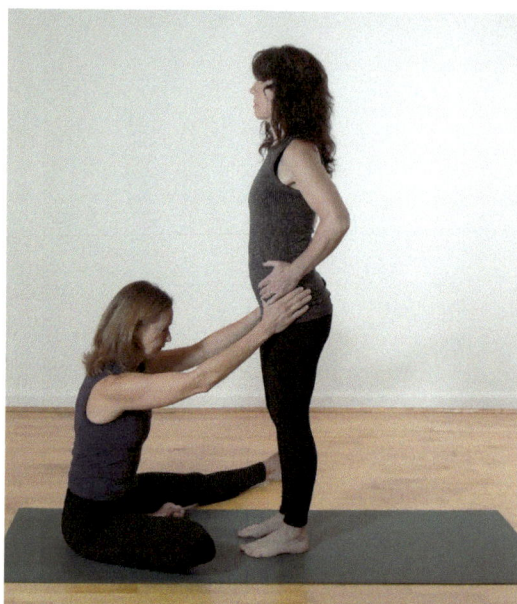

Figure 5.5A

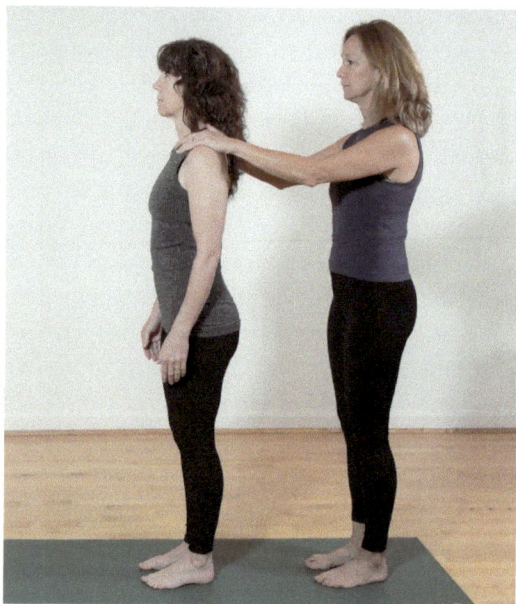

Figure 5.5C

▸ Client sensing how they are weighted in their whole foot.

▸ Developing Central Core awareness—shoulder blades to low belly suspenders.

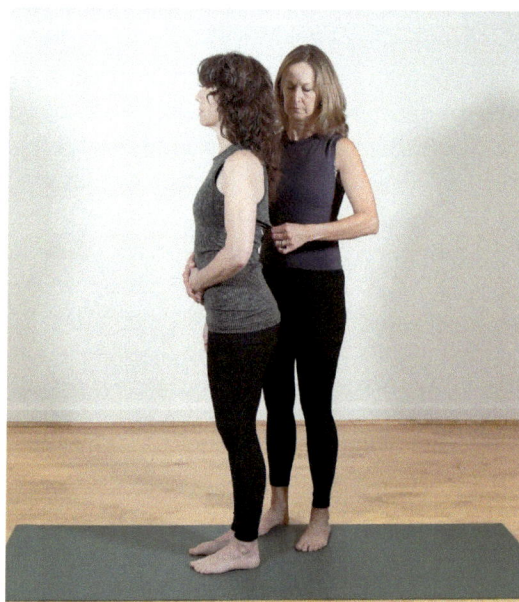

Figure 5.5B

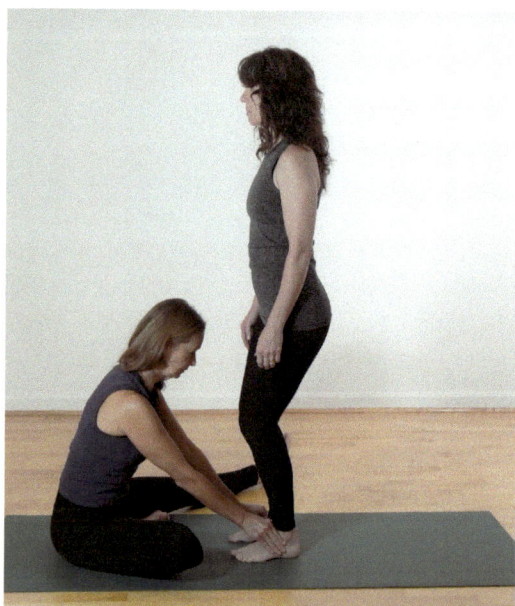

Figure 5.5D

▸ Client sensing breath awareness.

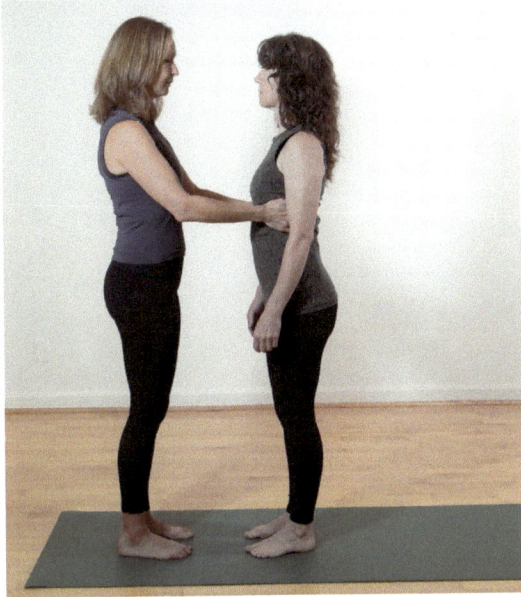

Figure 5.5E

▸ Developing Upper Core awareness—soft occiput related to sacrum and talus.

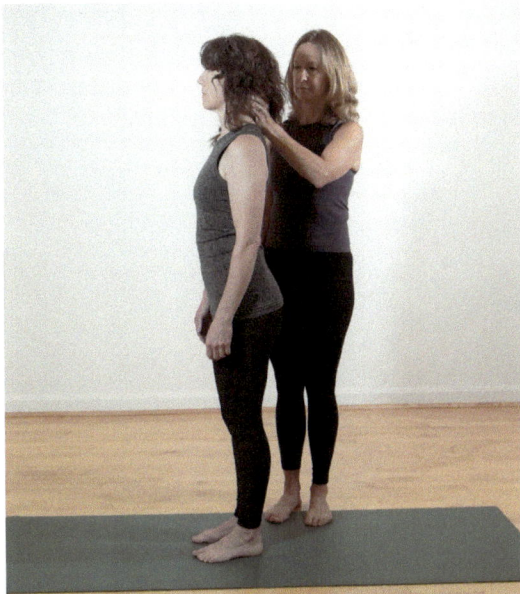

Figure 5.5F

▸ Embodied gravity press body assessment—post-test.

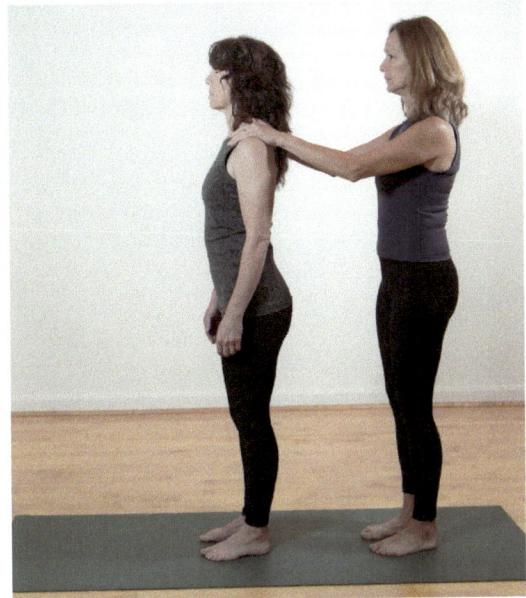

Figure 5.5G

Footwork at Wall with Partner as Guide

There is a powerful recalibration relationship through Domes of Uplift—from inner arch of feet to pelvic diaphragm, respiratory diaphragm, thoracic inlet to palate and domes of hands. This sets up a whole person Core-to-Core touch. **See Video 5.6 for deeper exploration**.

▸ Client is standing facing wall, with hands gently touching wall, sensing waterfall Down the Back, with a squishy ball between their heels.

▸ Guide is sitting behind client on the floor, near client's feet.

▸ Setting up Core-to-Core touch by guide:

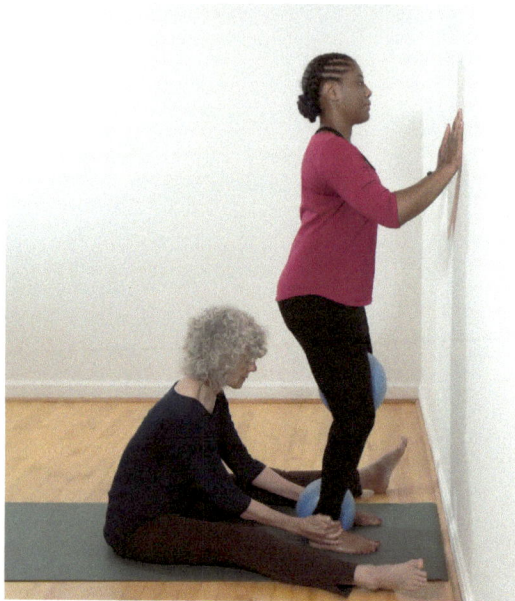

Figure 5.6A

- Guide gives just enough contact to support softening ankles, as client softens knees.

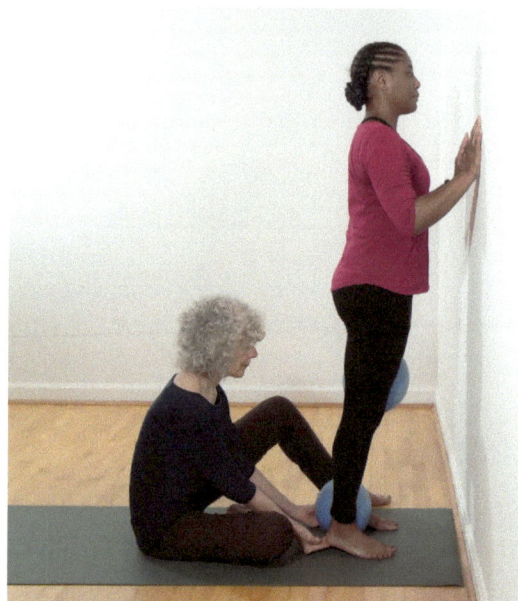

Figure 5.6B

- Guide places first two fingers under client's heels to support heavy heels feeling.

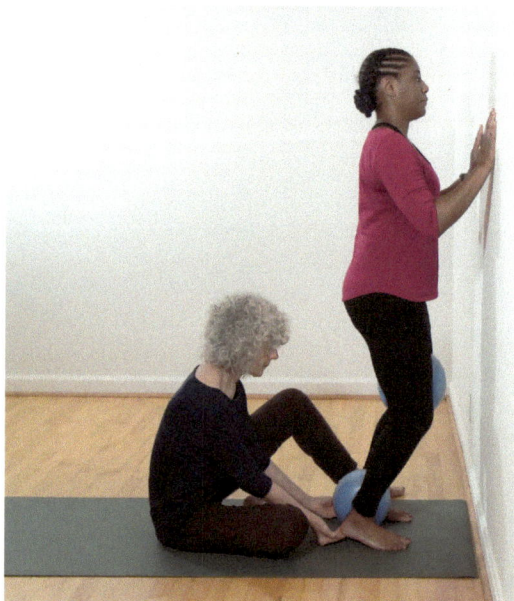

Figure 5.6C

- Guide gives just enough support, as client straightens legs.

Core-to-Core touch establishes pre-movement awareness prior to making contact with client, enabling the hands to come from a deeper place of embodied touch—whole person to whole person—where both parties grow in awareness. This is a very different experience from just putting your hands on someone's body to fix.

Bridge with Partner as Guide

Embodying Core Coordination from feet to head and hands—meeting others and being met.

▸ Client notices when they feel met by Guide and in collaboration with movement awareness.

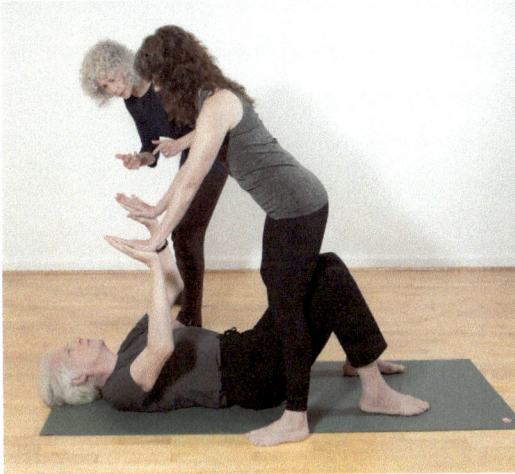

Figure 5.7A

▸ Guide makes contact with client's hands.

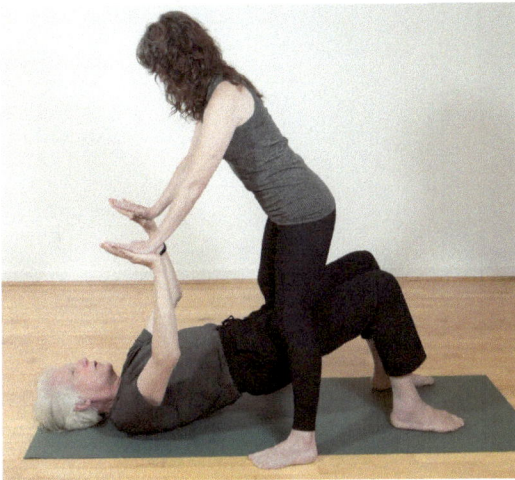

Figure 5.7B

▸ Guide supports client's bridge with waterfall down back from hands.

Guide and client keep checking in to see what feels nourishing to client. Notice that in order for your Lower Core to curl your breathing spine up from pelvic diaphragm to respiratory diaphragm, your Upper Core needs to feel grounded yet spacious, so that your head and neck can feel free and able to orient with your feet. **See Video 5.7 for deeper exploration.**

Heavy Head in Hands with Partner as Guide

Embodied Preparation for Pilates 100s, Rollup, One-Leg Rollup, etc.

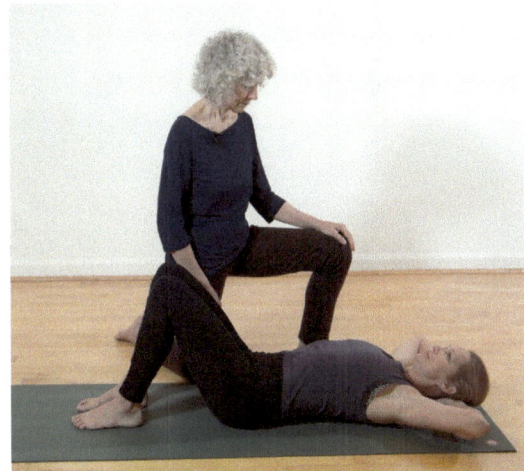

Figure 5.8A

▸ Guide is on client's side, comfortably positioned so your arms can feel free to touch and guide your client's movement awareness.

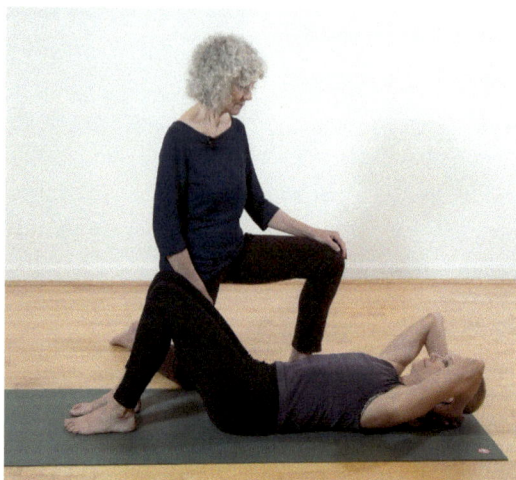

Figure 5.8B

▸ Client laces hands together, making a basket for head to rest into, so head can rest in hands.

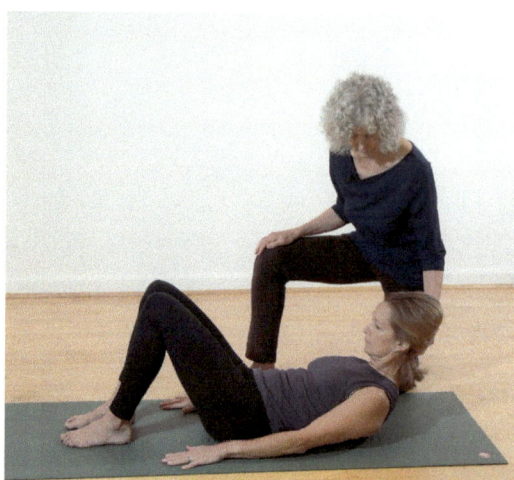

Figure 5.8D

▸ Client allows your inhale into back, sensing *backing*, and as you exhale, gently press into your feet to curl forward, with the support of your Guide.

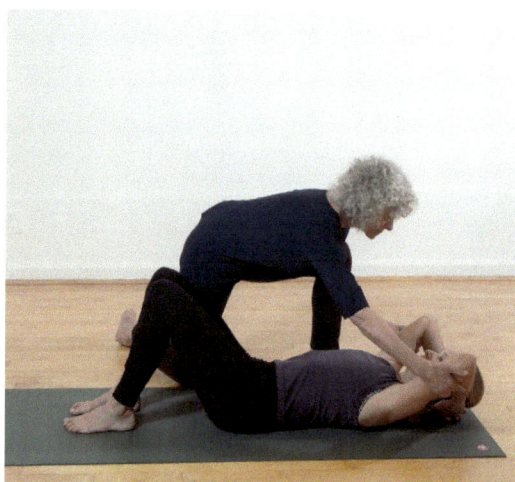

Figure 5.8C

▸ Guide places hands inside your client's elbow fold so you can support their rounding forward on the exhale.

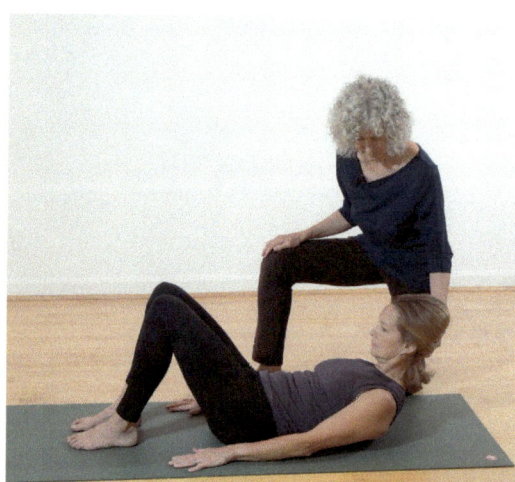

Figure 5.8E

▸ Guide places hand behind client's head to support their head float (check in to see you have your own waterfall supporting your hand) in order for them to release their arms (Down the Back) to pump arms gently or play with moving arms away from body on inhale and bringing arms close to body on exhale to sense elastic recoil breath.

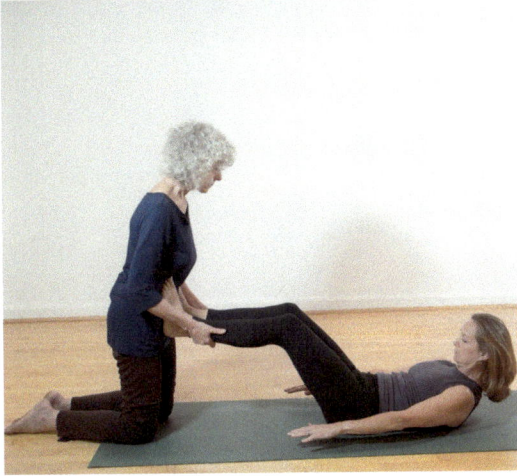

Figure 5.8F

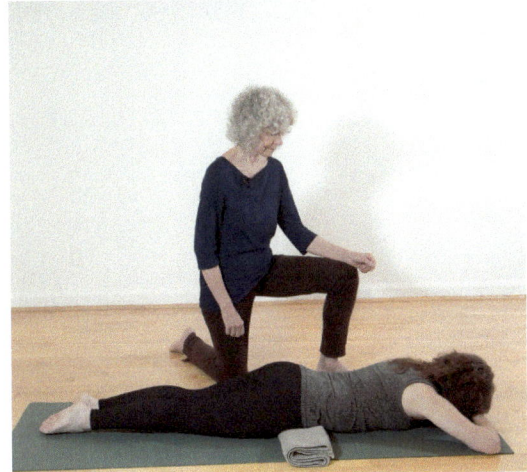

Figure 5.9A

▸ Guide moves their body to meet client's feet on Guide's abdomen, pressing gently into your Guide's support to feel uplift.

Play with the Pilates Matwork with feet on the wall, using weights in your hands/wrists, on your ankles, etc., to gain more *rooting, reaching, and backing* through your upper body as your shoulder blades waterfall Down the Back to your sacrum and feet. **See Video 5.8A for deeper exploration.**
    See Video 5.8B for exploration of One-Leg Rollup, Climb a Tree with Pilates Cadillac Push Thru Bar.

Swan or Cobra with Partner as Guide
Remembering how your embryonic yolk sac/front body supports your back body in softening, widening, and lengthening—freeing up your shoulders and head and neck when you extend your spine.

▸ Client lying prone on a mat, pillow, or pad under front of pelvis and above pubic bone to support uplift through low belly suspenders, head resting on the backs of your palms.

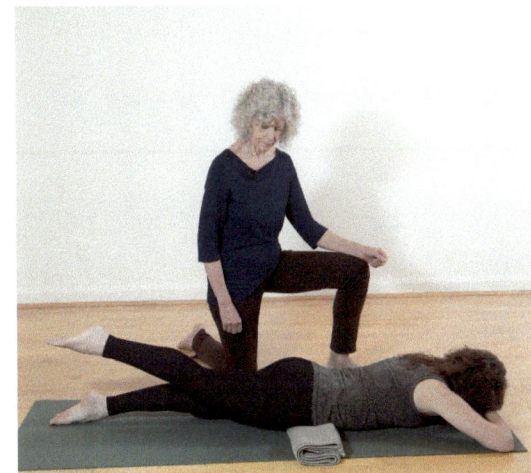

Figure 5.9B

▸ Reach long through each leg to enliven your Lower Core/legs, rooting from hamstring to inner thigh to the front of your pelvic diaphragm (low belly suspenders).

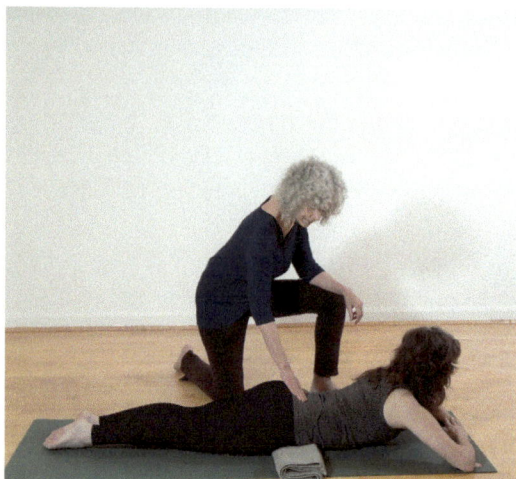

Figure 5.9C

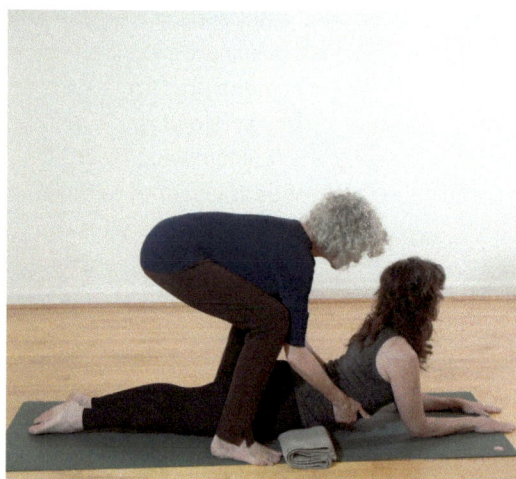

Figure 5.9E

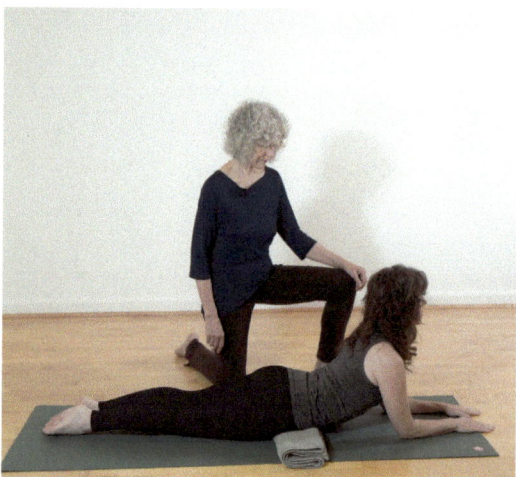

Figure 5.9D

▶ Then watch an ant crawl along the floor, up the wall, sensing your pelvis taking more weight as your arms spiral your elbows under your shoulders—coming onto your forearms.

▶ Reset your body so you are straddling your client's pelvis, facing forward toward their head. Place your hands in front of their low belly suspenders, inside each of the ileums, slightly below their navel.

As you are more comfortable in the fluid movement onto your forearms, look further up the wall and rise onto your hands. This is the foundational understanding of Pilates Swan Dive—arms in relationship with spine and fully able to extend and reach. **See Video 5.9A for deeper exploration.**

See Video 5.9B for Swan with Guide on Pilates Cadillac Push Thru Bar. This rootedness of the legs in the Lower Core to the front of the spine is often what is missing to free the shoulders for full extension in Pilates Swan Dive on the Cadillac Push Thru Bar.

Lying Spiral with Partner as Guide

Core Coordination from foot to head and hand—a powerful recalibration of your fascial matrix from foot to head and hand, supported by a Guide, which unravels fascial restrictions and provides a clear felt sense of grounding, centering, and uplift.

▶ Client—on your back, left side close to your Guide, with enough space so you can roll to your left side, with right knee bent with foot on floor; left leg is elongated on floor, left arm extended up next to your head. Place your right hand on the Guide's right shoulder and allow your left arm to release up on the floor so you can roll into your left armpit, if that is comfortable for you, or just do what is most comfortable.

▸ Client—you will be sensing this movement three times, and each time you will go deeper, so take your time. As you press into your right foot and begin to roll to the left, imagine you are pouring sand from left foot and hip to right hip.

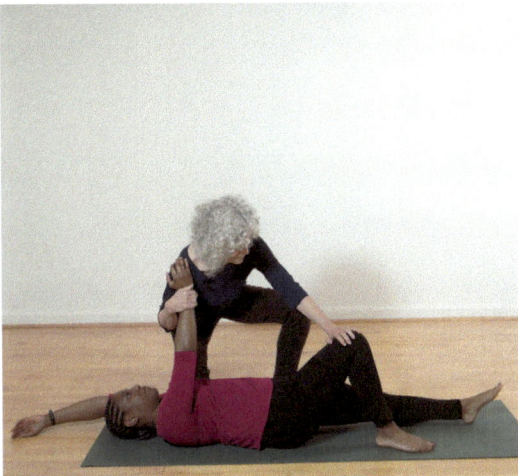

Figure 5.10C

▸ Guide—keep noticing how you can reset your awareness to be supporting rather than inhibiting client's roll from right to left side.

This simple yet profound act of rolling is a reset for our fascial matrix perineural nervous system, which supports our central nervous system. When we sense the weight shift of pouring sand from one foot to the opposite hip, we awaken a cascade of myofascial releases from foot to head and hand. **See Video 5.10 for deeper exploration.**

A great pre-test and post-test for the Lying Spiral with Partner is for the client to sense what a Pilates Rollup feels like before and after this fascially releasing movement sequence.

Squat with Partner as Guide

A powerful experience of breathing feet and spine through talus release and interosseous membrane softening and widening. **See Video 5.11 for deeper exploration.**

▸ Client stands barefoot and senses their unsupported squat, then Guide places the inner arch of each foot at the front crease of client's ankles. Client opens both palms to Guide, and Guide makes contact with client's palms

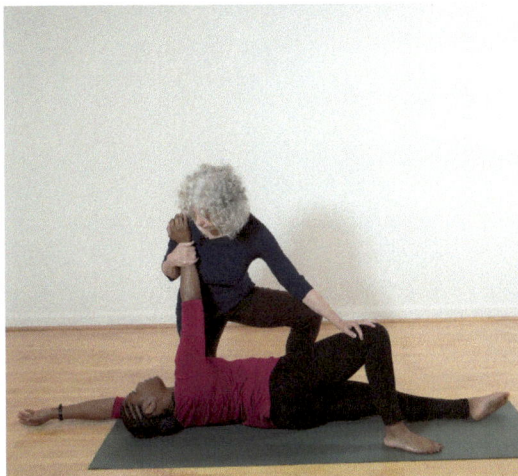

Figure 5.10A

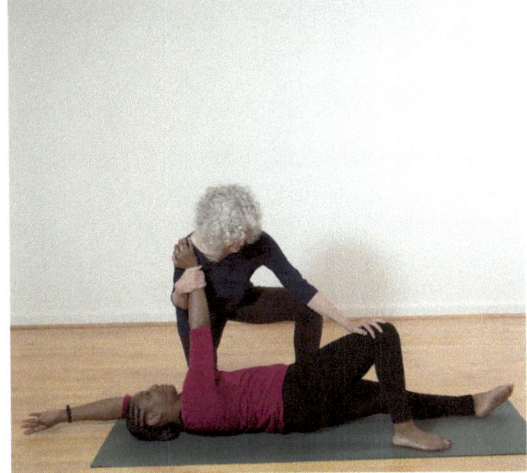

Figure 5.10B

by holding each pinkie between their thumb and first finger—so you have a solid contact between your palms.

▸ Client begins to squat down, sensing inner ears floating up. Guide presses gently into client's ankles, straightening Guide's legs and arms, in the same tension-compression timing with client moving, which supports client's squat.

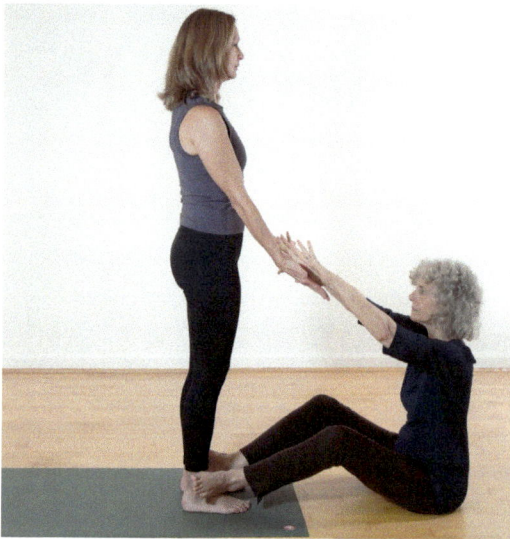

Figure 5.11A

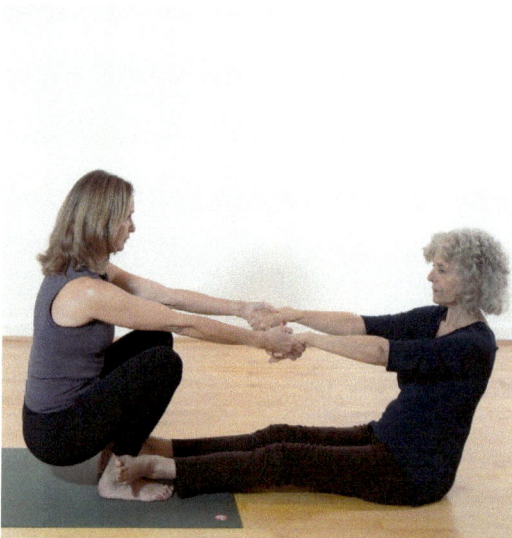

Figure 5.11B

Then in order for client to stand up:

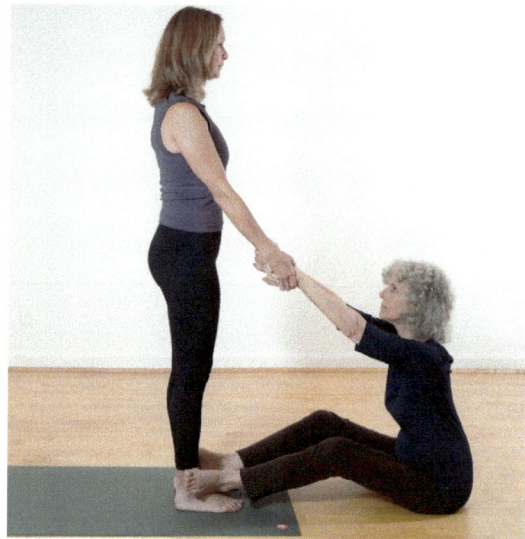

Figure 5.11C

▸ Guide keeps legs and arms extended, leaning back, with just enough time for client to feel internal lift from foot to head, then Guide bends knees, keeps hips where they are, and reaches arms up from sitting bones to support client standing up.

– The sensations of Down the Back, Up the Front, of sensing lifting-while-grounding, will be coequal partners supporting one another as you begin to squat.

– If you squat down too far too early, your knees will take all the weight. As you begin to squat, can you sense what is going too far down, where you lose uplift? Allow your knees to sense the bidirectional support of ground and lift, so they can feel the spacious connection with internal lift through your spine and arms.

– Can you sense the distribution of the load of your body through your fascial flossing spine through the core coordination with your feet and hands?

This chapter continues *Moving Beyond Core*'s discussion of biointelligent approaches to movement and bodywork by focusing specifically on the dynamic of teaching or meeting someone in a private session or class. Ultimately, the most important aspect of the teaching relationship is more than how masterfully you execute or relay movements. It is how your way of being in life expresses itself through your teaching work. If our way is grounded in perfectionism, being the expert and being "right," or having our clients perform for us rather than develop their own awareness of what they need, then fear of failure or excess tension will likely show up in our teaching. This fear will even be palpable in the way we touch a client and guide them through a particular movement. By reframing the practitioner–client relationship as one based on a wholehearted communication practice, and by recognizing how that communication practice flows from one's way of being in the world (and vice versa), we reveal yet another facet of "whole-body movement." Communication ceases to be a mode of conveying whole-body and/or the "right" biointelligent cues to a client and becomes an embodied exchange between teacher and student which opens doors to unexpected ways of being that can be life-changing.

With this deeper awareness, we are prepared to move on to a chapter devoted to self-care, since there can be no authentic teaching or communicating if there is no nurturing of self.

Use the following QR code for all videos in this chapter:

REFERENCES

Blakeslee, M. and Blakeslee, S. (2007) *The Body Has a Mind of Its Own*. New York, NY: Random House.
Juhan, D. (2003) *Job's Body: A Handbook for Body Workshop*. Barrytown, NY: Station Hill Press.

CHAPTER 6

Self-Care as Context for Community Service and Resilience

I was once told a wonderful story about an efficiency expert who visited a chocolate factory and carefully watched how the women hand-dipped the chocolates. They had each developed a particular gestural style of spiraling and twirling a strawberry out of the chocolate after dipping, in order to prevent drips as they placed them on the paper. The efficiency expert realized they could save time by discontinuing their gestural patterning and instead taught them to make more direct in, out, over, and down pathways. Within a week, most of them were complaining of carpal tunnel symptoms. Their actions had become machine-like as they had lost their innate self-care gestural patterning, which included a creative, social way of being with one another, and instead became tunnel-visioned and prone to fatigue and injury.

I read this story as a parable for self-care. When a social and collaboratively formed movement sequence was swapped out for a supposedly "more efficient" style of movement, not only was efficiency *not* achieved, but the individuals supporting the work of the factory began to suffer. They had, without telling themselves or anybody else, found a way to care for their bodies within the repetitive movement requirements of the factory. When this self-care regimen was removed, everything fell apart. Sometimes maximizing mechanical efficiency can be contrary to self-care.

We arrive at the practice of self-care by beginning with cultivating our Inner Guide. Much of this book offers a foundational approach to our own self-care and our understanding of ourselves as a Soma, a living organism in relationship with the natural living world. In this chapter, I invite you to consider that a cared-for self is a prerequisite for all the main insights we've explored. Chief among those insights is a refining of the familiar catch phrase "Be in the present moment" toward an ever-emerging awareness of *listening for those moments* when our body needs our full presence.

I didn't start the book with an explicit conversation of self-care because I wanted to map the complex relationships that make up our human core, our biointelligent self. For self-care to occur, it is important to attend to:

- how we back ourselves

- how we find earth's support by yielding into gravity

- how we find our orienting center from inner ankle to inner ear

- how we move from striving for perfection and control to process-oriented movement and an empathetic way of being in life.

By learning to decrease the effort we exert in our movements and to increase our sensitivity level, we can feel more of what we need to take care of ourselves and become more responsive and adaptable.

This chapter builds on the relational framework that has been constructed throughout *Moving Beyond Core* to engage with the by-now well-known notion of self-care. By establishing a more personal conversation with your body, you cultivate a practice of tending to the ecological diversity that each one of us is. The language of ecological diversity helps us not only care for ourselves as individuals but also enhances our awareness of and interrelationship with the well-being of others in our personal lives and in our communities, so we all thrive.

Moving to the lush Blue Ridge Mountains of Asheville, North Carolina, from the urban sprawl of Austin, Texas, was definitely about self-care. We had lived in the city center for our entire lives and now longed for a deeper nurturing relationship with Mother Nature. The ecology of Austin was missing the diverse ecology that we so longed for and found in Asheville. I can still remember being wide-eyed, meandering down the drive of the two and a half acres of our future home, an oasis of trees, with a pond and two streams running through it. Stepping onto the mounds of moss and lichens immediately touched my heart. I love the smell and feel of the ancient mosses and lichens, which represent such an enchanting miniature interconnectedness of our natural living world, our symbiotic world. Mosses feed my soul. I could feel their nourishing impact as I learned a great lesson from this natural, lush environment—something about slowing down, about growth, decay, and regeneration. This was, of course, metaphorically important, but it was also

literally manifested in our daily lives. My husband, Michael, began opening to a new kind of self-care that was more somatically based, being gentler with himself in his movement practice, which created more intimacy between us. We were learning new lessons from Mother Nature about treasuring the limited time we have in our later years. We could see and feel the change of seasons before our eyes and within our hearts. We have met so many extraordinary people here in Asheville and are particularly grateful to Aditi Sethi, a dear friend and hospice doctor, who had a vision of community-focused end-of-life care, which has blossomed into the Center for Conscious Living & Dying (CCLD). We are grateful to be supporting the growth of this visionary center and the "death as part of life" awareness that has deepened our love for and cherishing of one another, and our community, as we walk hand in hand toward our dying time.

I mention all of this to emphasize the literal and metaphorical aspects of the term "ecological diversity" that is alive in the notion of self-care that I'm exploring with you in this chapter. When I think of my practice of self-care at this stage in my life—which I'll talk more about further on—I cannot separate the small acts of self-care from the natural environment in which I live. I cannot separate my self-care from that of my husband. I also cannot separate our unified care of self from the acts of care that extend into our community from organizations like the CCLD. The intrapersonal, interpersonal, and communal are all interwoven into the notion of self-care. Even when I do not explicitly mention each of these aspects in the practices below, they are present in the smallest details of our living bodies.

A SENSE OF PLAY AND CURIOSITY

These days, we frequently hear the term "self-care." More than that, we hear that we *must* do

self-care, that self-care is necessary. However, consider replacing the *mandate* of self-care with the playful responsiveness of a sustained self-care practice.

I invite you to consider that when your movement practice is grounded in somatic principles that evoke loving support, orientation, awareness, and attention, you can more easily adapt to challenging circumstances, as you are accessing the language of your body. For instance, if you are injured, is your instinct to slow down, rest, and be gentle with yourself? Or if you are aging and can no longer do the "sit-to-stand" movement without using your hands, is that a problem, or can you adapt by spiraling down and up, using your hands where appropriate, to continue developing and strengthening your whole-body continuity by playing with gravity? I would answer those questions by saying that self-care only arises when a given activity is approached with a befriending curiosity and a willingness to adapt any "set" framework to suit your needs in each given moment. Otherwise, any so-called "self-care" activity may turn into something that doesn't benefit you at all.

We will approach this conversation with our body through a playful, curious way of being with *what's just enough support* that facilitates or motivates self-care practices, so they are constantly teaching us. Often, using "props" allows a deeper sense of fascial unwinding and support that invites effort with ease. What I have noticed over these years is that there is a tendency to think of "props" as quick solutions to acute problems. For example, if my hamstrings are tight when I'm attempting a triangle pose in yoga, I may feel that I'm not able to "do the pose correctly," because I need to reach for a block or a chair to extend the length of my arm to the ground. Instead of this judgmental thinking, we want to think of the prop as *an integral part of our whole-body fascial continuity.* We might even use the prop forever, each time we do triangle pose, as our body changes over time. Nothing is wrong with that. The prop is basically an extension of

my body schema, my physical self. In this way, we approach props through an embodied, felt sense direct experience—as a relationship which deepens our ability to yield to gravity that, in turn, supports us in befriending our bodies. Props guide us to *self-tune our self-care* and nourish our bodies, minds, and spirits. Remember, all of this work is about you attending to *how* you befriend yourself and respond to your body's needs. Begin noticing how you can use a ball, foam roller, your sofa, kitchen sink, etc. to more deeply remind your body that it is in relationship with the grounding and uplift of earth's support. Doing this requires a shift from thinking about what is wrong to a mindful approach of being with your body as a living process, sensing weight shift, and asking for support any time during the day or night.

Effective use of props relies on deep listening to what your body needs. To determine if a prop is beneficial, ask yourself: Am I forcing my body to stretch an isolated muscle, or am I encouraging whole-body restorative movement? For example, the difference between a hard foam roller and a MELT method soft foam roller is significant. The soft roller's texture aligns with your body's contours, allowing you to relax, release tension, and restore your body's natural balance. In contrast, a hard foam roller may resist your body's ability to release tension, especially in tight areas.

A true self-care prop integrates seamlessly into your movement, becoming part of you and aiding in relaxation, rebalancing, and self-healing. If the prop feels foreign or corrective, it may hinder your ability to let go of old patterns.

In your daily self-care, you "remember" and release what disrupts your body's tensional balance, responding to breath, gravity, and developmental patterns of movement. Simple props like Stretch-eze®, Tye4 body bands, Therabands, and balls can help your body soften, widen, and balance. This is different from forcing a stretch, as we are not rubber bands. Instead, we rebalance our interconnected, elastic nature, termed "Fasciategrity" by my colleagues John Sharkey and Joanne Sarah Avison.

Approach self-care playfully, shifting from judgment to curiosity. Curiosity overcomes fear and encourages trying new things. Just like a playground with various apparatuses, your self-care practice includes tools and props that bring a playful spirit to your routine. In the following sections, I'll guide you through these tools and props, drawing on insights from previous chapters. Remember to allow yourself to be playful, as scientists have discovered that it takes 400 repetitions to create a new habit, unless it's done in play. In that case, it only takes 10–20 repetitions.

In the visionary method of Joseph Pilates, the matwork and spring-based apparatus of his method, along with chairs, mattresses, and V-shaped beds he designed for home use, are highlighted in his books *Your Health*, published in 1934, and *Return to Life*, published in 1945 (Pilates 1998, 2003). In reading his books many years ago, I was inspired to note that his "exercises" always lived for him in a much larger vision—that we discover our own inner wisdom, our ability to self-heal and reconnect with the vital forces that constitute our true nature. In these books, he encourages postural awareness, skin brushing, deeper breathing, and healthy spinal movement. His genius, and that of other pioneers like B.K.S. Iyengar, was to support whole-body movement, although they often used more effort than necessary to tap into the deeper fascial matrix awareness that supports the whole person.

BEGINNING YOUR SELF-CARE PRACTICE: *CHECKING IN*

Our first orientation in the playground of life is an awareness to *checking in*. The invitation here is to evaluate your environment and reflect on your habitual postures and movements in that space.

Checking in is a reminder, for example, to take breaks after sitting or standing in place for a long time, a reminder to change positions, which allows us to "re-tune" our fascial matrix body.

When we check in, we tune in to our body's comfort or distress and can take action. The benefit of checking in is especially important for workers who spend all day either on their feet or seated at a desk. The more I've thought about the benefits of checking in, the more I see how the practice is beneficial for all people who find themselves either primarily seated or standing, or those who can feel locked into habitual movements by the nature of their work.

We remember that we are a living process, guided by embryological forces that enable us to constantly regenerate our health and healing through the ecological cycles of creation, maintenance, and repair. Checking in and reconnecting with grounding, centering, and uplift is essential.

> You don't have to look far in the natural world to observe the geotrophic (earth) and heliotrophic (sun) sensitivity of all vegetation. When a tube-grown seedling is placed outside the container, its stem will turn upwards and its roots downwards. Bipolarity illustrates a tensional interplay which organizes the growth of all living beings. Just like the seedling, as our spine is growing in the womb space, our sacrum is considered to be the negative pole and our head is the positive pole. Attention to two directions in our physical body is multi-directional and in relation to our centers of gravity. (Agneessens 2001, pp.66–67)

As Carol Agneessens says, all natural beings will orient themselves according to polarities. When we compress our bodies through habituated sitting/working, we counteract our natural buoyancy toward grounding, centering, and uplift.

Checking in allows us to reconnect with our natural orienting tendencies and enables growth through regenerative movement.

CHECKING IN AT WORK, HOME, OR WHEREVER YOU MAY BE

Have you been sitting for a long time? Take a moment to check in with your *body's posture*—does it feel effortless or effortful? How does your body feel?

▸ If you sense that you are *collapsed* and/or feeling tired, then reset your grounding, centering, and uplift.

– Come up to standing, feel your feet, and look up, while letting your shoulders and arms be heavy.
– The subtle act of looking up invites uplift, while feeling your feet helps you to ground.
– You might reach your arms out to the sides and gently yawn.
– Or reach up and yawn, feeling your feet support you as you weight-shift from left foot to right foot—feel better?

▸ Or if you are continuously standing a lot, and feel like you are *propping* yourself up, sit down and gently arch and curl with breath support, sensing your sitting bones and your feet.

– Place your hands on your desk, table, or a wall for more support and move in any way that makes sense to you and gives you a deeper sense of your connection between your feet and sitting bones grounding you and your inner ear and Domes of Uplift helping you to feel suspended and spacious with breath support.

▸ Notice that any combination of spiral motions, awakening peripheral vision, looking around the room, and pausing to awaken your fascial matrix body's connectivity from foot to head and hand will serve to revitalize you during a brief check-in.

GOLDEN NUGGETS FOR SELF-CARE AWARENESS

Here are some *golden nuggets* that speak to your body's ecology and language for co-regulating your nervous system and resetting grounding, centering, and uplift.

Golden Nugget One: Postural Reset
See Video 6.1 for full exploration.

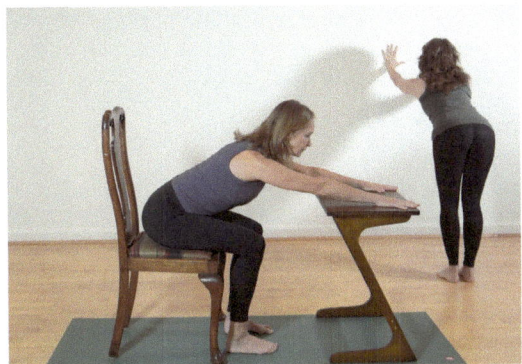

Figure 6.1 Postural reset

Golden Nugget Two: Small Ball Massage

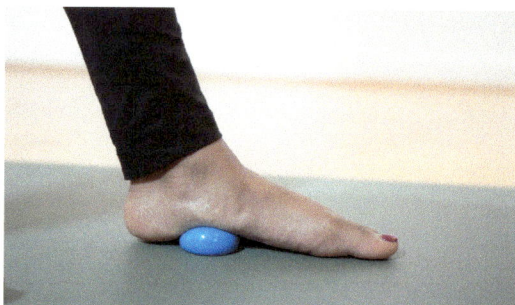

Figure 6.2 Small ball massage—energizing whole-body fascial awareness

The next stop is to notice how your feet feel. Are they in shoes that feel comfortable to your whole body? Are you able to spread your toes and move your feet internally and externally? Can you feel the helical nature of your feet from the inside to the outside of your feet? Answering these questions will shift your body's ability to release tension from your body through the grounding of your feet. Here is a simple practice that can help.

Get a humble small ball to energize your feet and hands. Remember that your feet and hands are portals to energizing the "domes/diaphragms of uplift" for your whole body. How amazing that gently stepping onto a small ball or massaging each foot and hand can awaken your entire body's vitality—yet we are remembering that our fascial matrix is a communication pathway for the energy of the meridians which are a continuity from foot to head and hand, and that self-care is a conversation with our body, which is always asking for support! **See Videos 6.2A and 6.2B for full exploration.**

Golden Nugget Three: Cervical Pivot

▶ Lie down and allow gravity to support you!

▶ Place the Cervical Pivot at the base of your neck so you feel you are addressing the

tension at the suboccipital muscles that support your eyes to whole-body relationship, which:

– tractions and massages your neck, shoulders, and spine
– co-regulates your nervous system and provides deep release by centering your breathing spine from sphenoid to sacrum.

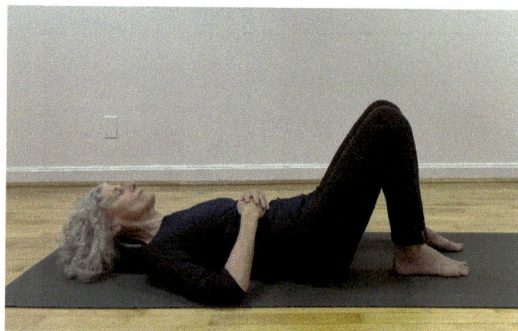

Figure 6.3 Cervical Pivot

See Video 6.3 for full exploration.

Going Deeper with Eye Orbits

Rolfer and craniosacral therapist Stanley Rosenberg also works with supporting vagal tone through gentle co-regulation. Here is a foundational exercise he teaches, using eye movements, which he calls Basic Exercise. It resets C1 and C2 vertebrae. He has noticed that a "rotation of C1 and C2 can put pressure on the vertebral artery, which supplies the frontal lobes and the brainstem, where the five nerves necessary for social engagement originate" (Rosenberg 2017, p.410).

▶ Pre-test: Sitting up, notice what it feels like to turn your head to the right and left. Just notice the level of tension in either side.

▶ Lie on your back the first time you explore this exercise and then, after you are familiar with it, you can explore it sitting or standing, or continue lying on your back.

▸ Weave your fingers of both hands together.

▸ Gently rest your head in your hands.

▸ Keeping your head facing forward, look your eyes to the right, moving only your eyes as comfortably as you can—without moving your head.

▸ After a short period—30–60 seconds—you may want to swallow, yawn, or sigh (this is a sign that your autonomic nervous system is relaxing).

▸ Bring your eyes back to looking straight in front of you.

▸ Keeping your head facing forward, look your eyes to the left, moving only your eyes as comfortably as you can—without moving your head.

▸ Keep looking there for a short period—30–60 seconds—until you notice a sigh, yawn, or swallow.

▸ Come back to center.

▸ Take your time to come up to sitting.

▸ Post-text: Notice if there is any improvement in your neck mobility, or do you notice any changes in your breathing?

I would also highly recommend these brilliant pioneers of eye care for the whole body:

• Meir Schneider—https://self-healing.org
• Peter Grunwald—www.eyebody.com

Related to the title of this chapter, notice that "self-care" does not take place in some pocket of time set aside from your work life. You don't need "more time" for self-care. Instead, self-care happens within the spaces that you already occupy and within the parameters of your working hours (mini pauses or breaks from seconds to minutes). Self-care can be as easy as checking in with yourself, in the ways outlined here.

Golden Nugget Four: Embodied Swan Swim on the Ball

In the next embodied exploration, you are meeting the ball as in rounding over your embryonic yolk sac (how your front body can release tension in your back body), fascial matrix support of Domes of Uplift from inner ankle to inner ear, and empowering the relationships between your peripheral vision in the orbits of your eyes and your shoulders and hips. **See Video 6.4 for full exploration.**

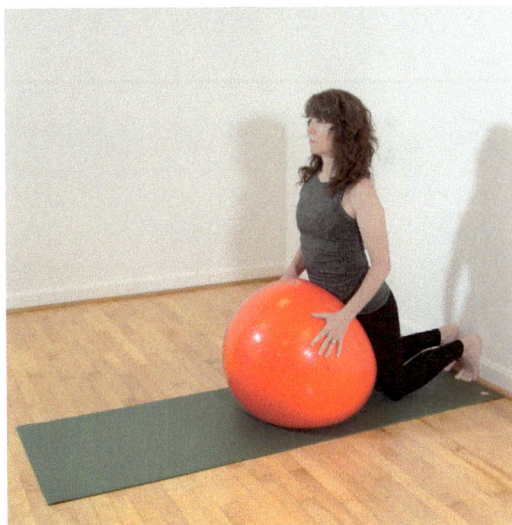

Figure 6.4A

▸ Pre-test for finding a ball that is the right size for your body: Can you kneel in front of the ball and open your hips as you relax over it? Is it too big (can't round over it and touch the floor comfortably with your whole hand), too small (feel cramped on it), or just right (it allows you to release around it and meet the floor and the wall)?

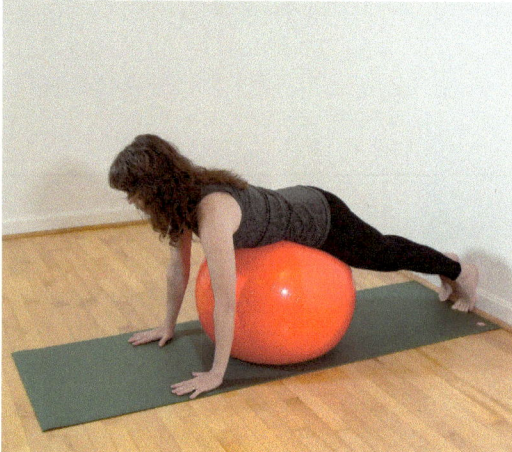

Figure 6.4B

▶ Set-up for Swan: Kneel facing away from the wall with the bottoms of your feet close to a wall and ball in front of you, hands on ball.

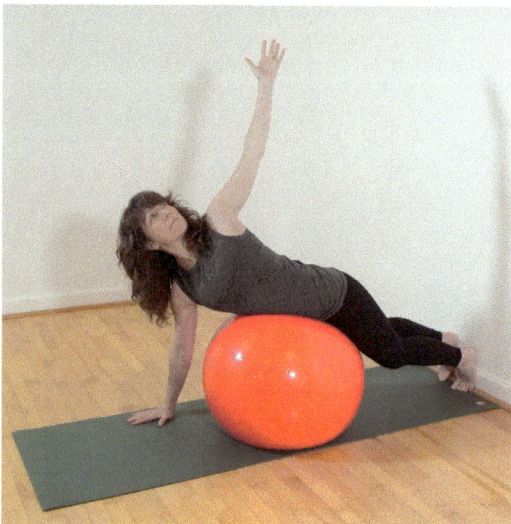

Figure 6.4C

▶ Meeting and Extending over the Ball, feet on wall.

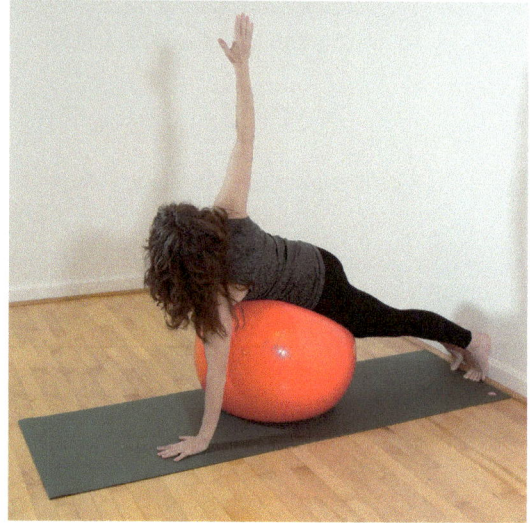

Figure 6.4D

▶ Sensing the Swim Spiral of Your Upper Core to left.
▶ Sensing the Swim Spiral of Your Upper Core to right.

Golden Nugget Five: Orienting in the Field of Gravity—Standing Balance

Reconnecting with effort with ease—internal support foot to head. **See Videos 6.5A and 6.5B for full exploration.**

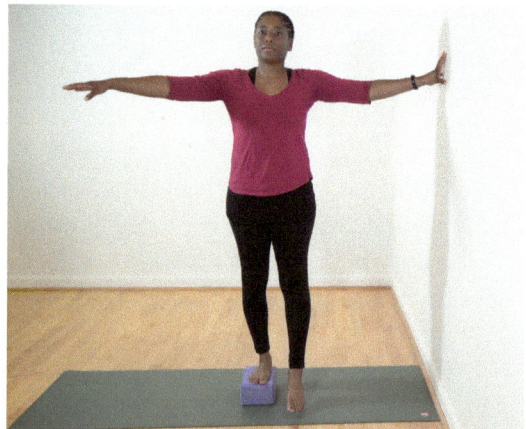

Figure 6.5A

Standing on yoga block (or solid books) on right foot, with five fingers of right hand reaching to touch wall, arm straight, in comfortable position and left arm reaching out from your shoulder for deeper lateral support.

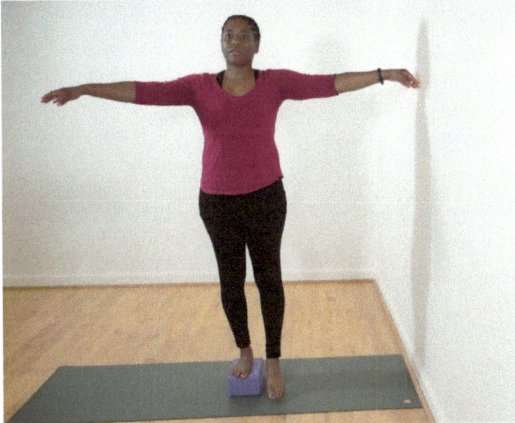

Figure 6.5B

Can you maintain that feeling without touching the wall?

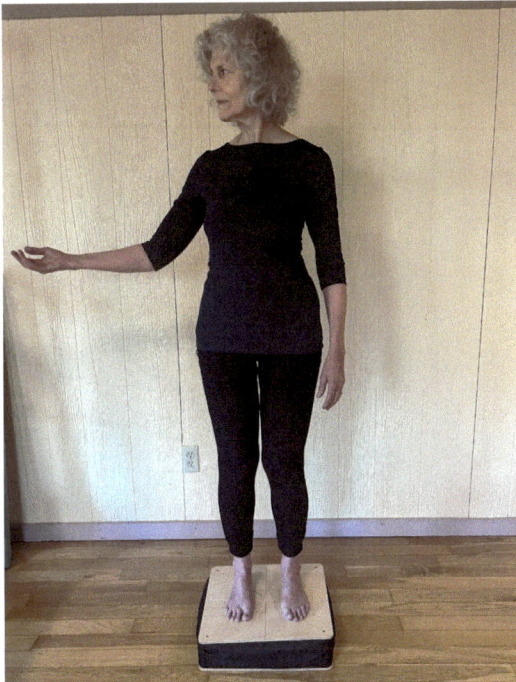

Figure 6.5C Standing Balance on the Tuning Board—orienting in the field of gravity

▶ Step off block and see what you notice.

▶ Change to left foot on block with left hand on wall and right arm reaching laterally.

Developed by Advanced Rolf Structural Integration Practitioner and psychotherapist Darrell Sanchez, the Tuning Board is a psychokinesthetic tool that I love. It is a standing platform with a gently moving surface that activates my feet and ankles and stimulates postural proprioceptors and the sensory and motor nerves that tone internal organs and my whole fascial matrix body. I find this self-tuning coordination and stimulation from foot to head cultivates deeper awareness, responsiveness, and a sense of wellbeing. Resource: www.rolfingboulderdenver.com/store

Golden Nugget Six: Embodied Squatting at the Kitchen Sink

If you are in a location (home or work) where there is a kitchen sink, your hands can "cup" the edge of the sink to allow a deeper connection with the waterfall Down the Back in this amazing reset of the biotensegrity spring-like relationship between your feet and ankles, knees, hips, spine, and hands, which tunes your internal organs.

▶ Breathing feet support the impact that strong, resilient legs can have on heart health and fluids in circulation with one another. **See Video 6.6 for full exploration.**

▶ Sense your hands' relationship to the waterfall of your shoulder blades, sit bones/tail, and tripods of feet.

▶ As you straighten your arms, sensing the waterfall, begin to sit down while allowing your inner ear to float up.

▶ Soften your elbows, allowing your pelvis to rest forward on the front of the sink and relax as you sense the ground through your legs.

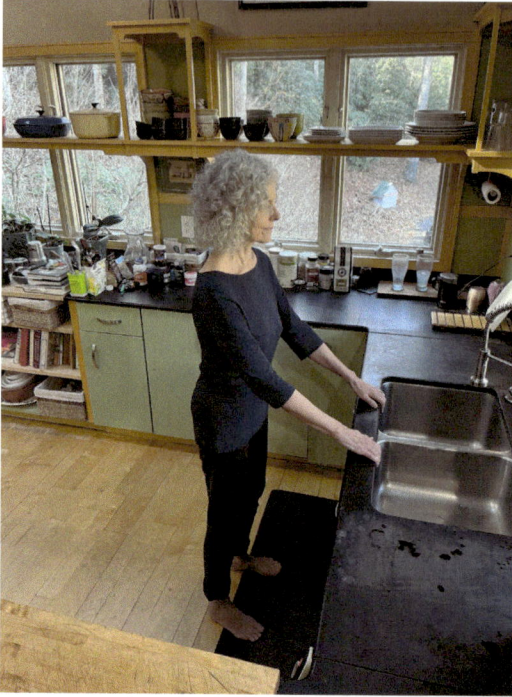

Figure 6.6A

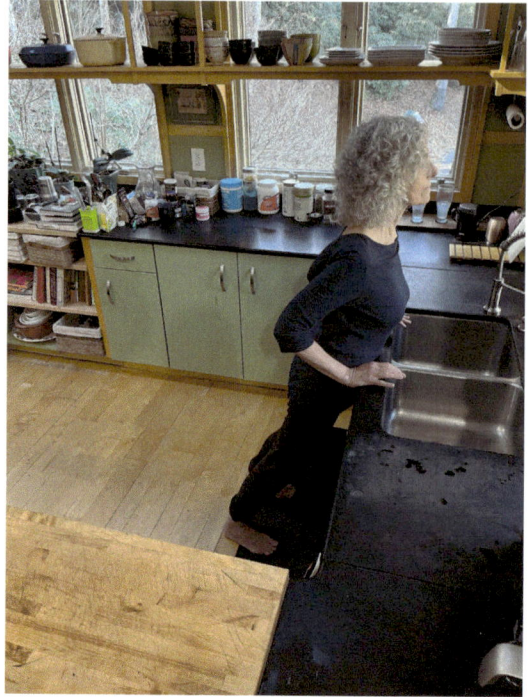

Figure 6.6B

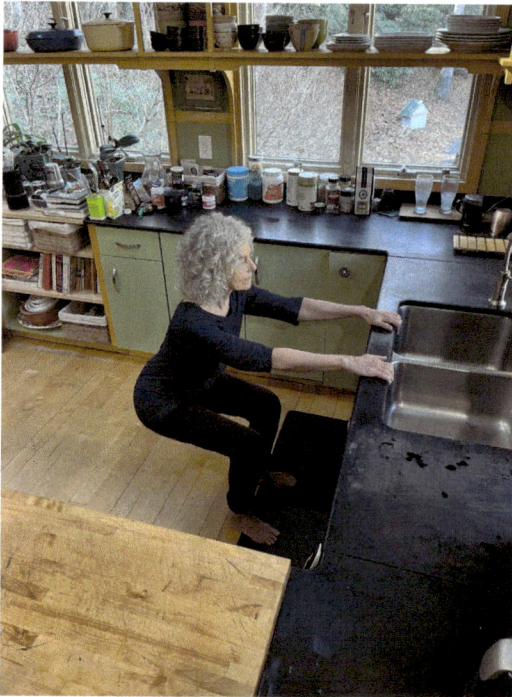

Figure 6.6C

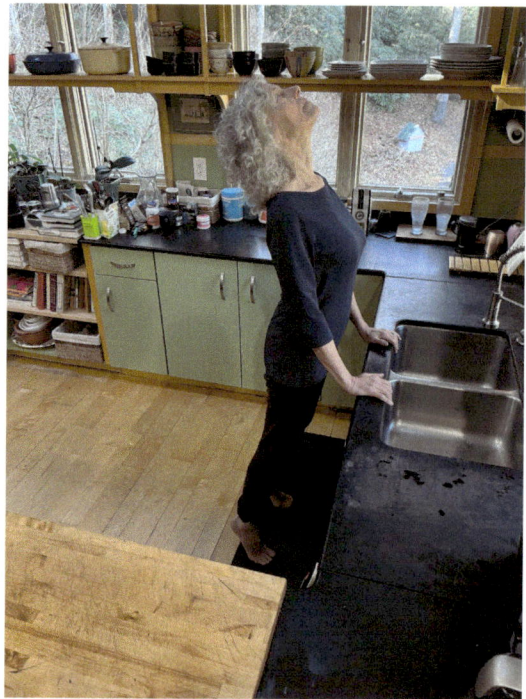

Figure 6.6D

▸ Then float upward onto the balls of your feet. You are waking up your low belly suspenders (front of your pelvic diaphragm—Up the Front—from inner ankles to inner ear).

▸ Notice if you are able to sense a deeper relationship from foot to head and hand through your fascial matrix breathing spine, awakening your Domes of Uplift from inner ankles to inner ears.

Your body is an elastic tensional-integrity fluid medium. You may find you begin to go deeper into your squat with minimal effort ("squatting-without-doing"). As the emphasis shifts from doing a squat to sensing your fascial breath's elastic relationship with the movement of squatting that opens the mechanoreceptors of your feet and hands to the play between grounding and uplift, you discover a more dynamic interplay of fluid movement. This fluid interplay wants to happen naturally, but too often we inhibit it through our notion of what a squat is supposed to look like or "how far we think we *should* go."

Golden Nugget Seven: Stretch-eze® Sensory Feedback Band

Sensory feedback whole-body bands are tools that enhance our proprioceptive and kinesthetic awareness of the important elastic continuity role that the proper tension-compression biotensegrity relationships play in regenerating our fascial matrix body.

The Stretch-eze® hand and the Tye4 elastic band (see Golden Nugget Eight) also support our midline postural awareness from foot to head and hand—orienting our upper center of gravity and lower center of gravity within the field of gravity through sensing Down the Back and Up the Front.

These bands are a powerful feedback tool for Pilates, yoga, Gyrotonic, etc., supporting clients in embodying their body awareness in a therapeutic setting, and for a personal reset of finding center in your own body. **See Videos 6.7A and 6.7B for full explorations**.

• Stretch-eze® band: To begin, purchase a band that meets your height. I have found that getting a taller band than my height gives me more movement variation as I can use it full length or shorten it by wrapping it around my feet to create more resistance and then spread by arms and feet away from center to widen my base of support, and create more laterality. Resource: https://dyenamicmovement.com/products/Stretch-eze®

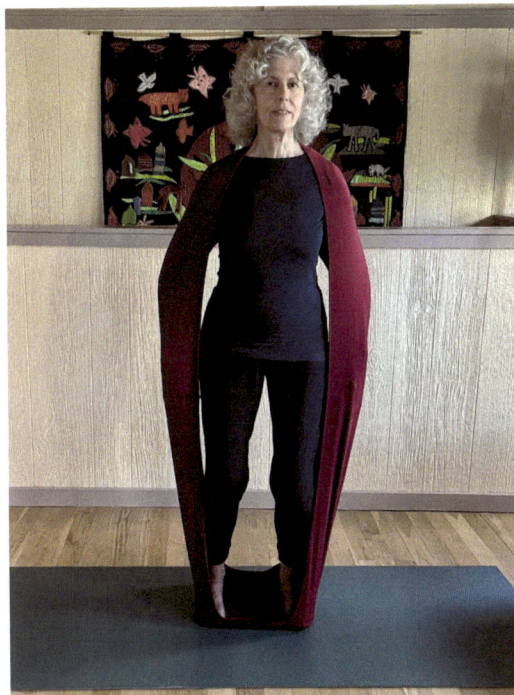

Figure 6.7A Standing in the Band—with weight shift and neck release

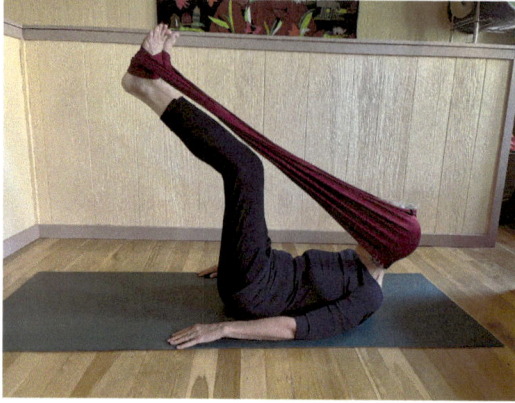

Figure 6.7B Heavy head resting in band with feet and leg support

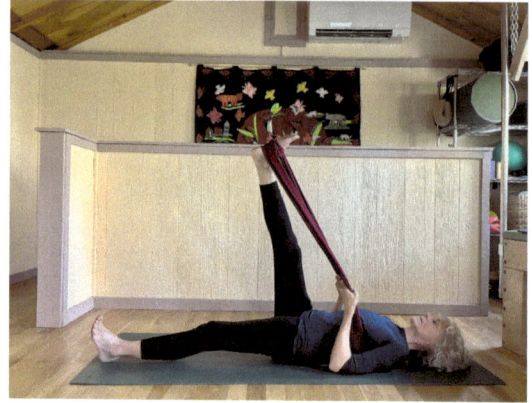

Figure 6.7E Leg circles

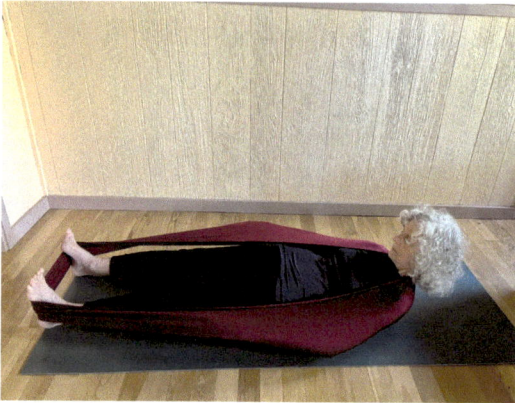

Figure 6.7C Rollup (band around shoulders) with lateral support (and feet wrap)

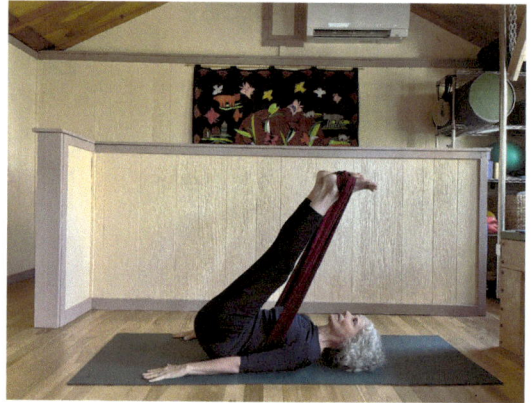

Figure 6.7F Rollover (band around midback and feet)

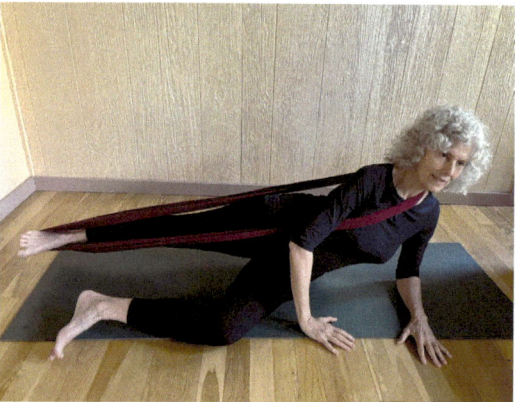

Figure 6.7D Sidekicks—opposite shoulder and foot

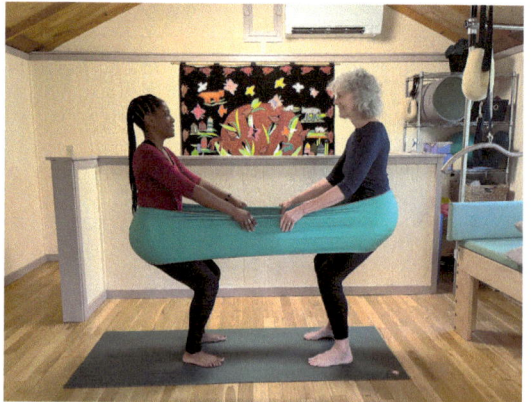

Figure 6.7G Squat with partner or self (twist around either side of doorknob to secure)

Golden Nugget Eight: Tye4 Sensory Feedback Band

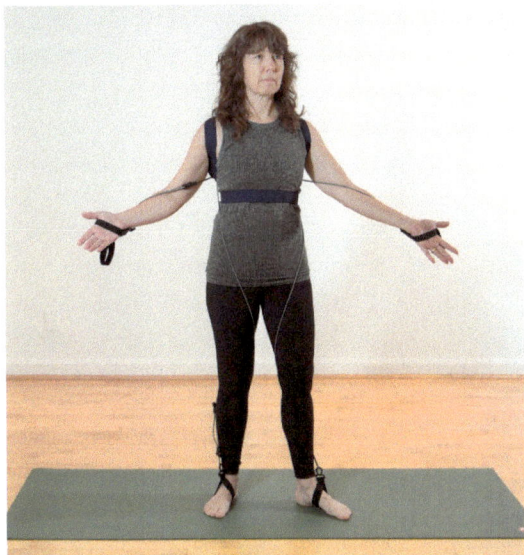

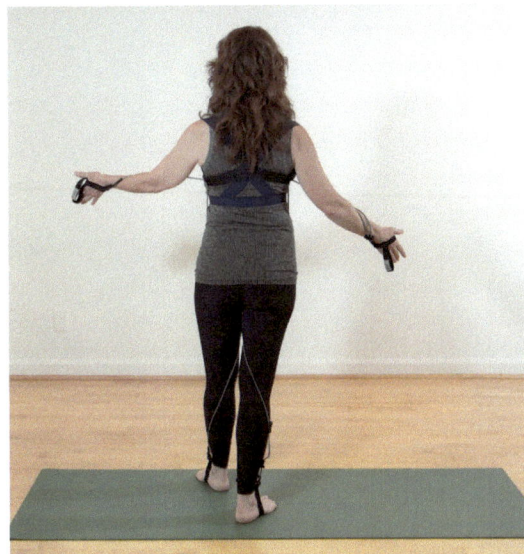

Figures 6.8A and 6.8B

This whole-body band gives a sensation like the springs on the Reformer. It can be wrapped around your arms (externally) and legs (internally) to deepen connecting to your midline and reach out from center to periphery. **See Videos 6.8A and 6.8B for full exploration.**

Golden Nugget Nine: Do-In Self-Massage as Self-Love

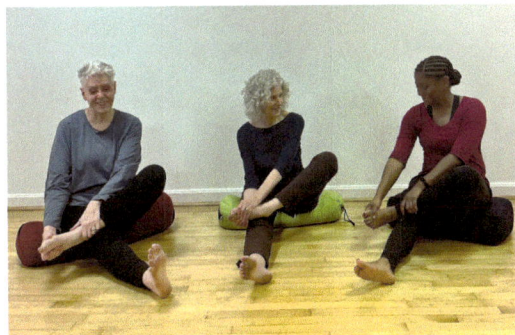

Figure 6.9 Do-In self-massage as self-love

Do-In (doe-een) is a traditional self-massage technique, which is a precursor to Qigong, originating in China and Japan, stimulating, toning, and co-regulating the nervous system and rebalancing internal organ energy through the meridians that originate and end at almost every finger and toe. I studied Do-In with Michio Kushi and Jacques DeLangre many decades ago and am so grateful for this weekly practice.

As we explored in Chapter 3 in our awareness-building practices, we are awakening our lived, daily experience of how we connect the visible and invisible worlds that sustain us. Notice how you feel before entering your Do-In practice and what you notice after your practice. *Energizing rather than exercising* can become a practice that is at the heart of any discipline. What we bring to our practice (our awareness, loving attention, and energy) determines how we practice. Equally important, by expanding our perceptual awareness, we will come to see and appreciate even the most minute undertakings. **See Video 6.9 for full exploration.**

Golden Nugget Ten: Good Morning Practice and Neti Pot and Skin/Body Care

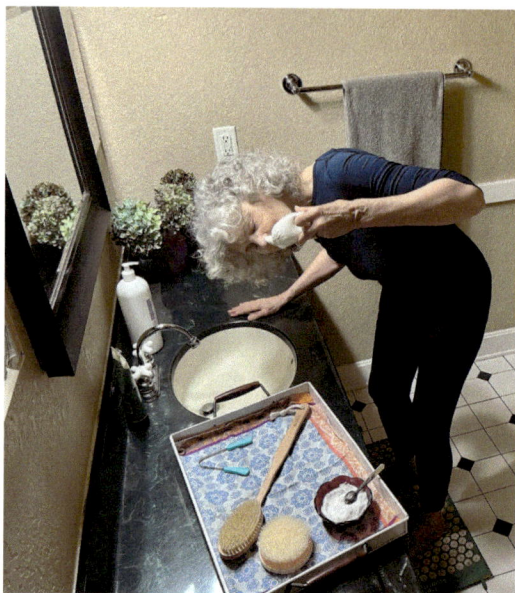

Figure 6.10 Good morning practice and neti pot and skin/body care

Each morning, my body enjoys entering the bathroom to invigorate itself, as I step onto an Acupressure mat in front of my bathroom sink to brush my teeth and massage my gums and use a tongue scraper to remove bacteria brought to the surface as the body is cleansing at night. This is the beginning of my morning routine, a real *waking up* of mind, body, and spirit.

Although there are many parts to my morning routine, which include a gentle movement and meditation practice, there are specific aspects of self-care I would love to share with you. First, skin care. We can easily forget that the skin is our body's largest organ. It is literally the place where the external world meets our internal world (through the pores). Skin brushing is important for fascial matrix health, stimulating the lymphatic system and exfoliating and rejuvenating the body's integration. It's been a major part of my hip replacement health practice.

A deeper awareness of my eyes' relationship with my whole body occurred for me several years ago. I was cleansing my face and gently massaged my eye orbits when my hips released on a deeper level. It was a visceral experience, where I felt my eye orbits supporting my hip orbits. This wonderful experience has morphed into a deeper conversation between my hip and shoulder orbits, which continues to feed an evolving movement practice. (Remember that lying on the ground and rolling can begin with looking in a direction to spiral!) Here's a happy accident of self care that speaks to our emergent, shape-shifting nature. If I didn't have this daily practice, I would not have found this connection. **See Video 6.10A for full practice.**

Second, the neti pot, which has supported my respiratory health daily for 40 years. This practice is rooted in ancient nasal irrigation awareness, an essential rebalancer for nasal and lung health. Often, when I ask if a client uses the neti pot, the answer is "Yes, when I feel I need it." Unfortunately, that is too late, as the problem is already in full bloom. Remember that we are an ecological body, embedded in our environment, so our nasal mucous membranes need support to keep our lungs healthy. Also, remember that as the salt water bathes and alkalinizes your nasal passage, it also bathes tissues that house your pineal gland—our third eye—so we are bathing this clarifying center of perceptual awareness with this grounding practice.

Even though I have done this practice daily for 40 years, remember that practice teaches us. During COVID, one morning I thought "Why am I not mouth washing and gargling with salt water?" as it is so alkalinizing and would support my immune system. I began adding that to my practice, and a year later, my dentist told me that the pockets in my teeth/gum health had improved. Alkalinizing the mucous membranes daily in your nose and throat is self-care which facilitates a regular conversation with your bio-intelligent body—plus it boosts immune support and promotes whole-body health. **See Video 6.10B for full practice.**

Golden Nugget Eleven: Guided Journey to Experience the Sacred Nature of the Elements

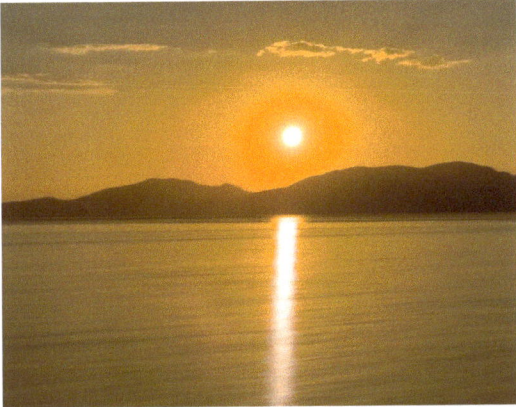

Figure 6.11A Paxos–Corfu sunset

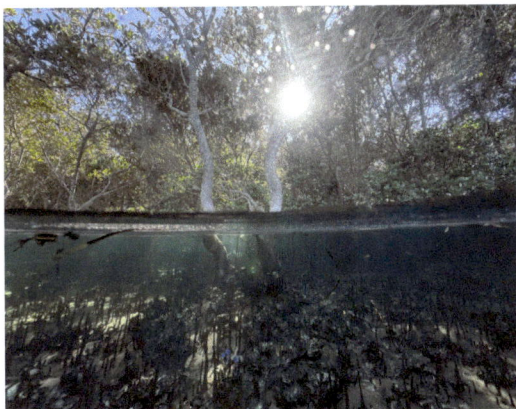

Figure 6.11B Mangrove
PRUE JEFFRIES, PHOTOGRAPHER, CONTINUUM TEACHER

This self-care practice is an invitation to befriend the elements that feed our body's soil—through body, mind, emotions, and spirit. These relational essences of transformation are easy to access and available to everyone. The goal of this self-care awareness is to greet and reap the benefits of Mother Nature's gift of sunlight/fire, air, water, earth, and growth.

Everything is alive and in relationship. This is true in nature and is reflected within our own miraculous bodies. For thousands of years wisdom traditions around the world have recognized certain archetypal expressions which we call the elements. These elements have energetic signatures that we can study and connect with to begin to experience their natures within us. In developing this awareness of these elemental energies within we can expand our sense of self to include all of nature. Being this we begin to step out of the dream of separateness and instead step into the dream of nature. This is the place of flow and connection, the place where wholeness begins. (Sheerin 2024)

I'd like to express gratitude to Prema and Scott Sheerin for the soulful meditation on how the elements support us as whole beings.

- Prema Sheerin, Traditional Spirit-Supported Healer, Life Coach, Dream Tender, After-Death Soul Guide: https://premasheerin.com
- Scott Sheerin, Musician and musical visionary behind the music on Healing Music Now: www.healingmusicnow.com/scott_sheerin

See Audio 6.11 for full meditation.

Golden Nugget Twelve: Food as Energy

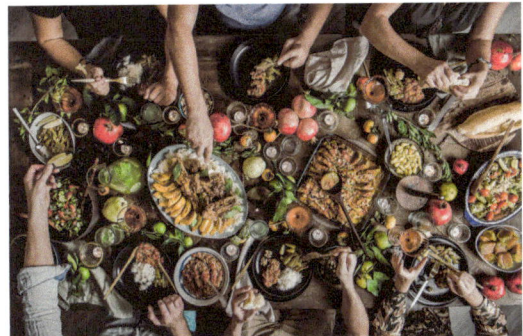

Figure 6.12 Food as energy

Modern-day eating is very confusing as we no longer are guided by eating with the seasons to support our internal organ health—everything is always available in the grocery stores, along with so many packaged, low-vitality non-foods or low-quality fast foods. We can easily boomerang between yo-yo-ing from one magic-pill diet to another, looking for a quick fix, or approaching food from vacation thinking—coming from scarcity of what we "shouldn't" eat and then letting it all go and eating anything at any time, or eating like children—pizza or dessert every day.

When we approach food as energy, we create awareness, bringing ourselves in touch with the basic needs of life—sunlight, air, water, nutrients, the life-giving habitats that grew our food, and the many people who helped to grow, harvest, and bring that food to our table. In this way, we are cultivating gratitude that feeds our cellular being. Food becomes a relationship that nourishes us deeply, and I have found that includes foods that are often thought of as "bad," such as sugar or salt. Sugar used to be an occasional food at special events. Now it's highly processed and put into almost everything, so our discerning taste for what our body needs daily is distorted. Sun-dried sea salt is full of minerals and aids hydration when used sparingly, whereas overly processed demineralized table salt can be problematic.

It is grounding for us to remember that we are a living process and that all processes are cyclical. For instance, the rotation of the earth around the sun allows for the change of seasons, which allows our ecosystem to replenish and re-energize. Our ecological body also responds to this change of seasons, and Traditional Chinese Medicine teaches us that we can harmonize and heal our internal organs by becoming aware that each of them is affected by the seasons (Lungs can be more challenged in their season, Fall), the colors we wear (wearing one color all the time, for instance, can be unbalancing), and the food tastes we eat regularly (too many sweet foods can imbalance the Stomach, Spleen, and Pancreas).

Table 6.1 How internal organs and their corresponding meridians are relational to senses/seasons/colors/taste/emotions

Organ/Sense	Season	Color	Taste	Emotion
LV/GB—eyes	Spring	Green	Sour	Anger
HT/SI—tongue PC/TW	Summer	Red/pink	Bitter	Joy
ST/SP/PA—mouth	Late Summer	Yellow/orange/gold/brown	Sweet	Empathy
LU/LI—nose	Autumn	White/gray	Spicy	Grief
KD/BL—ears	Winter	Blue/black	Salty	Fear

Legend: LV—Liver; GB—Gallbladder; HT—Heart; SI—Small Intestine; PC—Pericardium; TW—Triple Warmer; ST—Stomach; SP—Spleen; PA—Pancreas; LU—Lung; LI—Large Intestine; KD—Kidney; BL—Bladder.

Excellent resources for further study are:

- Pam Ferguson, *Take Five* (Dublin: Newleaf, 2000), p.41.

- Michael Reed Gach, *Acu-yoga* (Japan Publications, 2000), p.100.

To become more familiar with how this vital information works for us, you may feel tired in the afternoon around 3:00, when the bladder meridian is most active. The bladder meridian is located down the back of your head, along each side of your spine and low back, down the backs of your legs to your baby toes. If you feel any back discomfort, you can help yourself by moving—walking, standing on a tennis ball and rolling it under your foot, squatting using a stable surface, noticing how you can root through your feet and tail and create *space* in your body by reaching through your hands and head. Remember that your fascial matrix body is always listening and ready to respond to your self-care.

As Michael Pollan speaks about in his illuminating yet simple book *Food Rules*, what we do know that is important is that populations that eat the so-called Western diet—generally a lot of processed foods and meats, added fat and sugar, refined grains, everything except vegetables—suffer from high rates of Western diseases, like obesity, diabetes, cardiovascular disease, and cancer, while populations that eat a wide range of traditional diets often don't suffer from these chronic diseases. And most importantly, people who shift from the Western diet to more natural foods see dramatic improvements in their health and wellbeing—the negative effects of the Western diet can be improved surprisingly quickly. As we have been speaking about in *Moving Beyond Core*, many of us have relied on *experts*—doctors and diet books—to tell us how to eat. Remember that the more a food is processed, the more profitable it becomes to food company manufacturers and the unhealthier it becomes for our body to process—it doesn't register as food.

> The healthcare industry makes more money treating chronic diseases (which accounts for three-quarters of the $2 trillion plus we spend each year on health care in this country) than preventing them. So we ignore the elephant in the room and focus instead on good and evil nutrients, the identities of which seem to change with every new study. (Pollan 2009, p.xiv)

Choosing simple, easy-to-access foods enables us to feel supported in our deeper humanity within the living natural world and empowers us in moving beyond dieting to feeling deeply nourished.

STORY: I'd like to share a story with you about listening to my body and being flexible. My husband, Michael, and I were partners with several other couples in the late 1980s in setting up an international holistic health retreat in Colorado, which we all committedly did for two years till we had to close the doors. I was vegan when Michael met me, and here we were, six years later, having lunch at a little café, as we were discussing the end of the project, and I couldn't take my eyes off one item on the menu. It was the middle of winter, I was feeling cold, and my body wanted something that surprised me—so when the waitress approached to take our order, I went with it. "I'll have the rack of lamb," I said as Michael looked at me with shock. We still laugh about it today, decades later, because it was a defining moment in listening to my body, which was so grateful because that first bite felt like a blood transfusion that was so needed!

Golden Nugget Thirteen: Good Night Practice for Restful Sleep

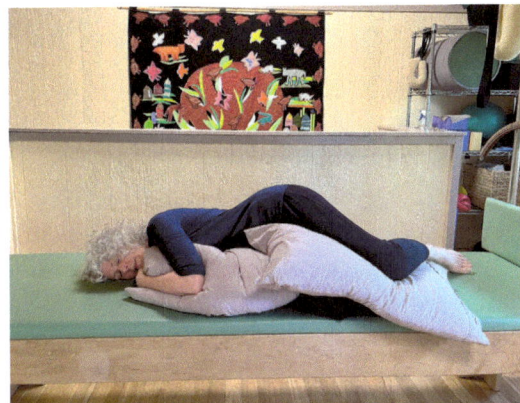

Figure 6.13 Good night practice for restful sleep

- Closing mouth with paper surgical tape, or

- MyoTape, developed by my teacher,

Patrick McKeown, which is placed around the mouth for those with sensitive lips.

We tell ourselves that we care for the self by attending to how we move, so we might be fooled into thinking that self-care only happens when we're awake. This is not true. All sorts of movements are transpiring in our sleep. Not only is sleep itself a form of self-care, but tending to the movements occurring while we sleep can add a whole new dimension to this perspective.

Going to sleep is not just about lying down. I have noticed over the years that it is a process of discovery and comfort for my body. To further support your sleeping movement, try adding a body pillow that has a thickness that feels just right to your body. I use two pillows, one that is not very full under my upper body and a fuller one between my knees or under one side of my side-lying body, and mold it to where I want support. You may also prefer lying on your back with legs straight, with support under your knees or thighs, which supports the flow of breath through the body. See what works best for you. So, instead of attempting to make sleep happen, try preparing for restful sleep by consciously positioning pillow(s) in your nightly nest.

If you find that you wake at night or in the morning with mucus in your eyes and a dry mouth, chances are your mouth was open all night (causing snoring and breathing problems), because, with your mouth open, your body got the signal that you were losing moisture and too much carbon dioxide, so it created mucus to compensate. You can help yourself with a simple remedy.

Use paper surgical tape or purchase MyoTape to cover your mouth and encourage nasal breathing during your sleeping hours. Doing this leads to more restful sleep. As discussed in Chapter 3 on breath, nasal breathing is necessary for optimal, whole-body health and for fully resting down. Mouth breathing during sleep stimulates the "emergency reflex," which tricks the body into thinking something is wrong. By using just enough lightly applied paper surgical tape to the mouth (loose enough so that you could push it off with your tongue), your body will retain moisture and circulate warmer air into your lungs during rest.

Going deeper:

- We now know that sleep has many benefits, playing a critical role in immune function, metabolism, memory, learning, and so many other vital functions.

- Remember that nasal breathing and slowing your breath relaxes your nervous system. Sense your exhale and allow it to be twice as long as your inhale. You are stimulating your parasympathetic, rest/digest/calming phase of your nervous system.

- In other words, you can sense, without efforting, how your exhale allows a gentle inhale. Relax into your body, letting go into support. Good night!

See Video 6.13 for a deeper exploration.

TRANSITION INTO COMMUNITY

It is important to remember that the ecological community has always been present throughout this conversation of *self*-care. When we choose food that is grown locally and organically, we are helping to rebuild the earth's soil. Self-care necessarily bridges individual wellbeing with community wellbeing.

When we touch ourselves with a loving way

of being and cultivate that as a practice, we plant seeds of loving kindness in the world that creates a ripple effect. This notion has been active throughout the book, but this moment presents an opportunity to explore where self-care emerged within each of the previous chapters.

Inner Guide

Consider how the Inner Guide understands stress. Contrary to common thinking, which sees stress as something to be avoided, the Inner Guide recognizes stress as something to meet, as a teacher. You can renew your ongoing conversation with your Inner Guide every time you check in.

> STORY: My husband, Michael, deals with tremendous stress every day, and has for the 38 years we have been married. He has a challenging neurological imbalance and PTSD which creates chronic pain that at times can be debilitating. As you can imagine, he has seen so many forward-thinking experts and participated in pioneering transformational and spiritual work that supports his ability to "hold" difficulty, and I have facilitated his process over the years with movement and bodywork that has been nurturing. In the early years of our movement practice together, Michael had difficulty slowing down and wanted me to just "tell him what to do." This challenged both of us as I wanted to do what I felt was best for him and satisfy his desire to work hard. So, we would move through some Pilates exercises or yoga asanas that felt good to him, with me coaching him to notice where he could help himself, and then he would do trampoline or some other aerobic workout. What surprised me was that about 15 years ago, he came up to me after his Pilates practice and said, "Honey, in my Rollup this morning, I noticed something." I immediately said, "Michael, this is not a small thing! This is a big thing that you are noticing something."

Then he shared something that was relevant to how he could help himself be more relaxed in his movement practice. And what is even more incredible is that from that day on, he approached his practice from a new place of awareness that has developed into a beautiful multi-discipline somatic practice that feeds him on so many levels.

Core as Relationship

When we approach ourselves as a relational being, movement becomes a potent way of resonating with our whole self, with one another, and with the environment that feeds us. Our self-care practices prepare us to hear the body's language and speak in that language so as to understand what the body needs to greet the day, greet others, and greet the natural world. My relationship with myself will naturally inform and shape my relationship with others.

Breath as Healing Bridge Between Matter and Spirit

Breath is like a bridge to everything we see, hear, smell, sense, and touch, as well as our relationship with the invisible and spirit world.

Movement Beyond Doing (Energizing Your Exercising)

When we allow ourselves to be fully present with lying, sitting, standing, walking, running, and any other movement, it becomes like a self-care massage.

Allow yourself to modify any given movement so it meets your needs and feels nourishing as an act of self-care. This is *Advanced Thinking* because it takes us beyond feelings of lack of self-worth and encourages us to listen to our Inner Guide. The Advanced Thinking Inner Guide will also ask you to reach for a prop that feels good to support your movement practice and emergent shape-shifting body.

Communicating from Our Way of Being

Many of us live in a culture of *busy-ness*, which challenges our ability to be present. But with the caveat that "self" is something more expansive. It isn't an identity that we possess. We are social beings, and if we are willing to connect and slow down, we begin to see that our interconnections with others makes our "Self" more porous and expansive than we previously thought.

Throughout this chapter, we have explored ways of being with ourselves that can be simple self-care check-ins that are profoundly healing and restorative. In *Moving Beyond Core*, we are challenging ourselves to see with new eyes and *take action*, because we need to take action and actually do what inspires us, igniting the process to shifting habits that creates life-changing growth and transformation.

SELF-CARE STORIES

Sharing their life-altering changes are the following inspiring self-care stories by people of various backgrounds who I have supported in their remembering how to help themselves.

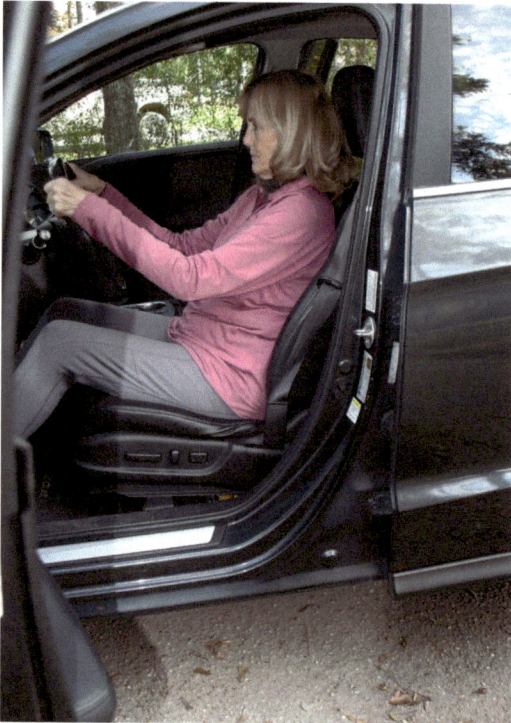

Figure 6.15A Jan Cranner, without Aston Pillows in car to support back and hip pain

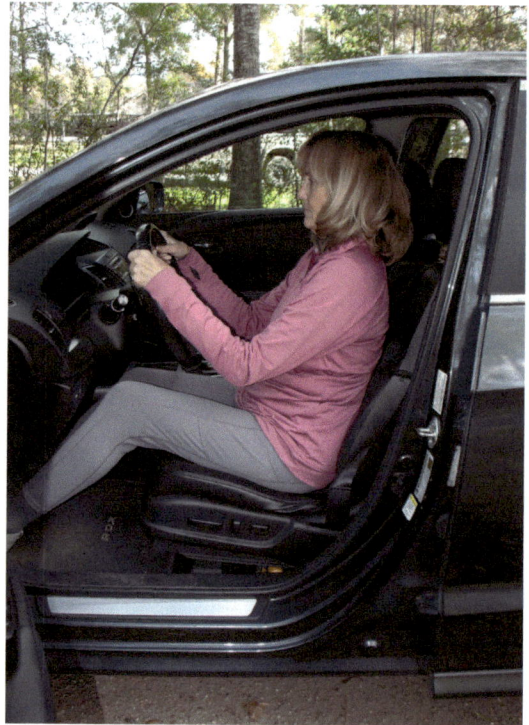

Figure 6.15B Jan Cranner, with Aston Pillows in car to support back and hip pain

I am a very active 66-year-old who, up until five months ago, played tennis and cycled three or four times a week. I had a bad fall and came down really hard on my hip. I went to an orthopedic specialist and got a steroid shot in my bursa after x-rays revealed no broken bones. It gave me some relief, but the pain and stiffness persisted. Started prolotherapy and began the healing process.

Driving in my car was causing a lot of pain in my lower back and hip, so Wendy suggested the Aston Kinetics back wedge and ergo triangle cushions. The difference has been amazing. The shift in my posture has taken the strain off my hip and back, and even long drives don't bother me.

or sturdy bench or table that is about chair height. The movement is called the Facial Dog Flow Series. It too aligns the spine and allows the muscles in my lower back to release.

The amazing thing is that these two simple exercises are easy to learn, accessible to anyone, and have given me freedom of movement that I thought I had lost!

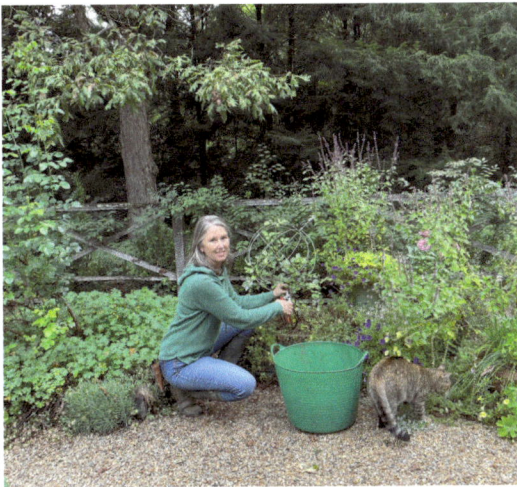

Figure 6.16 Nancy Duffy, garden designer—a healing story with no more back pain

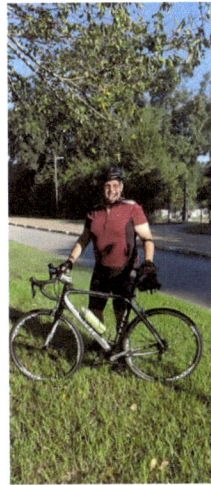

Figure 6.17 Bruce Cranner—nasal breathing transformed my biking endurance

I am a garden designer by vocation and gardener by avocation. I bend over a lot. Some years ago, I had a session with Wendy and she helped me to change my low back pain. I have continued to have no back pain since that session by practicing two exercises.

The first was very simple, and I call it the "waterfall." Wendy taught me to release the muscles in my lower back by adjusting my posture. I imagine water rolling over my shoulders and down my back. My shoulders and shoulder blades naturally drop and everything relaxes. I do this many times a day. I can do this anywhere and immediately feel my back muscles relax.

The second exercise is also very simple movements, although it requires a chair

Thank you for teaching me to breathe through my nose and use my diaphragm. As you know, I love road cycling but struggled with breathing consistently. A combination of asthma, allergies, and extra weight often left me panting and out of balance on the saddle. My posture, position, and cadence often devolved into a mess of sweaty effort. It's a downward cascade which I now understand began and ended with poor breathing.

The strain of a steep hill or long flat still puts pressure on my heart and lungs. That will always be true. But, instead of losing my focus, position, and discipline on the saddle, I focus on breathing through my nose and diaphragm in a circular manner. In through the nose with the mouth closed with my back extended, shoulders down, and elbows in and down. In this position, I can use my diaphragm to pull air deeply into my lungs. Then I exhale through my nose without changing position and slow down if I feel I want to open my mouth. With remarkably little practice, I have maintained this balance and discipline far deeper into the flats and hills than ever before. The mountain stage of the Tour de France is not calling this old lawyer, but the low rolling hills of my favorite cycling route are now less daunting and sometimes a real pleasure.

There is a beautiful quote by poet John O'Donohue that speaks to how our longest and most exciting journey is the journey inwards. Self-care is our deepest relationship with self that transforms how we can relate with others and the world in which we are embedded. Here is the end of John O'Donohue's quote:

There is a beautiful complexity of growth within the human soul. In order to glimpse this, it is helpful to visualize the mind as a tower of windows. Sadly, many people remain trapped in one window, looking out every day at the same scene in the same way. Real growth is experienced when you draw back from one window, turn and walk around the inner tower of the soul and see all the different windows that await your gaze. Through these different windows, you can see new vistas of possibility, presence and creativity. Complacency, habit and blindness often prevent you from feeling your life. So much depends on the frame of vision—the window through which you look. (O'Donohue 1997)

Use the following QR code for all videos in this chapter:

REFERENCES

Agneessens, C. (2001) *The Fabric of Wholeness: Biological Intelligence and Relational Gravity*. Ashland, OH: The Bramble Company.

O'Donohue, J. (1997) *Anam Cara: A Book of Celtic Wisdom*. New York, NY: Harper.

Pilates, J. (1998) *Your Health*. Incline Village, NV: Presentation Dynamics.

Pilates, J. (2003) *Return to Life*. Miami, FL: Pilates Method Alliance.

Pollan, M. (2009) *Food Rules*. New York, NY: Penguin Books.

Rosenberg, S. (2017) *Accessing the Healing Power of the Vagus Nerve: Self-Help Exercises for Anxiety, Depression, Trauma, and Autism*. Berkeley, CA: North Atlantic Books.

CHAPTER 7

It's All About Relationship

We now return full circle to the context of *Moving Beyond Core*, where the concept of "Core" is Core as Relationship, with gravity, ourselves, one another, and our living environment. As writer Anaïs Nin declared, "each friend represents a world in us, a world possibly not born until they arrive, and it is only by this meeting that a new world is born" (2015, p.10). With this statement, she speaks to the notion that we are aware that we each live our individual lives and that each life is also a collaborator in the birth of multiple worlds. These births happen every time we make friends, meet with another person, or take on a particular challenge. One life becomes amplified and connected to many lives spread throughout many worlds.

This world is made up of each of our songs. When you sing the song that lives in your heart, you contribute vital energy to the healing and renewal of the world. (Harper and Molin-Skelton 2023)

EMPOWERING YOUR SONG

In the world of movement and bodywork, this friend, as Anaïs Nin notes, or the song that Harper and Skelton speak of, may take many forms. We may befriend gravity, a special tool for self-care, a favorite exercise machine, another person, a client, student, a teacher, and even ourselves. A primary question prompted by the vision of this book is this: Are you, student and teacher/practitioner, cultivating an awareness of and attention to the creation of worlds that is taking place in each encounter? There is no extra effort needed, just being grateful for the encounter. Can we allow our hearts to lead our heads? What I mean by this is *when our head leads, we act from past knowing. When our heart leads, we act from a felt sense of the present moment of what is needed and what serves the greater good.*

For instance, if a teacher/practitioner seeks only to pass down knowledge of how to successfully perform an exercise, then what can be missed is the mystery of the world-making that is taking place, at the interface, with each touch and interaction. If, by contrast, the teacher/practitioner is attentive to the present moment of the encounter, a class, private movement, or bodywork session may become a portal to deeper growth and an entirely new *way of being*. In this way, it really is all about relationship.

I was inspired to write *Moving Beyond Core* to expand what we think of *movement* to include a whole-person way of being. This way of being invites us to sense Core as Relationship, a relationship with gravity, with ourselves, with one another, and with our living (natural and social) environment. As I see it, movement is not only about creating form; rather, it is the unleashing of creative intelligence, which grows our capacity for adaptability, resilience, and the forming of vital, life-giving relationships. When we view our bodies as living processes, rather than objects, we attune to the constant unfolding of our deeper self, one that reveals the "self" to be *porous*, always in relationship with other beings and the living environment. When we allow ourselves to become present to the living fascial web that we share with other beings and the natural living world, that presence changes our perceptual awareness of how we move in life. We are a living liquid crystalline fascial matrix, emitting and receiving energy from everywhere and everyone. This perceptual awareness allows us to sense our bioluminescence—a bridge between the sun's luminescence and the earth's electromagnetic field. We are light beings, coherent energy sources that have the capacity for self-regulation and dynamic relatedness.

I am so inspired by the research of evolutionary scientist Mae-Wan Ho and her pioneering work on the philosophy of organisms and sustainable systems. She shares:

> Our new philosophical position, Organicism, states that the universe and its various parts (including human societies) ought to be considered alive and naturally ordered, much like a living organism. It recognizes no boundaries between disciplines. It arises in the space between all disciplines. It is an unfragmented knowledge system by which one lives. It is a nondualist and holistic participatory knowledge system resembling those of traditional indigenous cultures all over the world. (Cited in Oschman 2003, p.309)

I have discovered that our living fascial matrix is an embodied process. We start by folding and unfolding in our embryonic environment, continuing to repattern and adapt throughout our lives. Our fascial matrix holds habitual patterns of emotional stress and trauma, influencing how we move and interact. These patterns can be unraveled by reconnecting with our primordial blueprint of health, which exists beyond cultural, familial, and personal expectations.

As explored in *Moving Beyond Core*, our relationship with gravity can be one of "fighting" or "effort with ease," depending on our approach. By discovering the minimal effort needed for movement, we learn to listen to our Inner Guide and connect with the universal field of life. This opens us to the alchemy of relationships, teaching us self-care, trust in our instincts, and how to turn challenges into growth opportunities.

The life experience of one colleague and student of mine exemplifies these ideas in practice. She had trained her body to excel in a certain type of athletic movement with overdeveloped (muscular) limbs. Everything about this was fine, until it wasn't. After a series of traumatic brain injuries, she realized that she could no longer rely on the familiar workout patterning that she had previously relied on. Furthermore, she found herself in need of forming a new relationship with herself because the injuries had disrupted her nervous system and introduced obstacles to balance and coordination. In this new arrangement with herself, she came to me for some sessions. Meeting her where she was, from a biointelligent approach, I invited her to sense a soft knee bend to help reacquaint her with her Lower Core. This one invitation unlocked a series of insights about how to access deeper support through the relationships in her body at the present, which were distinctly different from the striving for perfection and over-muscling relationships she had built previously through her training. Not only did this embodied approach help her to learn about herself and be guided by her own healing force—her Inner Guide—but the lessons also inspired her to approach teaching from a biointelligent perspective. This chain of realizations and life changes unfolded from the way I met her where she was and the simple invitation to soften and straighten her knees with gravity's support. Underneath that invitation, however, were the principles of practice of whole-body relationships that would have remained inaccessible if she had continued to compete with herself, fight gravity, and compare herself to others, while applying isolated muscular, biomechanical techniques to her body. She later shared with me that before our work together, she had approached movement as something she did separately from how she existed and moved through the world.

How we move in the world is dependent on our relationship with the world. I love to imagine that I am planting seeds of inspiration in working with clients or mentoring teachers. The soil we build together is based on principles of practice that continue to flourish far beyond our time together. My goal with teaching is to empower an awareness that we are connected through our living crystalline fascial matrix beyond ourselves to a wider world, and that our actions create a ripple effect.

In that spirit, with the movement explorations that I offer, I invite you to create Embodied Play Gatherings for self-study with others for support, growth, and empowerment, to explore nourishing movement, the shifting of old perceptions, and the unraveling of habitual patterns.

Here's a recap of key distinctions in order to learn principles of practice that reveal your authentic nature and *the song you were meant to sing*:

- Remember that you are a deeply intelligent organism, embedded within your living environment, who knows innately how to self-heal, adapt, and self-organize till the day you die.

- Remember that rather than collapsing or propping yourself up, you can instead build a tension-compression, orienting relationship with grounding, centering, and uplift, through your relationship with earth (tail and feet) and sky (inner ear)—what we call the fluid biotensegrity fields of "Down the Back and Up the Front."

- Remember that before you move, relationships are already happening. Sensing your pre-movement, by yielding to gravity, connects you to ongoing relationships and evokes your internal lift through the Domes of Uplift within your whole body—from foot to head and hand.

- Remember that we are *being breathed*. To sense this, feel into the waterfall. Down the Back and the internal lift. Up the Front through your low belly suspenders. How you breathe matters. Bigger and faster mouth breathing triggers your body into thinking there's an emergency. Softer, slower, and deeper, nasal breathing, to the contrary, connects breath to your body's metabolic needs. Allow peripheral vision to support a more receptive awareness.

- Remember that practitioners who invite collaboration and curiosity rather than perfection and competition create safety and support, which enables the discovery of authenticity and aliveness.

- Remember that there is no neutral touch. How you touch someone (through your eyes, heart, hand, and speaking) and how you receive their touch creates a ripple effect.

- Remember that props are a way we befriend ourselves. More importantly, though, you benefit from thinking of props as tools for change and transformation. How can your feet, hands, a pillow, ball, etc. become a *fulcrum/balance point* and energetic bridge for your orienting, omnidirectional body? Are the props *meeting and inviting* you to explore shape-shifting internal organ and fascial matrix health and vitality?

- Remember that *reorienting* is more important than "perfect posture"—it is awareness of your sphenoid/occiput to sacrum to talus relationship, your midline's relationship between earth and sky, which leads to dynamic fluidity.

MOVEMENT EXPLORATIONS AND FLOWS

As we move forward into familiar and unfamiliar movements, we have the opportunity to move beyond just doing "exercise" to find an enlivening, "energizing" conversation with our bodies. As we move in the flow of our fascial matrix, an electrical, tensional, fluid communication system, the quality of our movement can determine how we water our tissues, as if we were irrigating a garden. Below, I offer several movement flows—

- Biotensegrity-Inspired Myofascial Release Series Flow
- Embodied Pilates Matwork Flow
- Embodied Pilates Matwork with Props
- Embodied Yoga Flow

— to invite you to sense and play with your tensional-integrity body flow in new ways. This will help you sense micromovements, the power of a fulcrum to support omnidirectional spinal awareness, and the rootedness of our arms and legs. You will also explore several "Primal Poses." With our culturally acquired mode of chair sitting and aversion to going barefoot, most of us have lost flexibility through the fascial matrix of our feet, knees, hips, and spine. These postures are ones which encourage a retuning of our biointelligent architecture to be able to "rest down," using support that recalibrates the full spiralic coiling of our foot and leg's fascial matrix with our breathing spine, allowing tension to melt from tight neck and shoulders. Let your

biointelligent body guide you as you explore the magnificence of your living architecture.

Biotensegrity-Inspired Myofascial Release Series Flow

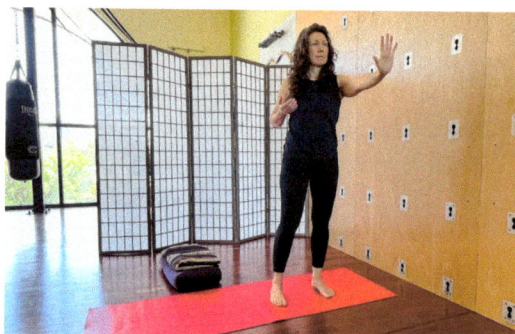

Figure 7.1 Biotensegrity-Inspired Myofascial Release Series with Jenny

Props needed:

▸ Soft rolled towel, pillow, or a bolster to function as a fulcrum.

Move with Jenny as she explores an embodied approach to moving from a biotensegrity-inspired perspective.

See if you can stay supported by the bolster/fulcrum as you roll to each side in your flowing practice and explore "embryo to adult" sequences on each side of your body.

1. STANDING, SENSING RELATIONSHIP BETWEEN EARTH AND SKY—DTB AND UTF

1. Sensing your pre-movement relationship between your grounding feet and the space around you through peripheral vision…

2. Allow your *inhale* to be received through your feet and sense your *exhale* gently exiting through your nostrils.

2. STANDING HELICAL FEET SPIRAL WITH PUSH/PULL HELICAL HANDS

1. Gently weight-shifting back and forth from right to left foot…

2. Play with a push/pull gesture that begins with weight shift to the left foot as the left hand pushes forward and right hand pulls back toward shoulder. Weight shifts to the right. Sense weight shift into the right foot as the right hand pushes forward and the left hand pulls back toward the shoulder.

3. Notice, as you weight-shift to your left foot, your breathing spine spirals to the right.

4. Allow your hands to spiral naturally and sense how your body *knows* this movement as a playful gesturing—pulling toward and pushing away.

5. Sense and play with how your breath supports the movement.

3. LYING OVER FULCRUM (A CURLED BLANKET OR PILLOW THAT GIVES YOU A SENSE OF ARCH WITHOUT LOSING YOUR HEAD-TO-TAIL CONTINUITY WITH MELTING RIBS)

1. Rest your head in your hands.

2. Can you sense you are "backing yourself" lying on the fulcrum?

3. Can you sense the two directions of your spine (DTB and UTF) and your front ribs melting so your eyes, jaw, chest, neck, shoulders, and hips can soften and widen?

4. If the blanket is too high or the fulcrum is too hard, you may need to find another surface that feels "welcoming" and supportive so you don't lose that head-to-tail continuity with melting ribs.

4. ARCH AND CURL WITH BUTTERFLY ELBOWS AND KNEES WITH BREATH (STILL LYING ON THE FULCRUM)

1. As you inhale, allow your tail to gently roll toward your feet, so your waist slightly floats off the mat.

2. As you exhale, press gently into your feet, so your tail curls toward you and your waist gently floats toward the mat.

3. Play with this movement to sense your breathing spine leading.

4. Once you feel the rhythm of this movement:

   a. As you inhale and gently arch your breathing spine, allow your elbows and knees to butterfly open.

   b. As you exhale and gently curl your breathing spine, allow your elbows and knees to butterfly closed.

   c. Sense what is just enough effort for the movement, so you are allowing your elastic fascial matrix body to tell you the range of motion that feels nourishing.

5. KNEE SWAY WITH HEAD SWAY CONTRALATERALLY

1. Sense your head in your hands and your backing on the fulcrum.

2. As you exhale, allow your knees to gently sway to the right as you look to the left.

3. Inhale, returning to center.

4. As you exhale, allow your knees to gently sway to the left as you look to the right.

5. Which side feels more difficult? You may wish to pause and breathe into the tightness and know that change can happen over time when we listen for guidance.

6. ROLLING TO EMBRYO ON RIGHT SIDE

1. As you roll your knees to the right again, allow your upper body to follow and spiral in the same direction so your right armpit is supported on the fulcrum.

2. Stay lying on fulcrum, if possible for you, and just roll to one side.

7. HEAD TO TAIL—ARCH AND CURL WITH YOUR BREATHING SPINE

1. Allow yourself to "sense" the womb-like shape of your embryo by allowing your head and tail to curl toward one another as you exhale, and then inhale as your head and tail curl away from one another.

2. Gently sense the exhale and inhale fluid resonance of your breathing spine.

8. EMBRYO TO ADULT

1. Finding axial elongation between earth and sky, come to "standing." ("Standing" refers to a full-body extension standing-like posture achieved while staying connected to the floor.)

   a. From your experience as "embryo"...

   b. Sensing your pre-movement, yield into the fulcrum.

   c. Allow your head to find its backing into your hands—sensing the waterfall Down the Back (DTB) holding your head.

   d. Sensing your pre-movement yield into the fulcrum, extend your top leg, elongating into standing, hip height—keep your bottom leg bent.

   e. Flex both feet to sense standing—foot to head awareness.

   - Inhale, allow right upper body and left top leg to release over fulcrum toward mat.

   - Keeping both feet flexed to sense DTB and UTF—tensional continuity...

   - Exhale, sensing pre-movement into fulcrum, yielding into side body on mat, as extended left top leg (hip) and upper-body sidebend toward one another.

   - Sense this movement three times on this side. Sense the inhale releasing right upper body and top leg to mat, and exhale, supporting left top leg and upper body curling toward one another.

9. BIOTENSEGRITY SPIRALS—ROOTING AND REACHING

1. Inhale, top leg (or knee) sweeps forward as upper body spirals contralaterally.

2. Exhale, eyes move spine into extension to the right as left leg releases behind.

3. Sense the contralateral flow of this movement with breath and sense what feels good to your body.

10. COME TO CENTER AND ROLL TO EMBRYO ON YOUR LEFT SIDE

11. REPEAT #6–10 ON YOUR LEFT SIDE

12. COME BACK TO CENTER

1. Lie on your back over fulcrum.

2. Hands behind head, with both legs bent and feet on floor.

13. LEG SLIDE AND UPPER CORE LIFT FROM DOWN THE BACK, UP THE FRONT

1. Sensing rooting of legs into primordial midline—DTB and UTF.

   a. Inhale, slide right leg out, flex foot, as upper body arches over fulcrum, back softening and widening, with hands behind head—DTB.

   b. Exhale, press gently into opposite foot, and float your head in hands as your ribs melt over fulcrum, allowing extended leg to lift and be received and rooted toward your midline—UTF.

c. Bend the extended leg and slide it out again, repeating a and b.

d. Can your back soften and widen as you inhale and exhale, and can your belly wall drop back into your wide back and primordial midline, allowing your leg to be received by your psoas?

e. Play with each side 3–5 times.

f. Come back to center.

2. Place both hands inside above knees to sense the cooperative polarity support of DTB and UTF to curl forward and come to sitting with knees bent—feet reaching.

   a. Sense the internal lift that happens from reaching through your feet and sensing the tension-compression of your hands to support UTF.

   b. Upper Core and Lower Core meeting Central Core in Bent Knees Teaser.

14. PRIMAL POSTURES

1. One Knee Balance on pillow—with widening clavicles and reaching arms.

   a. Place a pillow on the floor.

   b. Kneel on one knee and bring the other foot close in front of the knee on the pillow to balance.

   c. Place the top of the back foot on the floor.

   d. Extend your arms wide for fascial matrix support, sensing DTB and UTF from foot to head and hands.

e.   Count to 30—if easy, you can close your eyes.

f.   Also good to do with sandbag on head to support tonic function of the two directions of your breathing spine.

g.   Repeat on the other side.

2.   One Knee Balance to Standing up from Back Foot Push Off

   a.   Extending the toes and placing the balls of the feet on the floor is a "'ready position' which primes the whole extensor pattern of the body for standing up" (Beach 2010, p.27).

   b.   Extend the toes of your back foot so the balls of your foot are on the mat.

   c.   Place your hands on your front knee and push off the back foot, reaching through your spine and head to stand up and walk.

   d.   Repeat on each side three times.

3.   Toe Sit

   a.   This is a posture that many traditional cultures around the world use as a "resting" pose for sitting, cooking, weaving, etc.

   b.   Extend your toes and sit down with your sitting bones next to your heels.

   c.   Use a pillow or rolled-up mat to allow your body to fully "rest," as it is counter-productive to fight the tension by not giving yourself the support your body needs.

d.   Can your heels release back, by walking your knees back, so your heels are not in front of the balls of your feet?

e.   If your heels are too forward, it's like lifting your heels in squat, preventing your back body from finding ground.

f.   Don't spend too much time in this pose, as you can easily over-stretch ligaments in the joint spaces.

4.   Hero

   a.   This posture may be more familiar as a meditation posture and is also one called "seiza" used by Japanese people, which I experienced while eating at a traditional restaurant in Tokyo with hosting teachers.

   b.   Sit on the tops of your feet, resting your sitting bones on or inside your heels.

   c.   Place a pillow between your calves and thighs to relax your knees if needed in order to "rest down."

   d.   Sometimes a small, rolled towel under your ankles can feel good if there is too much pressure in that area at first.

   e.   Release your legs forward for Long Sitting with extended legs on the floor, if you need a release before proceeding to the next exploration.

5.   Looking Far to Near and Near to Far

   a.   Notice how breath supports curling in and extending out. Can you pause, rest, and wait for your inhale to *invite* extension of your eyes, head, and breathing spine?

b. Still sitting in Hero position, with hands resting on your knees, look into the distance with peripheral vision.

c. *Exhale* and begin watching an ant crawling down the wall, along the floor toward your knees as you round your spine to follow the ant (pause on your inhale, and allow your exhale to support the full curling in of your eyes and spine toward your knees).

d. Then reverse the movement.

e. *Inhale*, as you follow the ant along the floor away from you, up the wall (pause on your exhale, allowing the inhale to support your full extension of your eyes and spine overhead).

f. Still sitting down, pausing on your exhale, allow your inhale to support you following the ant along the ceiling, as your eyes lead your spine into deeper extension, while sitting down.

g. Then just drop your chin to allow your head and eyes to look forward again.

h. Repeat three times.

i. You can also explore the same sequence spiraling to the right or left, looking down and up in either direction. Staying seated, allow your gaze to sweep up as you inhale, pausing to allow your breath to support your movement.

6. One-Leg Hero

a. Still seated, one leg is in Hero and the other is in a squat position.

b. Can you stay level in the center,

allowing the floating hip to have weight, rather than falling toward the seated side?

c. Notice which side is more challenged and what changes over time.

7. Z Sit

a. Sit down in a Z position, which we use often in Rolf Structural Integration movement sessions.

b. As you sit down, one leg is externally rotated and the other is internally rotated.

c. Put a pillow under the sitting bone that allows your pelvis to feel more centered, rather than leaning to one side.

d. Eyes, Spine, and Breath Awareness:

Let's explore how breath moves our body, through our eye movement. Can you allow your inhale or exhale to be the natural mover of your body? When you let go, your inhale naturally extends your spine and your exhale naturally rounds your body into a C curve; however, the expansion and condensing of breath in the body can happen in any position. Notice what allows you to feel your fluid body moving and what breath awareness feels nourishing.

i. If your left leg is in front, externally rotated, place your left hand on the floor beside you and your right hand on your left shoulder.

ii. While breathing gently through your nose, begin spiraling your eyes, spine, and right hip to the left, so your right hip might be off the mat as you look left.

iii. And then gently sit back down.

iv. Repeat this movement three times and on your last time:

a. pause as you are extended over your left hand

b. and, just moving your head, look back—then look over your left shoulder again—then look back over your right shoulder—three times

c. then allow your head and torso to move oppositionally, so you look over your left shoulder as you sit down on your right hip and then look back over your right shoulder as you extend out to the left.

- Explore this movement three times.

- Then *stay extended out* and play with your peripheral vision:
  - Look down as your nose moves up.
  - Look up as your nose moves down—three times.
  - Look left as your nose moves to the right.
  - Look right as your nose moves to the left—three times.
  - Look down to the right as your nose moves up to the left.
  - Look up to the left as your nose moves down to the right—three times.
  - Look down to the left as your nose moves up to the right.
  - Look up to the right as your nose moves down to the left—three times.

v. Repeat Z Sit flow on the other side.

15. SPIRAL FROM SITTING TO STANDING

If you are like me, I could easily cross my feet and, without using my hands, stand up a few years ago. However, since having some serious microbiome issues and a hip injury, that approach is no longer nourishing for my body, so I have adapted to help my body. Phillip Beach calls standing up from sitting "erectorcises" and says they are imperative to be done regularly and are profoundly tonic to the overall tuning of our living architecture.

1. Play with standing up from sitting with your spiraling, helical feet.

2. Sitting on your left hip with your hands on the floor, press into the floor and spiral your hips up as your feet spiral to support you, and sit down on your right hip.

3. Spiral back and forth from one hip to the other, pressing through one or both hands in order to lift your hips.

4. Play with this movement 3–5 times in each direction—coming up to standing each time.

16. SPIRAL TO DOWNWARD DOG WALKBACK—POURING UPPER CORE THROUGH CENTRAL CORE INTO LOWER CORE

1. Come into Downward Dog, resting your shoulders in your standing hands and allowing your head to release toward your hands and your tail to lengthen away from your hands.

2. As you *inhale*, soften your knees, and as you *exhale*, walk your hands back a few inches, sending your tail back.

3. Feel the rhythm of inhaling and softening your knees, and exhaling and sending your tail back in order to walk your hands back.

4. You are pouring yourself into your feet with this recalibrating movement.

5. Notice if it serves your spine more to come up to standing by staying rounded till your head floats up.

6. Or, if your spine has some kyphosis in standing, place both hands on knees, relax your tail, and, pressing gently into your feet, come to standing looking up.

17. WALKING WITH NEW AWARENESS

1. Weight-shift walking—notice what feels new as you walk.

2. Can you allow your back heel to have weight as you weight-shift through that foot to pour your weight into your front foot?

See Video 7.1 for full exploration.

Embodied Pilates Matwork Flow

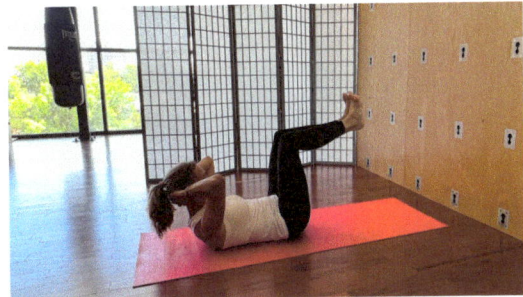

Figure 7.2 Embodied Pilates Matwork Flow with Sybil

Move with Sybil as she explores the flowing transitions of Pilates Matwork through an embodied lens. **See Video 7.2 for full exploration.**

Embodied Pilates Matwork with Props

Props:

▸ Stretch-eze® band (small, medium, or tall— what works best for your height) or elastic band—wrapped around thighs to relax rooting of legs to breathing spine.

▸ Pilates Push Thru Bar, or ankle weight (2½lb) or wall (for Arms Coming Alive in Small Bridge).

▸ Towel or pillow.

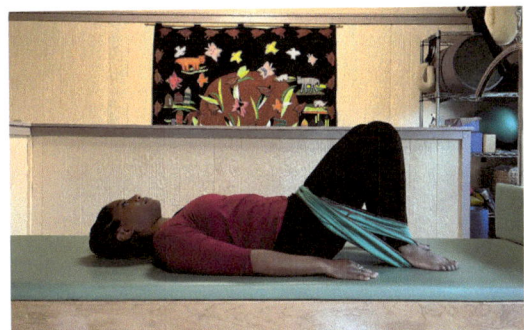

Figure 7.3 Embodied Constructive Rest to Arch and Curl with Amanda

Prop: Stretch-eze® band or elastic band.

Constructive rest is a nourishing somatic aware-ness exploration which can provide a baseline of where your body is with tension, discomfort, etc., and creates an ability to transform that experi-ence through a conversation with your self-heal-ing biointelligence.

Be sure your Stretch-eze® (small, medium, tall) or elastic band is knotted or tied to a tension that allows your legs to feel centered and grounded with your feet, sensing whole-body support—Down the Back and Up the Front. **See Video 7.3 for full exploration.**

Embodied Small Bridge
Prop: Stretch-eze® band or elastic band.

▸ Check in with a gentle press of your feet sensing the mat, which creates a small bridge through sensing the Down the Back from the collar bone, scapular, tail bone, sit bone, and then to the feet, and Up the Front from the inner ankle, inner thigh, back of the thigh, front of the spine, and then to the inner ear.

▸ Sense the hamstring connection from the back of the leg to the front of the spine (soft-ening lower ribs).

▸ Sensing the back yield to the support of grav-ity supports a fascial flossing small bridge which is vital for all inversions.

Embodied Arms Coming Alive with Small Bridge
Props:

▸ Stretch-eze® band or elastic band.
▸ Push Thru Bar or ankle/wrist weight (2½lb).

The arch and curl fascial flossing movement ener-gizes the arms to come alive. The Upper Core is energized from the pre-movement of the Lower Core, feet pressing into the mat, reaching the

knees over feet, so the breathing spine awakens the arms and opens the chest, which allows the arms to move and open out.

▸ Sense the weight of your arm moving from the waterfall Down the Back.

▸ You could gently move with just the weight of your arms or:
   – hold the Pilates Push Thru Bar (without springs) or reach to a wall, both of which act as weights to enhance the upper arms rooting to the breathing spine when arms reach out from the back
   – or use a small weight in your hands.

Embodied Arms Wide with Knee Sway
Prop: Stretch-eze® band or elastic band.

▸ Soften your eyes, to support your arms reaching wide as your helical feet roll to one side, thereby supporting your legs and lower breathing spine in rotation.

▸ By doing this, your legs and hips are supported by the lemniscate counter-rotation of your upper breathing spine, head, and shoulder to the opposite side.

▸ Sense the waterfall down from the scapular area to your feet, which connects to your breathing spine and your arms reaching out.

Embodied Heavy Head in Hands, Arms Open-Close, and 100s
Prop: Stretch-eze® band. If you don't have a Stretch-eze® band, place your interwoven hands behind your head and let your head rest heavy in your hands. Both the band and your hands enhance the feeling of Down the Back, Up the Front—providing a fulcrum of polarity to support the two directions of your spine, which increases the feelings of grounding and uplift. **See Video 7.4 for full exploration.**

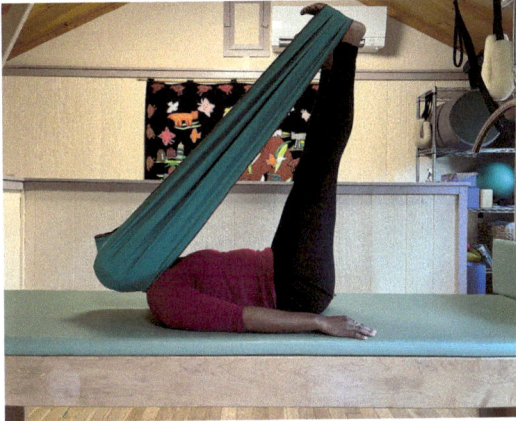

Figure 7.4 Down the Back (Lower Core) floats the head and Upper Core for embodied Pilates 100s

STEP 1

▸ Place the band behind your head and around the dome of each foot (or use your hands behind your head).

STEP 2

▸ Press gently into the band (or your feet on the mat) to begin widening your feet and slightly straighten your legs *just enough* so that your head begins to float off the mat.

▸ You'll have the sensation of "holding your head, heavy in your hands."

Arms Open-Close

▸ Sense your head heavy in the band, which curls you forward and frees up your arms for movement.

▸ Open your arms (as you inhale) and then close your arms (as you exhale), sensing how your arms are connecting to the waterfall, Down the Back, and the lift of your inner ears, Up the Front.

▸ Reach your arms from the waterfall Down the

Back to sense how you can move your arms from your chest, staying soft and wide, and breathe into your back.

Embodied 100s

▸ Reach your arms forward, alongside your body, from the waterfall Down the Back.

▸ Gently pump your arms up and down from the waterfall, inhaling for 5 pumps and exhaling for 5 pumps, as you allow breath into your back and whole-body connection from foot to head, and hand.

Embodied One-Leg Rollup, One-Leg Circle, Climb a Tree, Twisting Teaser

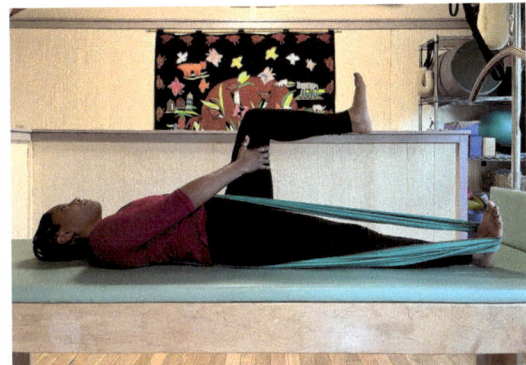

Figure 7.5A One-leg rollup

Props:

▸ Stretch-eze® band—on left shoulder and around right foot.

▸ Ankle weight on left ankle—approx. 2½lb (optional)

▸ Pad (or folded towel) under right thigh.

This is a great way to deepen your understanding and access to the traditional Pilates Rollup. The invitation is to find deeper support through grounding through feet (DTB) and to encourage UTF from inner ankle to inner ear. Typically, people have problems because of locking the knees and gripping the hips and back, which causes your legs to overpower your breathing spine. Instead of doing that, you'll begin by finding a lengthened and widened back, which creates your hammock-like spine and enables your belly wall to gently fall back toward your primordial midline as you curl up. **See Video 7.5 for full exploration.**

Embodied One-Leg Rollup

▸ Lie on your back and place the Stretch-eze® band over left shoulder and around right foot with your right leg extended on the mat.

▸ Place a thick pad under your right thigh that supports the opening of that extended hip, softens your knee, and creates connection of the hamstring to the front of your spine in movement.

▸ Then press the left thigh into your hands as you curl up to sitting. Keep pressing the leg into your hands as you roll back down. Repeat 3–5 times.

Embodied One-Leg Circle

▸ After completing One-Leg Rollup, place hands on low belly suspenders, keeping the left hip heavy, and straighten the left leg to find the back of the leg to the front of the spine connection for Leg Circles.

▸ Inhale as you circle your leg in one direction 5 times and then the other direction 5 times.

▸ Play with the ankle weight in your One-Leg Circle and then create a contrast, feeling how your leg moves without the ankle weight, with more grounding, centering, and uplift and connection from head to foot.

Embodied Climb a Tree with Ankle Weight

▸ After completing One-Leg Circle on left side, keep the left sitting bone long and connected to right foot. Press that leg into your hands and away from you and walk up that leg towards your foot from a heavy hip.

▸ You may notice you are rebalancing your body from foot to head and hand.

▸ Walk back down your leg to lie on the mat and repeat 2–3 times.

Embodied Twisting Teaser with Ankle Weight

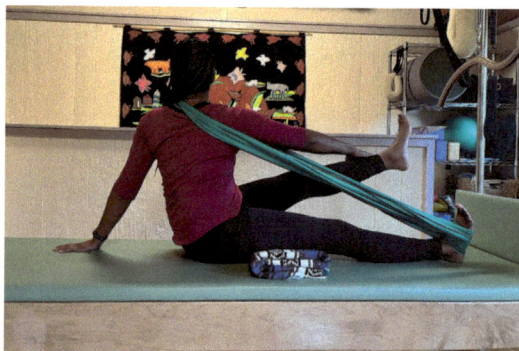

Figure 7.5B Embodied Twisting Teaser with or without ankle weight

As you Climb a Tree on your left leg, pause at the top and place your right hand on the lateral side of your ankle and your left hand on the mat behind your body. You may sense that both upper arms and thighs are rooted to the spine.

▸ What do you notice on each side of your body as you play with Twisting Teaser, inhaling to soften your knee, and exhaling to straighten your leg and move deeper into your twist—with and without an ankle weight?

Embodied Rolling Like a Ball, Embodied Rollover, Downward Dog Walkback

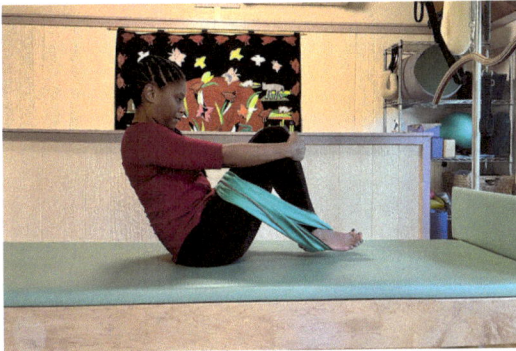

Figure 7.6A Embodied Rolling Like a Ball

Props:

- Stretch-eze® band
- Ankle weights (optional)
- Pillow, small blanket, or pad

These movements will help increase your fascial elasticity throughout your body. It's important to allow the way in which you breathe to give you a sense of grounding, centering, and uplift. **See Video 7.6 for full exploration.**

Embodied Rolling Like a Ball

- Use the Stretch-eze® band under the feet and over the knees to sense the action of the feet reaching and inner ear lifting through the two directions of the fascial flossing spine.

- The Stretch-eze® band or ankle weights support the seated round back, hammock-like—two directions of the spine position—without collapsing.

- Inhale as you roll back to your shoulders. Exhale as you roll forward to balance your feet off the mat. Repeat 3–5 times.

Embodied Single-Leg Stretch

- Transitioning from Rolling Like a Ball, remove the Stretch-eze®—you may notice a deeper internal connection in your body from foot to head and hand.

- As you curl down to the mat, place your left hand on your right inside knee and your right hand on your outside right ankle.

- Then press your left leg away from you to curl your upper body forward to the base of your shoulder blades.

- Alternate the movement by switching leg and hand positions.

- Repeat 3–5 times on both sides.

Embodied Double-Leg Stretch with Ankle Weights

- Transitioning from Single-Leg Stretch, bend both knees toward chest and place hands on your shins.

- Lying on your back, curl towards your shoulder blades. Inhale as arms and legs reach up and out. Exhale as you hug your knees towards your chest.

- Can you sense the reach through the waterfall Down the Back and the internal lift Up the Front?

- Repeat 3–5 times on both sides.

Spine Stretch with Stretch-eze® Band

- Transitioning from Double Leg Stretch to Spine Stretch, come to sitting.

▸ Place the Stretch-eze® band around your feet and behind your back.

▸ Be sure to sit up on or in front of your sitting bones, not behind your sitting bones, as you are lengthening from foot to head. Sitting behind your sitting bones will compress your lumbar and thoracic spines as you round forward.

▸ Inhale as you sit tall. Exhale as you round and reach forward.

▸ Repeat 3–5 times on both sides.

Embodied Saw with Stretch-eze® Band

▸ Transitioning from Spine Stretch to Saw, sense the grounded pelvis, reaching legs, and lifted spine as you reach both arms out to the side at shoulder height.

▸ The Stretch-eze® band enhances the relationship between the midback and feet, supporting the two directions of your spine, encouraging just enough effort to sit tall and allow a more spacious rotation in each direction.

▸ Inhale and sit tall. Exhale as you spiral to the right and reach the arms away from one another, left palm facing down, right palm facing up.

▸ Inhale and sit tall. Exhale to spiral to the left, left palm facing up, right palm facing down.

Embodied Swan

▸ Transitioning from Saw to Swan, move to a prone position on the mat.

▸ Place your pad or small blanket, on your pelvis,

above your pubic bone. Do not place pad or blanket under your legs.

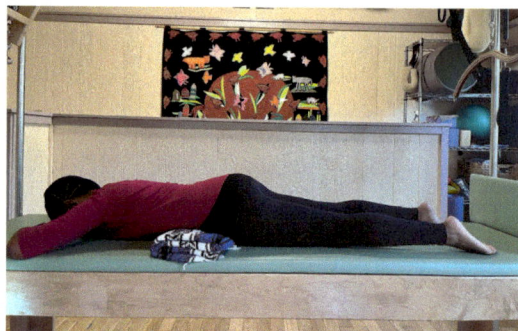

Figure 7.6B Embodied Swan

▸ When your tail can relax and rest down, your low belly suspenders can find uplift by connecting with your adductors and their relationship to your hamstrings and the front of your spine; you are accessing your embryonic primordial nature, where your front body (yoke sac) supports your back body.

▸ Breathe naturally as you look forward, curling up, resting on your forearms and allowing your elbows to come to rest under your shoulders.

▸ Gently curl back down. Repeat 3–5 times.

Embodied Sidekicks

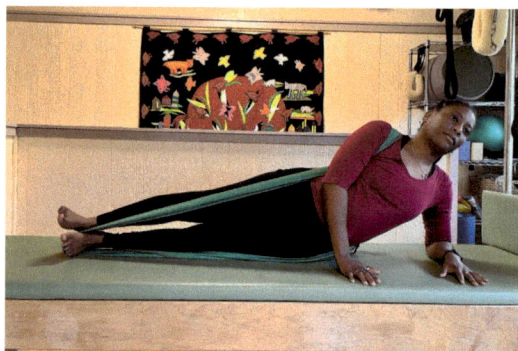

Figure 7.6C Embodied Sidekicks

▸ Transitioning from Swan to Sidekicks, lie on your side with the Stretch-eze® over your shoulder and around your opposite foot. The wrapped foot is your standing foot.

▸ The pre-movement, yield to gravity, through your standing leg from foot to head, allows your other leg to move more freely.

▸ Your free leg lifts and lowers, moves front and back, and circles in both directions.

▸ Repeat 3–5 times, then switch to the other side.

Embodied Seal

▸ Transitioning from Sidekicks to Seal, come back to sitting up on the mat and remove Stretch-eze®. Can you notice the benefit of whole-body connection from your experience in Sidekicks?

▸ Bring your feet toward one another with your knees wide and reach your arms from your waterfall support to hold each heel.

▸ Clap your heels together three times. Inhale to roll back, clap your heels together three times, and exhale to roll forward and balance.

▸ Repeat 3–5 times.

Embodied Teaser with Soft Knees

▸ Transition from Seal to Teaser with Soft Knees. As you come back to sitting balance with bent knees, move your hands to the back of your thighs, keeping that sense of Down the Back and Up the Front.

▸ Pressing the left leg gently into your hand, sense your heavy hip and, with soft eyes,

straighten your leg from the sensation of a heavy hip and a soft knee, yet straight leg.

▸ This internal lift helps to not stiffen your body as you straighten your leg.

▸ If straightening your legs feels easy for you, play with releasing your hands from behind your legs and reach your arms toward your extended feet for a full Teaser.

Embodied Rollover with Stretch-eze® and Ankle Weights

▸ Transitioning from Teaser to Rollover, lie on your back and place the Stretch-eze® around your midback and around each foot so you feel a supportive tension from foot to head— use ankle weights for more grounding and uplift.

▸ What is most important is to set up your Upper Core so your back, shoulders, and arms can take the weight of your legs and lower spine curling over your chest.

▸ Set-up for Upper Core Double Spiral Platform:
  – Widen your arms on the mat, shoulder height and palms up, so your chest widens.
  – Then slide your arms alongside your body, keeping your chest wide and your palms facing up.
  – Have an elastic band ready near your sitting bones so you can grasp it when you are ready and pull gently out for lateral support.
  – This is your Upper Core Double Spiral Platform—set-up for any Inversion.

▸ Allow your legs to roll back, supported by the ankle weights, Stretch-eze® band, and the Upper Core. Roll back down.

▸ Repeat 3–5 times.

Embodied Downward Dog Walk Back

▶ Transitioning from Rollover to Downward Dog, come up to standing and bend forward into an inverted V with palms and feet weighted evenly, tail reaching back.

▶ Notice that you are lengthening your spine and rooting your legs to the front of your spine by pouring your Upper Core through the Central Core into the Lower Core to feel your grounding feet receive your upper body as you stand up and orient in the field of gravity.

Embodied Upper Core Awareness Bridge Series

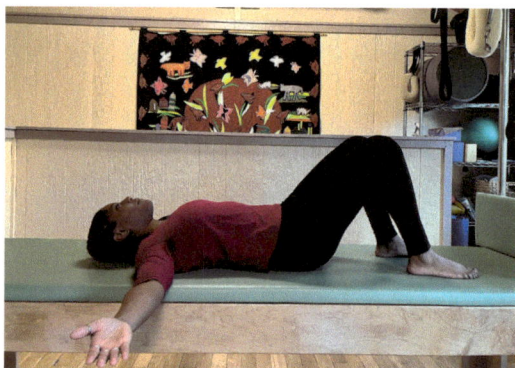

Figure 7.7 Set-up for Upper Core awareness bridge series

You may notice that in the Pilates Matwork, there are few *arm-balancing* exercises until the Advanced Matwork. For this reason, I have added these arm-balancing movements to the Basic Matwork which continue to progress through the Intermediate to the Advanced Matwork, strengthening the fascial matrix of the Upper Core and its relationship with the Central and Lower Core continuity. This series can be explored on its own, or integrated into your Pilates Matwork or another flowing series. **See Video 7.7 for full exploration**.

Embodied Shoulder Bridge with Leg Extension to Kicks with Hips Up
STEP 1

▶ Transitioning from Downward Dog Walk Back, lie on your back with knees bent, arms wide, allowing chest to open.

▶ Press gently into feet to support the arch and curl, with soft eyes.

▶ Keeping palms up as you bring your arms by your side, you may notice your back widening. Then turn your palms down to support your double spiral arm platform.

STEP 2

▶ Press gently into your feet and arms to curl your tail off the mat and sense your knees going over your feet, to support the bridge lift from inner ankle to inner ear.

▶ Slowly curl back down.

STEP 3

▶ Press gently into your feet and arms to curl the spine off the mat into a bridge.

▶ Can you allow the fascial flossing to ease through your spine, which allows you to extend one leg?

▶ Lift and lower the leg, as you press gently into the other foot. Repeat 3 times. Roll back down to the mat and repeat on the other side.

Suspension Bridge on Knees to Full Plank
STEP 1

▸ Transitioning from Shoulder Bridge, turn over to Child's Pose, sitting back toward your heels, with the toes curled for support on the balls of your feet and arms extended and reaching forward.

STEP 2

▸ Keep reaching the heels back as you move forward to a Kneeling Plank.

STEP 3

▸ Float your knees off the mat to Full Plank with soft knees and support of your shoulder blades to internal belly suspenders.

▸ Going deeper: If you have difficulty weight-bearing on the balls of your feet, place a small, rolled towel under your toes, so you can bear less weight on your toe tendons and more weight on the padding of the balls of your feet. This small but important difference will change the flexibility and strength of your feet and how they relate to giving support to your upper body.

Reverse Spinal—One Hand Position to Three Hand Position

▸ Transitioning from Suspension Bridge, start with sitting on the mat with hands behind you, feet parallel, and knees bent.

▸ Place your hands in the position that feels best for your shoulders to feel relaxed in movement.

▸ Straighten the arms as you press gently into your feet on the mat, so your tailbone curls up and breathing spine begins to lift.

▸ Reaching your knees towards your toes, come to Tabletop, sensing the DTB from your widening collar bones, gliding scapular, tailbone release, to your feet.

Side-Lying Inner/Outer Spiral Twist with Wall
STEP 1

▸ Transitioning from Reverse Spinal, lie on your side, side-lying on the left hip, yielding weight into the forearm, creating shoulder blade to low belly suspender internal support.

▸ Let the left foot reach to the box or wall. Put the right foot on the mat, in front of the left knee, with knee bent.

STEP 2

▸ Sensing the support of the left side from foot to head and hand, spiral the right arm open as you inhale, and exhale as you spiral and close.

▸ You can spiral open and closed several times to sense an Outer Spiral and look in the opposite direction to sense Inner Spiral.

▸ Going deeper: Press gently into your left foot on the wall and lift your pelvis off the mat as you spiral your arm to the right, opening your chest, and then spiral your arm back under your ribs.

Control Balance: Explorations from Pilates Rollover to Control Balance
Control Balance is an advanced Pilates exercise that challenges the body's ability to find grounding, centering, and uplift in an inverted position. By embodying the principles that allow a fluid Rollover, where your legs are rooted to your breathing spine and your tail is floating to support your legs reaching from Down the Back and Up the Front, the Rollover becomes *effort with ease*. **See Video 7.8 for full exploration.**

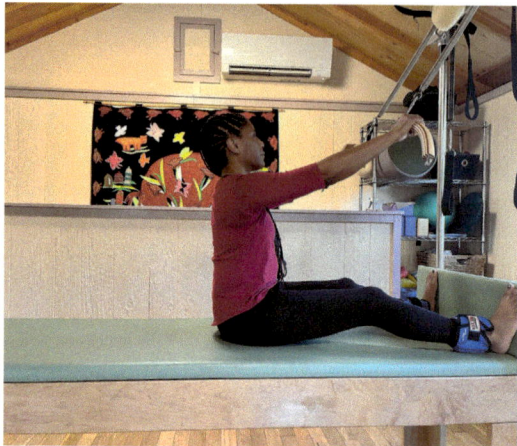

Figure 7.8A Embodied Pilates roll down

Props:

▸ Ankle weights.
▸ Pilates Roll Down Bar.

We are beginning with the Pilates Roll Down Bar and ankle weights to support reaching through the legs and internal lift through the front of the spine, head, and arms.

▸ Sensing uplift through the inner ears from inner ankles, and the ankle weights reaching the feet from the waterfall of your shoulder blades Down the Back, let the sitting bones and tail release toward your feet as you curl backwards.

Embodied Bridging

▸ Transitioning from Rolling Down to Bridging, stay in the supine position from the previous Roll Down and sense your breathing spine and the weight of your sacrum.

▸ Bend each knee, so your feet sense their grounding.

▸ Press gently into each foot so you can gently curl your tail, as your scapular glides Down the Back, supporting your bridging.

▸ Notice that the Roll Down Bar supports your hands' connection to your scapular in sensing their relationship Down the Back into your feet, which allows uplift along the front of your spine from inner ankle to inner ear.

Embodied Pilates Rollover

▸ Transitioning from Bridging to Rollover, using the Roll Down Bar and ankle weights helps your body feel the reach of your arms from the waterfall Down the Back and the rootedness of your legs Up the Front of your spine.

STEP 1

▸ Bring each leg in front of the Roll Down Bar, so the ankle weights help the thighs to go deeper into the hip socket, connecting each foot to your breathing spine.

STEP 2

▸ The ankle weights will help your legs feel weighted and connected to your spine, and as you allow the weight of your legs to begin rolling and reaching over toward your head, notice that your reaching arms from the waterfall Down the Back are assisting your tail in curling deeper to support your legs and spine moving into Rollover.

STEP 3

▸ Your shoulder blades waterfalling Down the Back connect with your low belly suspenders lifting Up the Front, which is the internal support you need for Pilates Rollover, Jackknife, and a successful Control Balance, which are all intermediate to advanced Pilates exercises.

Embodied Control Balance with Roll Down Bar

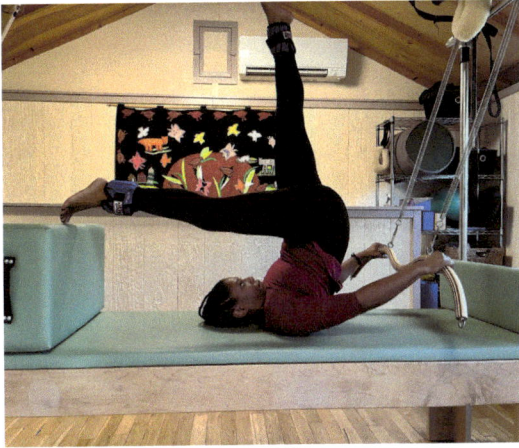

Figure 7.8B

▸ Transitioning from Rollover to Control Balance with a Roll Down Bar, stay in the supine position, sensing the Down the Back and Up the Front, shoulder blades to the deep belly connection.

▸ Your legs are still in front of the Roll Down Bar, with ankle weights on, so you can feel the value of the Rollover that you just completed.

▸ Control Balance is a deeper Rollover, with more of a lift, like Jackknife.

▸ With the reach of your arms and the reach of your tail, can you reach one leg toward the ceiling and release one leg toward a box behind your head (unless you can release your foot to the floor without losing the height of your tail)?

▸ Your challenge is to not lose the Down the Back and Up the Front (grounding, centering, and uplift) as your legs move up and down.

Embodied Control Balance with Elastic Band

▸ Transition to Control Balance without the Roll Down Bar and with an elastic band support for hands reaching.

▸ Place an elastic band in front of your hips, where your hands can contact the band and "pull out" for reaching support through your arms and hands when Down the Back support is needed.

▸ You are now challenging your body's understanding of Control Balance with less support of the Roll Down Bar reaching your arms with the elastic band "pull out," widening your back, and the ankle weights rooting your legs to the front of your spine and reaching with your tail.

▸ Can you keep your tail and one leg lifted and slowly lower one leg toward the floor, or to a box to limit your range of motion and give deeper quality of movement that allows you to keep your tail and the other leg reaching up?

▸ Can you let go of the elastic band and, staying centered through your shoulder blades and internal belly suspenders, with a long neck and your tail and one leg reaching toward the ceiling, can your hands reach back toward the leg moving down?

Embodied Downward Dog Walk Back

▸ From a position of being on hands and knees, begin to straighten your arms so your shoulder "receives" the weight of your upper arm and sends your spine and tail back, away from your hands, as you straighten your legs.

▸ Notice that your neck is free to move when the shoulder blades to deep belly suspenders are supported by your breathing spine.

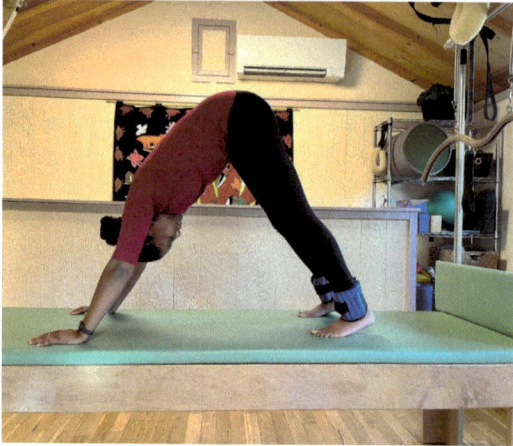

Figure 7.8C Embodied Downward Dog Walk Back

▶ Keep repeating this relational balance between your hands, spine, and legs to walk your Upper Core back to being unweighted and pouring yourself into your Lower Core through your Central Core.

This approach to Pilates movement awakens the spring-like tension-compression that is our natural, pre-tensed fascial matrix nature. Those who are familiar with the springs of the Pilates apparatus will sense the resonance between those springs and our biotensegrity body. In this chapter, we are sometimes using the Pilates apparatus. We are also using sensory feedback tools like Stretch-eze® bands, weighted sandbags, ankle and wrist weights, pillows, and pads. For many, these tools help the body feel the interplay between gravity and ground reaction force more viscerally.

Embodied Yoga Explorations with Wendy

With our embodied yoga focus, we are not just inhabiting positions but exploring the process of our living architecture through these movements. "Movement beyond doing" is crucial for yoga since yoga can become such a familiar practice of over-stretching or self-judgment about "doing it right." The danger of studying yoga as "perfect forms" is that practitioners can start simply "doing" yoga to perform, rather than exploring and growing through the process and challenges of movement. In other words, asking, "What do I need today in order to be present with the guidance of my body?" Once we cease that exploration, we disconnect the movements from life and the process of living.

You will notice that I am in a constant conversation with my Inner Guide to support an injured hip and how my whole-body fascial matrix can "share the spatial biotensegrity load," from foot to head and hand, to provide support and guidance. I will be using a chair, the height of which feels more nourishing to my body. Feel free to place your grounding hand on a yoga block or the floor, if that feels like a more nourishing challenge for you. **See Video 7.9 for full exploration**.

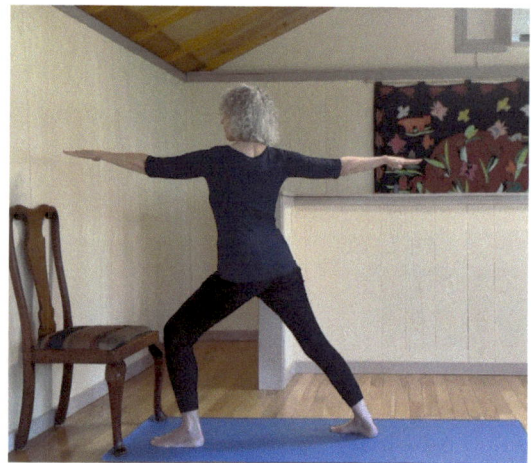

Figure 7.9 Embodied yoga explorations

WARRIOR I

▶ Place a chair in front of a yoga mat with the seat facing toward you—be sure the chair is secure.

▶ Open to breath moving your body.

▸ Begin in a lunge position, left leg forward, with knee bent and right leg behind.

▸ Sense your feet opening as you inhale while softening your left knee, arms spiraling forward in a lemniscate, figure-eight pattern.

▸ Exhale as you straighten your leg with a soft knee, as arms spiral back in a lemniscate, figure-eight pattern. See what pattern feeds your movement—I like to explore inhaling as I circle my arms forward with a bent knee and exhaling as my arms circle back as my front leg straightens and deepens awareness from foot to head and hand.

WARRIOR II

▸ After sensing that movement a few times, transition to Warrior II by inhaling, softening your left knee, opening arms, and spiraling your torso to the right, with arms reaching away from one another at shoulder height, as your torso remains twisted to the right and your head looks forward. Bending and straightening of the knee is again paired with inhale and exhale as you spiral each hand internally and externally to sense a deeper relationship with whole-body fascial matrix movement from foot to head and hand.

TRIANGLE POSE—WITH CHAIR OR YOGA BLOCK

▸ Transition to Triangle, placing your left hand on the chair in front of you and your right hand behind, resting along your back.

▸ On the inhale, soften your left knee as you open space to spiral your torso on your exhale more deeply to your right, gently straightening your leg.

▸ As you inhale softening your knee and exhale straightening your leg, notice how deeply your

body wants to spiral to the right in order to feel a deeper conversation with your left hand on the chair, which invites your right arm to reach up and out.

SINGLE LEG FORWARD BEND

▸ Bring your hands into prayer position behind your back, or hold elbows or reach hands down and back with an open chest (whichever feels more comfortable to your shoulders).

▸ Sensing your feet and your head-to-tail midline uplift, inhale and then exhale, and gently fold forward from your hips, just to where you can stay connected to grounding, centering, and uplift from foot to head.

▸ Then look up, sensing your feet, and begin to breathe gently, softening your front knee, while reaching your arms down and then forward and up. Return to a standing position with arms reaching wide to open your chest and heart to the sky.

REVOLVED TRIANGLE

▸ Transitioning to Revolved Triangle, place your right hand on the chair (or yoga block).

▸ Breathe spine spirals to the left, with your left arm behind your back, still with your left leg forward in lunge.

▸ The inhale softens the left knee. As you exhale, extend left leg with a soft knee, spiraling more to your left.

▸ Continue to inhale, soften knee, and exhale spiral to your left.

▸ Deepen your Revolved Triangle by extending your left arm up toward the sky, or place your hand behind your head and open your chest toward the sky (so your spine is in relationship with the range of motion of your arm).

▶ Be aware of the power of sounding as you exhale and discovering your shoulder blade to deep belly suspenders support.

RETURNING TO STANDING BALANCE IN MOUNTAIN POSE

▶ Returning to center, bring your right foot forward to meet your standing left and come back up to Standing Balance, with hands meeting at your heart center.

▶ Repeat the whole flow with your right leg forward and left leg behind.

– As is common, one side will feel different from the other. In my case, I have a right-side hip replacement, and so I deepen my whole-body relationships by keeping both hands on the chair in front of me at first and then begin the flow, modifying to stay in a conversation with my body guiding me.

CONCLUSION

This book started with a discussion of the Inner Guide, and I'd like to end with some stories that deepen that discussion, which continues to reveal how discovering our authentic inner song creates a ripple effect to a healthy global community.

In sharing about listening or not listening to our Inner Guide, I was speaking recently with my dear friend and colleague, Victor van Kooten, senior Iyengar yoga teacher and artist, living on the beautiful island of Lesvos, one of the largest Greek islands. Victor and I were sharing stories of how we learned to listen to our Inner Guide, by experiencing moments when we didn't and each wound up with damaging results:

I, Wendy, shared that I had an experience about 25 years ago where I didn't listen to my Inner Guide, while exploring with a fellow yoga colleague. We were in a rich exploration of asana flow when he suggested we use a yoga block for pelvic support and our feet on the wall for a plank pose. This was when there were no soft yoga blocks, so we were using the old wooden blocks. After a while, I felt I needed to come out of the pose, and he said, "You can do more!" I didn't listen to my

body and continued. When I came out of the pose and released to the floor, I had no feeling in my legs and couldn't stand for at least 30 minutes. What I discovered later was that I had compressed my femoral artery and could have severely damaged my body. It was a very good lesson about deep listening to my Inner Guide.—WLA

I, Victor, had an experience in a demonstration where I was assisting Iyengar and I allowed him to push me over the 4x4 after I resisted him twice before, and now was lying over it with my mid-thoracic as my calf muscles were held over a half-moon shape topping a similar 4x4 by someone assisting. When he put his hands on my shoulders to press them down, I heard myself making this ridiculous remark: "If I cannot trust men, I will never be able to trust God," and he pressed down in my surrendering... I landed in a fog and was sobbing as he triumphantly said, while he asked me to hold a rope extended from the ceiling, grabbing my right leg in a dancing Shiva pose backbend, and placing my foot onto my head: "See what you can do now?" It all did not mean anything to me, for I was far away from feeling my body...and when I walked home, that inner voice told me loud into my left ear, three times: "No yoga for three days."

And since I felt good the next morning, I decided that being here with the best yoga teacher in the world (yes, we all believed him when he said he was the best), I ignored the inner voice for the first time in my life, and it never came back as an audible sound after this! After three days, I became paralyzed during the night and got a high fever and enormous pains in my shoulder and hip joints, and for over two weeks lost the peristaltic movements in the food pipe, stomach, and intestines, and lost my voice and my ability to write or draw. But when I recovered after half a year and retrained my body into a reasonable asana practice, I had discovered to use SPACE as a stimulation for energy flow and told Iyengar I was unable to teach his method anymore... But he wanted me to stay as one of his yoga teachers and promoted me as the healer through yoga practice and told me that I was like his younger brother, but nothing could win me over, mainly because I was told many years before by this loud voice that I should: "Take Iyengar as your Guru, not for what he can teach you but for what he can't teach you."

And this all comes back to what I wrote to you about the space I always felt as a child and still...the outer world can show you things, promises and disasters, but your Inner Guide will make the choices, and even when you ignore the choices, you will have to walk your own way and see where it leads you...

Resource: https://angela-victor.com

When I process my story and Victor's, I reflect on how a certain blind adherence to a particular discipline muted the volume of our Inner Guides. The insight Victor shares is that honoring the messages that come from the Inner Guide is more vital than the perfection of any given discipline. His insight was an illuminating moment in what would become a long career of demonstrating the power of biointelligence that he explores with communities around the world.

As we know, life is a journey that challenges us to meet ourselves, sometimes face to face. The ability of our human bodies to function in the ways they do and repair themselves has been a constant source of wonder to medical science. As we studied in Chapter 2, biotensegrity, our living tensegrity through the forces of tension-compression, is the physical representation of the invisible forces, between structure and energy, that allows us to function as a self-organizing organism. While study of the fascial matrix in relation to health and disease has been an integral part of manual therapies for a few decades, I have explored the value of biotensegrity for manual and movement therapies and principles of practice, which are often misunderstood and yet fundamental to a deeper understanding of our Inner Guide and how to help ourselves.

I so appreciate this quotation by biologist and osteopath Graham Scarr, because it says so much about how our bodies are relational organisms and that we gain access to helping ourselves through the ways we listen and respond.

Living tissues [...] operate in exactly the same way in a healthy body as in a dysfunctioning one, in the sense that their underlying physiological processes always follow the same principles and are constrained by the same rules of self-organization. Even though homeostasis is built into the system, a change in the balance of forces in one region can shift it away from its normal operating parameters, with the tissues now acting within a different set of constraints and displaying a different pattern of behavior.

However, it is us who really make the value judgment about health and disease, not the biology. Whether we have a cut finger, chronic arthritic joints, or invasive cancer, the body always responds in the most energy-efficient (and only) ways that it can, and the same fundamental principles of biotensegrity always apply.

So while it is the responsibility of the practitioner to understand the client's problem, it is equally important to recognize that treatment is about initiating changes, and then allowing the body's inherent self-organizing mechanisms to respond to this as it moves towards a different state of health. The resolution of a local condition can then require a whole-body approach to treating it, or vice versa, particularly if tissues some distance away have become chronically adapted to changes in the structure balance, and an understanding of biotensegrity provides the rationale for this. (Scarr 2021)

It is my hope that this idea, and all the ideas in this book, plant seeds that continue to foster growing ourselves and strengthening our communities through collaborations across disciplines, encouraging Embodied Play Gatherings—to experiment with, reshape, and transform ourselves and our clients through the principles of practices I've introduced in *Moving Beyond Core*.

Please be in touch to share your discoveries and insights, along with your questions and comments that support our continued growth as a co-creative, adaptive global community functioning within a web of relationships.

Use the following QR code for all videos in this chapter:

REFERENCES

Beach, P. (2010) *Muscles and Meridians: The Manipulation of Shape*. London: Churchill Livingstone.

Harper, S. and Molin-Skelton, M. (2023) "Wild Heart of Imagining" [workshop].

Nin, A. (2015) *The Quotable Anaïs Nin, Collected and Compiled by Paul Herron*. San Antonio, TX: Sky Blue Press.

Oschman, J. (2003) *Energy Medicine in Therapeutics and Human Performance*. Oxford: Butterworth-Heinemann.

Scarr, G. (2021) "Biotensegrity: The Structural Basis of Life." *Massage Magazine*. www.massagemag.com/biotensegrity-the-structural-basis-of-life-129777

Glossary

Advanced Thinking: Term coined by the author of *Moving Beyond Core*, which encourages us to adapt any given movement so it meets our needs, is an act of self-care, and encourages us to listen to our Inner Guide.

Anthroposophy: an early 20th century formal education, therapeutic, and creative system established by Rudolf Steiner, centering on the theory that we are spiritual beings living a physical existence.

Backing into the womb: Term used by Dutch embryologist and anthroposophist Jaap van der Wal. He is particularly recognized for his integration of anthroposophical perspectives into the study of human development. Van der Wal's phrase "backing into the womb" is associated with his ideas about embryonic development and the orientation of the embryo in the womb, referring to the idea that the early embryo exhibits movements that appear to actively position itself moving backward into the uterus. This concept is part of van der Wal's broader exploration of embryonic movements and their significance in our lifelong actions and behavior. (Gratitude to clinical anatomist John Sharkey for contributing to this distinction.)

Biointelligence: The body's way of knowing, which emerges from the innate fluidity of each person's somatic architecture and relationship with the field of gravity, other beings, and our living environment.

Biotensegrity or **living tensegrity:** A term introduced by orthopedic surgeon Stephen Levin. Most literally, it names a regenerative, *spring-like* integrity and a tensional balance within the fascial matrix that forms the living architecture of our whole organism.

Breathing spine: Our primordial relationship between earth and sky that comes into material reality as our structural spine. The adjective "breathing" helps remind us of the spine's fluid, wave-like nature from sacrum/pelvic diaphragm to sphenoid/inner ear/palate.

Breathwave: The fluid, naturally occurring rocking motion of breath that coordinates the body's movement between sphenoid (head) and sacrum (tail).

Chakras: Originally coming from the Hindu worldview, these are centers of spinning energy that support our physical, emotional, and mental experiences and resonate with our neuroendocrine glands.

Connective tissue consciousness: Responsible for wound healing and injury repair, it resides in the living matrix of your fascial matrix body's perineural nervous system.

Core: Beyond a muscular holding pattern, Core as Relationship in *Moving Beyond Core* is a dynamic, biointelligent expression; an effect of sensing earth's energy through the gravitational field; and a spatial, enlivening, social, and physical relationship with ourselves, one another, and our living environment.

3CoreConnections: A perspective of embodied awareness through whole-organism core coordination developed by Wendy LeBlanc-Arbuckle that refers to the body's internal relationship between grounding, centering, and uplift through the body's interrelated Lower, Central, and Upper Cores.

Domes of the Body or **Domes of Uplift:** Dynamic centers within your primordial midline consisting of inner ankles, pelvic diaphragm, respiratory diaphragm, thoracic inlet, palate/occiput, and cranium—connecting feet, head, and hands. They are resonant with the relationship between your body's tensional-compression forces and the forces around you, and are the true fulcrum or axis of your human body, which creates grounding and uplift.

Down the Back (DTB) and Up the Front (UTF): A term for *befriending gravity* used by Wendy LeBlanc-Arbuckle to refer to the weight shift and force transfer through the body from foot to head and hand of the fluid-dynamic, tension-compression forces of gravity and its partner, ground reaction force.

Elastic recoil fascial matrix breath: The body-wide balance of tension-compression that is felt elastically through the fascial matrix of the rib basket, pelvic diaphragm, respiratory diaphragm, and palate.

Embodied awareness: A felt sense of what the body knows—pre-verbally.

Embodiment: The conscious knowing of the body, achieved through breath, sound, and movement awareness through listening to one's biointelligence.

Fascial matrix, also **extracellular living matrix:** Physically, the fascial matrix is the fiber-optic support throughout our body that weaves everything together and coordinates whole-body relationships. It is a continuous, crystalline, oscillating communication system, from the dural covering of the brain and spinal cord, through the periosteum of living bone, to the connective tissue wrapping of every visceral, internal organ to the nucleus of every cell.

Felt sense of breathing: A phenomenological perception originating inside breath itself. A direct experience of our body's natural breathing patterns.

Field of influence: Refers to the effect of the midline on our orientation in space, and serves as a reference point for the biological development of other structures and functions.

Fluid intelligence: A term that refers to the primordial intelligence of water. Since the body is predominantly fluid intelligence, we embody that deeper knowing.

Ground reaction force (GRF): Gravity's partner. The force exerted by the ground on a body in contact with it, evoking internal uplift.

Inner Guide: Our biointelligent self that learns through sound, breath, and movement, and communicates through awareness to our body/mind/emotion/spirit.

Interoception: Our ability to sense our internal workings and our sense of self in the world.

Kinetic centers: A sensory term coined for the tension-compression biotensegrity of elbows and knees that highlights the response of those areas to the interplay of gravity and ground reaction force. They act as centers of communication through your fascial matrix, where elbows and knees amplify or inhibit movement. Resonant with clinical anatomist John Sharkey's "fascial listening pegs."

Lemniscate: A figure-eight pattern that is non-linear, multi-dimensional, multi-directional, and ever-changing. It is a pattern by which formative forces create living organisms.

Letting go: "Restful resilience." Not a collapse. It affects perception, emotions, and behaviors.

Meso: The third, "in-between" dimension of the body, which embryologist, MD, and anthroposophist Jaap van der Wal considers our proprioceptive innerness. He uses the term Meso to emphasize that the body is not matter made of three layers, but a triune body with an inner dimension.

Perceptual field: Linked specifically to Rolfer, Rolf Movement practitioner, and researcher Hubert Godard's usage of the term, *perception is an action*, where our perceptual state affects our motor patterns and behavior.

Perineural nervous system: Orthopedic surgeon Robert O. Becker's dual nervous system concept, which challenges the neuron doctrine of the classic (all or none) nerve network. The evolutionarily more ancient but important direct current analog system resides in the perineural connective tissues, which supports the classic central nervous system, and is responsible for wound healing and injury repair.

Phenomenologist: A person who studies how we experience things as a participant, rather than an observer, from the first-person, lived experience perspective.

Pre-movement: Rolfer, Rolf Movement practitioner, and researcher Hubert Godard's term that identifies the body's preparation for movement. Referring in *Moving Beyond Core* to the activation of our context for embodied movement in relationship with the world as the medium through which our perception and expression flow.

Primary respiration: A term used by Dr. William Garner Sutherland to describe the original pulse of life. The foundational movement of all life that expands and contracts.

Primordial midline: The pulse of our primitive streak emergence as an embryo. That emerging, energetic phenomenon from which we self-organize and shape ourselves.

Proprioception: The body's ability to sense movement, action, and location.

Proprioceptive innerness: A term coined by embryologist and MD Jaap van der Wal to describe a kind of bodily seeing and sensing from the inside.

Psychosocial: The influence of social factors on a person's mind or behavior, and the interrelationship between behavioral and social factors.

Resonance: A fluid-vibrational connection within and between bodies.

Self-knowing: Pre-verbal total awareness of our fluidic nature.

Self-tuning: A term for how we sense and coordinate the body's concert of relations, from micro- to macromovement, through the crystalline, semi-conducting energy of the fascial matrix, through listening, open awareness, and core coordination, which allows us to self-tune within the gravitational field.

Somatic approach: A way of being which develops perceptual, kinesthetic, interoceptive, and proprioceptive awareness, with the vision of developing a relational sense of self (with and between all beings and the natural world).

Tensegrity: A term developed by Buckminster Fuller that speaks to tensional integrity, or the dynamic interplay of tension and compression within a structure.

Tonic: Refers to the intrinsic muscular support of our primordial midline structure and function, through the head-to-tail's relationship between earth and sky.

Tonic function: A term developed by Rolfer, Rolf Movement practitioner, and researcher Hubert Godard, referring to gravity-based organization of inherent tone in the body, which is expressed through our coherent relationship with earth and sky through our orientation with focal and peripheral vision, inner ears, and feet.

Torus: More than a donut-shaped surface generated by a circle rotated around an axis, the torus serves as a visual depiction of energy flow, the intricate connections weaving through everything, and the harmonious equilibrium between the material and spiritual dimensions. The torus encapsulates the perpetual dance of creation and dissolution, the constant rhythm of beginnings and endings, illustrating the timeless essence of existence. More than this, the torus represents the fourth dimension of human development, as the embryo moves through itself reflecting the infinite nature of being while establishing chirality and the spiraling nature of our wholeness. (Gratitude to clinical anatomist John Sharkey for his contribution to this definition.)

Vectors of directionality: Sensory receptivity from the body's midline through the extremities of hands, feet, head, and tail.

Ventral vagus nerve: The part of the nervous system that helps us co-regulate through social interaction, safety and support.

Vibrational hum: Produced when two bodies resonate together, as in the human body and the natural environment that sustains it. Each body feels the other through the resonant hum.

Wholeheartedness: Being fully present, both for our own benefit and for the benefit of others.

Yield to gravity: Resting aliveness. Somatic educator Bonnie Bainbridge Cohen's term for the support of the earth that generates innate developmental patterns of push, reach, grasp, and pull, along with evoking uplift and spatial orientation.

Yielding to reach: Yield—as in the sense defined in "yield to gravity"—is the grounding support that allows reach to happen, in order to walk, from foot to head, and move with ease in all activities of daily living.

Resources

- Hoberman Sphere - Small and Large Breathing Ball (Image 3.6)
  - Small Breathing Ball: www.lakeshorelearning.com/products/science/physical-science/hoberman-sphere/p/ES130
  - Large Breathing Ball: www.lakeshorelearning.com/products/science/physical-science/hoberman-original-sphere/p/KT7793

- Swopper Chair (Video 3.17): https://www.aerismotion.com/collections/products/products/aeris-swopper-wool-blend

- Weighted Tools for Sensory Adaptation (Video 4.6)
  - Sandbags: www.theyogawarehouse.com/Kakaos-Sandbags (We fill ours with aquarium gravel, which molds to the body shape)
  - Ankle Weights: www.activerecoveryessentials.com/products/all-pro-adjustable-ankle-weights

- Thera-Band (Image 4.13A)
  - Medium Resistance: https://www.optp.com/Thera-Band-Latex-Free-Resistance-Band-75-Feet-Bulk-Pack?kw=theraband

- Blackboard Toe Bands (Image 4.17)
  - Set of Tensile Toe Bands: https://naturalfootgear.com/products/blackboard-toebands

- Soft Inflatable Ball (Image 4.21)
  - 9 Inch Diameter: https://www.optp.com/Soft-Gym-Overball?kw=ball

- Inversion Table (Video 4.25C): https://teeter.com/product/fitspine-x1-inversion-table

- Mini Balls (Image 6.2A)
  - Mini Balls For Feet: https://www.optp.com/Mini-Balls?kw=ball

- Cervical Pivot (Image 6.3)
  - OPxTP Cervical Pivot: https://www.optp.com/Cervical-Pivot

- Exercise Ball (Image 6.4)
  - Exercise Ball - 65cm: https://www.optp.com/Gymnic-Classic-Plus-Exercise-Ball

- Yoga Block (Image 6.5A)
  - Foam Yoga Block 4" X 6" X 9": www.yogadirect.com/foam-yoga-block-4-inch-x-6-inch-x-9-inch.html

- Tuning Board (Image 6.5C)
  - Original Tuning Board: www.rolfingboulderdenver.com/store/tuning-board

- Tensegrity/Sensory Feedback Band (Image 6.7A)
  - Stretch-eze: https://stretch-eze.com

- Tensegrity Feedback Band (Image 6.8A)
  - TYE4: https://www.physicalmindinstitute.com/tye4-and-tye4x

- Morning Practice Resources (Image 6.10)
  - Netti Pot: https://shop.himalayaninstitute.org/collections/neti-pot/products/ceramic-netipot
  - Tongue Scraper: https://www.grove.co/products/stainless-steel-tongue-cleaner
  - Acupressure Mat: https://www.amazon.com/ProSource-Acupressure-Pillow-Relief-Relaxation/dp/B00I1QCPIK?ref_=ast_sto_dp&th=1
  - Skin Brushes
  - Hand Held : https://manjeriskincare.com/products/body-brush
  - Long Handle: https://www.coopmarket.com/products/earth-therapeutics-far-reaching-back-brush-18

- Restful Sleep Resources
  - Paper Surgical Tape: https://www.amazon.com/dp/B0082A9EGQ?ref=nb_sb_ss_w_as-reorder_k0_1_9&amp=&crid=TF9GPW5MIWJ7&amp=&sprefix=micropore
  - MyoTape : https://myotape.com

- Ergonomic Support (Image 6.15B)
  - Aston Kinestics Standard Back Wedge: https://www.astonkinetics.com/ergo-supports/standard-back-wedge
  - Aston Kinestics Medium Egro Triangle: https://www.astonkinetics.com/ergo-supports/medium-ergo-triangle

- Resources for Five Element Study:
  - Pam Ferguson, *Take Five*, 2000, Newleaf, Dublin, Ireland, pg 41
  - Michael Reed Gach, *Acu-yoga*, Japan Publications, 2000, pg 100

- Sounding and Voice Resources
  - Continuum Teachers Association: www.continuumteachers.com
  - Susan Lincoln: www.susanlincoln.com/about-hilde-girls
  - Jeremy Mossman: www.singingwithjmoss.com/bbvp
  - Daniel Barber: www.danielbarber.com

Index

Sub-headings in *italics* indicate figures.